What Price Better Health?

What Price Better Health?

Hazards of the Research Imperative

DANIEL CALLAHAN

University of California Press

BERKELEY   LOS ANGELES   LONDON

The Milbank Memorial Fund

NEW YORK

The Milbank Memorial Fund is an endowed national foundation that engages in nonpartisan analysis, study, research, and communication on significant issues in health policy. In the fund's own publications, in reports or books it publishes with other organizations, and in articles it commissions for publication by other organizations, the fund endeavors to maintain the highest standards for accuracy and fairness. Statements by individual authors, however, do not necessarily reflect opinions or factual determinations of the fund.

University of California Press
Berkeley and Los Angeles, California

University of California Press, Ltd.
London, England

© 2003 by the Regents of the University of California

Library of Congress Cataloging-in-Publication Data

Callahan, Daniel, 1930–
     What price better health? : hazards of the research imperative /
Daniel Callahan.
         p. ; cm. — (California/Milbank books on health and the public ;
9)
     Includes bibliographical references and index.
     ISBN 0-520-22771-9 (cloth : alk. paper)
     1. Medicine—Research—Social aspects—United States.   I. Title.   II.
Series.
     [DNLM: 1. Research—United States. 2. Ethics, Research—United
States.
     3. Morals—United States. W 20.5 C156w 2003]
     R853.S64C35 2003
     610'.7'2073—dc21   2003002459

Manufactured in the United States of America
11 10 09 08 07 06 05 04 03
10 9 8 7 6 5 4 3 2 1

The paper used in this publication meets the minimum requirements of
ANSI/NISO Z39.48–1992(R 1997) (Permanence of Paper).∞

For
Perry Ann Turnbull Callahan
Who has brought lightness and joy to my life

Contents

Foreword

The Milbank Memorial Fund is an endowed national foundation that engages in nonpartisan analysis, study, research, and communication on significant issues in health policy. The fund makes available the results of its work in meetings with decision makers, reports, articles, and books.

This is the ninth of the California/Milbank Books on Health and the Public. The publishing partnership between the fund and the press seeks to encourage the synthesis and communication of findings from research that could contribute to more effective health policy.

Daniel Callahan is a profound and provocative participant in debates about appropriate health policy. He has observed, analyzed, and advocated at the intersection of moral philosophy and journalism throughout a long and distinguished career.

In this book, Callahan argues that a biomedical "research imperative" has for many years pervaded American culture. This imperative has both positive and negative effects, he writes. Positive effects have included the relief of considerable pain and suffering and the expansion of scientific knowledge. Negative effects have included unrestrained pursuit of profits and knowledge; the former has caused unnecessary costs, the latter has placed many research subjects at unnecessary risk of harm.

Callahan emphasizes that negative or questionable aspects of the research imperative are not the result of "nefarious researchers, narrow self-absorbed interest groups, or a benighted public." The research imperative, and therefore any benefits and harms that result from it, derives from our culture. He champions changes in policy that, he believes, could ensure that the benefits exceed the harms that result from it.

Daniel M. Fox
President
Samuel L. Milbank
Chairman

Acknowledgments

This is a book I simply could not have written without the help of people who tutored me at the start and then read the results of my efforts at the end. I have lived long enough to understand that experts and gurus disagree, often flamboyantly. But I was lucky to find experts who welcome an exchange of views and who worked hard to make clear to me where they stood in the various battles described in this book.

I will single out first of all my splendid research assistants, all of whom were pursuing their own educations but helped as well to advance mine: Liza Abeles, Barbara Binzak, Emily Feinstein, Michael Khair, and Samantha Stokes. Debra Aronson plumbed the depths of years of congressional testimony on the annual NIH budget hearings, and Courtney Campbell and Gregory Kaebnick brought their critical skills to the whole manuscript. Others who read most or some of the manuscript or sent me in the right direction include George Annas, Marcia Angell, Robert Baker, Allan Brandt, Joseph P. Newhouse, John Broome, David Cutler, Leon Eisenberg, Albert Jonsen, Diane Meier, Jonathan Moreno, Sherwin Nuland, John Evans, Erik Parens, David Alan Ehrlich, Stuart Newman, Bruce Jennings, Raymond deVries, Mary Ann Baily, and Thomas Murray.

As is the custom with the Milbank Fund/University of California series, the fund brought together a group of people from various backgrounds to review a manuscript of the book. They were of immense help to me. Some were very supportive of my overall argument, and some were highly critical. But from each of them I learned something, and the book would have been much poorer without their help. The group included Irene W. Crowe, Roger Herdman, Sheldon Krimsky, Gilbert C. Meilaender, Herbert Pardes, Dorothy P. Rice, Leon E. Rosenberg, Stuart O. Schweitzer, Samuel C. Silverstein, Haldor Stefansson, and Arthur C. Upton.

Raymond S. Andrews, Jr., and the Patrick and Catherine Donaghue Research Foundation were most helpful with a grant to support my work on priority setting in medical research. My secretary of twenty-seven years, Ellen McAvoy, worked with me, as she has done so often in the past, to prepare the manuscript—which can be the worst kind of stoop labor—and never complained.

Finally, I must thank Dan Fox and the Milbank Memorial Fund for the financial support that helped make this book possible. I am proud to be part of the series published jointly by the Milbank Fund and the University of California Press.

Introduction

An Imperative?

Recent years have seen an almost unprecedented level of excitement about medical research. The dramatic increases in the annual budget of the National Institutes of Health (NIH), running 10 to 15 percent a year, even as many other federal agencies' budgets are being cut, reflect that excitement. So do reports of striking research progress and improved health traceable to research, along with the public's enthusiasm over medical advances. Americans seem to have a special predilection for scientific progress, technological innovation, and better health. Hardly a doubt is voiced anywhere about the likely benefits of an ever greater commitment to research.

Aristotle defined the basic human instinct behind research in the fourth century B.C. in the opening line of his *Metaphysics,* "All men by nature desire to know." In the sixteenth century Francis Bacon applied it to the power of science to improve the human condition. Medical research has been one of the most glorious of human enterprises and grows stronger every year. I am entering old age in relatively good health, undoubtedly in great part because of its success in relieving pain and disability and in forestalling death. Why should the public not be enthusiastic about research since it brings such patently valuable human good?

Langdon Winner has suggested that it is plausible to think of technology as a "form of life," which has power to reconstruct social roles and relationships.[1] Because of technology, we think differently about the world and live in it differently. Something analogous can be said about medical research: it gives us a fresh view of the possibilities of living our lives and managing our miseries, of shaping our bodies and our minds. Medical research has become as much a "form of life" as the technology it creates. It gives us a new means of thinking about life itself.

Yet within its praiseworthy activity lie some shadows that require a

1

closer look. My aim in this book is not to halt research, much less to impugn its great contribution to our common good, but to enhance the possibility that it will move forward in the most socially sound way possible. Precisely because of its value—social, medical, economic—medical research tempts us to invest too much hope in it as a way of relieving the human condition or leads us to excessively commercialize it, to cut moral corners in pursuit of therapies and cures, or with human research subjects, or to divert attention from the social and economic sources of sickness. This is only to say that medical research has hazards as well as benefits.

I call these hazards "shadows" to stress the interplay of light and shadows on the body of medical research. It has no fundamental flaws or dread disease. On the contrary, medical research is an essentially healthy, valid, and vitally important activity. Most medical research raises no problems whatever. The shadows are hardly the whole story, nor are most of the abuses I mention dominant and widespread. Yet the shadows can do great damage if we ignore or minimize them. They emerge from larger cultural attitudes and values that have had a powerful impact on medical research. By tracing them to the larger American culture, I want, at the least, to put aside two possible responses to my analysis. One of them might see it as an attack on the researchers, an accusation that their values create the shadows. On occasion that is so, but usually the societal counterpart to their values has been brought into play.

The other possible response would read my critique as a veiled denunciation of the whole enterprise of medical research. One longtime and insightful commentator on science, Daniel S. Greenberg, has written along these lines: "Ethical concerns are a sideshow of science, providing grist for the press and moralizing politicians, though with little actual effect on the conduct of the research enterprise. . . . More money for more science is the commanding passion of the politics of science."[2] I do not share that judgment. The full reality of that politics reveals an enterprise marked by drama, by great human benefits, by unbounded ambition, by selfless altruism, by flagrant cupidity, by excess in the pursuit of the good, by moral sensitivity and moral obtuseness—and by still uncharted possibilities for progress in the relief of pain and suffering.

I want to examine that mixture of the good and the bad, the light and the shadows, by focusing on the idea of a "research imperative." Though unfamiliar to most scientists and the general public, the term expresses a cultural problem that caught my eye. It occurs in an article written by the late Protestant moral theologian Paul Ramsey in 1976 as part of a debate with a Jesuit theologian, Richard McCormick. McCormick argued that it ought to be morally acceptable to use children for nontherapeutic research, that is, for research of no direct benefit to the children themselves and in the absence of any informed consent. Referring to claims about the "necessity" of such research, Ramsey accused McCormick of falling prey to the "research imperative," the view that the importance of research could overcome moral values.[3]

That was the last I heard of the phrase for many years, but it informs important arguments about research that have surfaced with increasing force of late. It captures, for instance, the essence of what Joshua Lederberg, a Nobel laureate for his work in genetics and president emeritus of Rockefeller University, once remarked to me. "The blood of those who will die if biomedical research is not pursued," he said, "will be upon the hands of those who don't do it." It also captures the meaning of such commonly heard phrases (which I cite as the book moves along) about the "necessity" of research, or the "moral obligation" to pursue certain kinds of research, or the overpowering "promise" of research to relieve suffering, a goal not to be denied; or the "need to relieve suffering" as a justification for the high price of pharmaceuticals.

Some scientists see no evidence of any such imperative at work, and perhaps others remain skeptical. But I believe that such an imperative pervades our culture, finding reflections within science, politics, research advocacy, and public sentiment. It parallels the more familiar "technological imperative."[4] That imperative, as I understand it, holds that if technologies exist, they ought to be used and usually will be used. They cease to become psychologically optional.

I define the "research imperative" as the felt drive to use research to gain various forms of knowledge for its own sake, or as a motive to achieve a worthy practical end. As with technology, where an attractive innovation generates an interest in finding an even better version, research has a similar force. Research generates not only new knowledge but new leads for even more future knowledge; and that is a major part of its excitement. Research has its own internal imperative, that of learning still more, and more.

The research imperative has a continuum of uses and interpretations, each of which I have drawn from many years of reading about research, from listening to its advocates talk about it, and from observing its uses in the public arena:

> the drive to gain scientific knowledge for its own sake (to understand the human genome)

a felt moral obligation to relieve pain and suffering (to find a cure for cancer)

a rationale for pursuing research goals that are of doubtful human value or potentially harmful (as some would argue, research to achieve human cloning)

a public relations tool to justify the chase after profit (the pharmaceutical industry's defense of high drug prices)

the pursuit of worthy goals even at the risk of compromising important moral and social values (hazardous research on competent human beings without their informed consent)

Those are five possible meanings of the phrase, and its underlying concept, that are central to my inquiry. On occasion I refer to a "benign" or a "hazardous" imperative if I think my meaning may be unclear. Though I have worked to keep those different senses of the phrase clear and distinct in the rest of the book, on other occasions I may fail. The reason for that will not necessarily be sheer carelessness on my part (which can happen), but two other confounding reasons. At times the different senses run together, creating an admixture of good and bad that is a part of research just as it is a part of the rest of our lives. And pervasive disagreements about the appropriate goals of research and the morally valid means to pursue them cause one person to judge a particular line of research highly appropriate while another rejects it.

Some, for example, view research to achieve human reproductive cloning—which might offer insights into the relief of infertility—as the research imperative in its most noble manifestation, and others find the idea repugnant. Some social scientists believe that it is legitimate to deceive research subjects if there is no other way to carry out the research and if the reason for deception is scientifically valid. Medical researchers would reject such reasoning out of hand. So, too, one person might believe a particular line of research is morally imperative while others might judge it as important and helpful, but not imperative. In any event, I try to be reasonably consistent in my use of the term and hope, as the book moves along, that the idea's complexity and power become clear.

RESEARCH IDEALS

If I have placed a somewhat elusive concept at the heart of this book, I also bring to medical research a set of animating ideals. Some are commonplace, others perhaps less so, and all (whether I mention them or not) are there just below the surface. I call them "ideals" because they represent high aspirations, not always or easily achievable. But that is no reason not to entertain and hope to achieve each condition:

Safe. Both the means and the expected aims or results of research must be physically safe for all parties involved. This does not in principle rule out risk, but when risk is reasonably possible, the burden of proof—which ought to be strong—should lie with those who want to carry out the research, not with those who will be endangered. There may, naturally, be reasonable disagreements about what constitutes a threat to safety and the degree of that threat. Of the various ideals I suggest, this one is the most accepted, usually defined as a duty, expressing the principle of nonmaleficence, the Hippocratic rule to "do no harm."

Socially beneficial. Medical research should aim to improve and sustain human health, whether at the individual or population level. Medical research directed solely at meeting individual desires rather than genuine health problems should be discouraged as a poor use of research talent and resources.

Resistant to market determinations. For-profit research, aiming to make a contribution to health while also turning a profit, is part of American culture, not to be eliminated however strong the complaints against it. At the same time, the power of for-profit research should never become strong enough—in trying to create or meet market demands—to shape overall national research priorities, much less to discourage research that will bring no profit or to rob the research community of talented researchers.

Conducive to a sustainable, affordable medicine. Recent increases in health care costs can be traced in part—and not an insignificant part—to new technologies and an intensified use of both old and new technologies. Many if not most of these technologies are the fruit of research, sometimes NIH-sponsored basic research, at other times the work of pharmaceutical or biotechnology research. A sustainable medicine, a medicine that is affordable over the long run, ought to be an ideal of medical research. It is obvious that not all valid research can promise affordable medicine, but it should try.

Conducive to equitable access to health care. This point is closely related to the previous one: a sustainable medicine ought also to be conducive to equitable access. A research drive that ends by exacerbating the gap between rich and poor, insured and uninsured, makes a defective and even hazardous contribution to health care. It may come about if technological innovations (pharmaceutical or otherwise) that come from basic research drive health care costs to unaffordable heights (see a statement about this possibility by former NIH Director Harold Varmus on page 270).

Open to meaningful public participation in setting priorities. Nothing is so important for good science as allowing researchers to follow their own leads and ideas. Good research cannot be bureaucratically programmed. Yet the public should be heard and its needs and interests taken seriously. Advocacy groups have always had an important role, but their interests are typically narrow, oriented toward their own constituencies. The voice of the general public needs to be heard as well, both about its urgent health concerns and about its views on controversial research.

Morally acceptable to the public, and sensitive to moral views held by the public. It is not enough simply to listen to a full range of public voices before setting research policy and priorities. It is no less important to avoid offending, so far as reasonably possible, the views of a minority. The research community, and its lay supporters, ought never assume that its moral principles are superior to the principles of those who dissent from various lines of research.

Consistent with the higest human good and human rights. There is no necessary correlation between a good life and good health: some healthy people are unhappy and some happy people are unhealthy. A long life is desirable, but a short life is not incompatible with a good life. Good health helps provide a foundation to enjoy the fruits of human rights—but a denial of basic rights sometimes cannot offset even a healthy life.

CONVERGING ISSUES

If my primary purpose is to assess the research imperative in its various manifestations, another aim is to link a variety of issues within medical research, issues ordinarily treated separately and commanding their own literature. What were in the past treated as discrete issues are coming to influence and overlap one another. The role of the pharmaceutical industry in funding clinical research bears directly on many problems of human-subject research. The setting of research priorities by Congress can have a potent effect on the future of health care delivery, influencing what therapies will be available for distribution and what their costs might be. The extent of any obligation to carry out research is highly relevant to determining what moral principles must bear on the use of human subjects to advance research, just as they must bear on research on embryos or germline therapy.

There seems, in short, to be a potential unity in the various aspects of medical research as a scientific and social venture. The term "research ethics" is now narrowly used to refer either to human-subject research or to scientific integrity in the conduct of researchers. That term should be expanded to cover the research enterprise as a whole, to encompass all the ends and means of research along with its social and political implications.

Ours is a period of great public, legislative, and media attention to medical research, a strong if sometimes overwhelming stimulus to any author interested in such matters. I began this book just at the moment of the completion of the Human Genome Project, mapping the human genome, and wrote much of it during the heat of the stem-cell research debate and the federal crackdown on many universities for violations of human-subject regulations. It was hard to keep up with it all, and I found myself swinging to and fro as new developments emerged, drawn to the power of medical research to change and enrich our lives but at the same time often troubled by the capacity of some professional and lay enthusiasts to skip over important moral considerations.

Yet even in those cases it was the mixture of the good and the bad, tightly bound together, that was most arresting. The capacity of good people with good motives to do unwitting harm is an old story, and one on display when the research imperative is pushed too far or in the wrong way. At the same time the impetus behind what we judge to be wrong or harmful or bad public policy often reflects our culture's way of pushing people one way or the other, not deliberate intent or moral carelessness. That is why I think of the research imperative as a cultural problem, not a problem of nefarious researchers, narrow self-absorbed interest groups, or a benighted public.

We are all in this together, and if fault is to be apportioned, there is enough to convict almost all of us. Some readers of an earlier draft of the book read it as a dissenting book. There is surely dissent here, mainly about a faulty response to, or understanding of, the research imperative. But I am trying to make better sense of a social phenomenon of a fascinating, sometimes troubling, kind: as valuable and cherished as research is, commanding a remarkable consensus of public approval, it still generates a wide range of controversies and disputes and sometimes does actual harm. Why is that?

The book moves through three phases: the goals or ends of medical research, the means used to pursue those goals, and the fashioning of public policy on research. One underlying question articulates each chapter, and I include it in each summary.

Chapter 1 traces the history of medical research in the United States. It aims to show the trajectory of research goals and how they gradually came to embody the research imperative, a note relatively absent from its earlier history. *How and why did a research imperative arise?*

Chapter 2 begins the the first phase, probing the goals of medical research. This chapter takes up the foundational issue, that of the goals and values of science, of which medical research is simply one expression, and then turns to the social obligations of scientists as well as recent threats within medical research to their scientific integrity. *What are the animating values of scientific research and what are the norms of social responsibility that should guide researchers?*

Chapter 3 narrows the discussion of goals to that of the goals of medical research, relating them to the goals of medicine, which should be the point of departure for socially valid research. The war of medicine against death and aging, two characteristic notes of contemporary research, serves as a test case of the validity of traditionally important research goals. *What are appropriate research goals, and how best should we deal with two traditional goals of research, forestalling death and relieving the burdens of aging?*

Chapter 4 more broadly takes on the goals of medicine in relation to the concept of "health," the cure of illness, and the relief of suffering, as well as the difference between a medicine oriented to preserving or restoring health and one aimed at enhancing human traits and the satisfaction of individual desires. *Should medical research focus solely on the prevention of disease and the restoration of health, or should it move on to the enhancement of human physical and psychological traits?*

Opening the second phase, chapter 5 assesses the problem of balancing risks and benefits in medical research. Both risks and benefits encompass social and cultural values, not simply physical safety. *What stance, and with what values, should the research community and the public take toward research that has both risks and benefits?*

Chapter 6 takes up a principal means of carrying out biomedical research, the use of human subjects for clinical research. Human-subject research, a longtime troublesome matter, is a central and necessary means for pursuing clinical knowledge and thus an unavoidable topic for this book: is a balance between subject protection and research needs possible? *Why has human-subject research been such a significant issue for medical research, and what are the history and values that have given it such practical and symbolic importance?*

Chapter 7 looks at the growing and difficult problem of using research methods that raise serious moral questions or offend a significant portion of the public. How is controversial research best understood and dealt with in a pluralistic society? Is it possible to achieve a consensus without eliminating valid dissent? *How should pluralistic societies deal with, and resolve, research debates that reveal great religious, philosophical, and ideological differences?*

Chapter 8 is the first chapter in the book's final phase, devoted specifically to important policy issues of biomedical research. The first, discussed here, is the place of the private sector, and specifically the pharmaceutical industry, in shaping the direction of research and its social impact on the costs of health care, on the pricing of drugs, on universities and their researchers, and on health in developing countries. *Because of its importance for health, can we hold the pharmaceutical industry to different—and higher—moral standards than other industries, and can the need to do research justify the industry's traditionally high profits?*

Chapter 9 switches the examination to the public sector, and specifically to the role of the NIH and the federal government in supporting and directing medical research. A central consideration is the role of Congress, the NIH leadership, the public, and the research community in shaping NIH priorities. *At present there is no well-organized system to set national research priorities: can we develop and justify such a system?*

Chapter 10 pulls together the varied and numerous strains in the argument of the book to present a picture of how medical research might better manifest the ideals of research sketched in the introduction. *How can we find a better fit between national research priorities and national health care distribution practices?*

1 The Emergence and Growth of the Research Imperative

My first visit to Monticello, Thomas Jefferson's remarkable Virginia home and enduring avocation, showed me far more than I expected. Like everyone else who has read about him, I was aware of the breadth and complexity of his mind: science, politics, history, law, agriculture, architecture, and philosophy just begin the list of topics that engaged him. Yet to see with my own eyes in his house the evidence of his range of theoretical and practical passions was still startling, books and gadgets side by side. At the center of it all was his bewitchment with science. "Nature," he said, "intended me for the tranquil pursuit of science, by rendering them my supreme delight." He believed science would bring the relief of all human ills. "The ingenuity of man," Jefferson claimed, "leaves us to despair of nothing within the laws of nature."

While there has been dispute about just how good a practicing scientist Jefferson was, the historian of science Gerald Holton notes that he had a sharp eye for problems that fall outside the scope of science's two strongest exemplars. One is Isaac Newton, who aimed at *omniscience*, a general explanatory theory for the totality of empirical facts. The other is Francis Bacon, who wanted science to serve power and human autonomy, even achieving *omnipotence*, "the enlarging of the bounds of human empire, to the effecting of all things possible." By contrast, Holton argues, Jefferson's style of science "locates the center of research in an area of basic scientific ignorance that lies at the heart of a social problem."[1] The result was a notion of science that looked both to the classical ideal of an expanded knowledge of nature for its own sake and to the more modern goal of "the freedom and happiness of man." It applies equally well to the spirit of medical research.

Yet Jefferson might have been shocked, even appalled, to observe the powerful twenty-first-century role of government in the promotion of science. Possibly a man noted for holding that the less government the better would bet on the market as an alternative to carry the burden of research today. Though medicine was one of the few scientific areas about which Jefferson wrote little, he no doubt shared Benjamin Franklin's Enlightenment faith in the power of science to overcome the ills of the body. "It is impossible to imagine," Franklin wrote to a renowned scientist of the day, Joseph Priestly, "the height to which may be carried, in a thousand years, the power of man over matter. . . . All diseases may be prevented or cured, not excepting even that of old age, and our lives lengthened at pleasure even beyond the antediluvian standard."[2]

Franklin's unbounded optimism resounds in a statement by the French philosophe Condorcet, published in 1795: "Would it then be absurd to suppose that this perfection of the human species might be capable of indefinite progress; that the day will come when death will only be due to extraordinary accidents or to the decay of the vital forces, and that ultimately, the average span between birth and decay will have no assignable value? Certainly man will not become immortal, but will not the interval between the first breath that he draws and the time when in the natural course of events, without disease or accidents, he expires, increase indefinitely?"[3] For the great American physician Benjamin Rush, it was the American revolution itself that "opened all the doors of the temple of nature . . . [making possible] a knowledge of antidotes to those diseases that are supposed to be incurable."[4]

Despite this cluster of beliefs in the promise of science in the service of health—echoing and more than exponentially amplified to this day—the United States fell well behind Europe in the cultivation of research aims and skills. Nearly a century passed before the medical sciences began fully to benefit from them. American pragmatism, the frontier spirit, and a lack of basic institutions were no help either. Yet once harnessed, the entrepreneurial spirit that flowered in the biotechnology industry during the 1980s and 1990s also has deep roots in American culture. As the historian Joyce Appleby has asserted, to fail to mark the early republic's "freedom to innovate, to aspire, to seek a range of individual satisfactions in the market . . . is to obscure a very important element in American history: the creation of a popular, entrepreneurial culture that permeated all aspects of American society."[5] In the early twentieth century, through the Rockefeller family and other wealthy patrons, that culture provided massive private support for medical research and the beginning of American research distinction. It helped as well to explain the influx of the market's language and practices into contemporary medicine, aiming to turn any good into profitable goods.

But I am getting ahead of the story here. Franklin's belief in unlimited scientific progress and the Jeffersonian blend of basic and applied science needed four ingredients to produce the medical research imperative: success in medicine's struggle against infectious disease during the first half of the twentieth century; an end to the bias against a strong federal role in support of science; a marshaling of lay activism to lobby for more research; and the prospect of enormous profits for corporate America from a medicine to enable us at once to fight disease and, in Franklin's phrase, attain "at pleasure" not just health but a great enhancement of our human nature.

None of these developments, however, quite explain the movement from medicine as a visionary, progress-driven enterprise, full of hope about the future, but still accepting human finitude, to one that by the twentieth century advanced the moral demand—unavoidable in its ethical necessity and reluctant to accept any practitioner's failure—to stamp out or radically limit death and disease. That fourth ingredient began to make itself felt in the second half of the nineteenth century and reached full force with the National Institutes of Health in the second half of the next century.

AMERICAN MEDICAL RESEARCH: THE EARLY STAGES

Four stages in the history of American medical research stand out.[6] From 1750 to 1820 the British influence was dominant, stimulated by aristocrats who formed the first scientific societies. The Royal Society for Improving Natural Knowledge, emerging in 1660, published its influential *Transactions*, which became the first important source of scientific publications. These developments did little for American research in the early days of independence, but they did provide an education in Britain for the most important early figures in American science, William Charles Wells in biology and medicine, and Benjamin Franklin and Benjamin Tompkins in physics. The first American medical schools, at the University of Pennsylvania in 1765, at Columbia University in 1768, and at Harvard in 1782, had advanced educational practices but little interest in research.

By the 1820s American wealth and population had grown rapidly, and the emergence of strong urban centers allowed the creation of hospitals, schools, and libraries. In that context, French developments in empirical research found a warm welcome, allowing American physicians to throw off the British influence and to turn to France for an advanced education. The Parisian empirical philosophers encouraged physicians to carry out large-scale clinical and epidemiological studies. More precise research methodologies became the model, emphasizing a search for correlations between symptoms and lesions and a focus on the physical diagnosis examination of patients. Parisian clinicians had the advantage of professional journals, close ties with mathematicians and other scientists, and strong academic institutions. The French focus on pathology was to provide a solid basis for research innovation while their strong medical centers and publications provided stimulating models of excellence.

While the Civil War contributed mainly to clinical developments—as is true of most wars—the period between that deadly conflict and the end of the nineteenth century saw the gradual flowering of serious and extensive medical research.[7] But the initial stirrings of greatness appeared first in agriculture: a combination of the first land-grant colleges financed by Congress and the agricultural experiment stations connected to them began to make significant research progress in agricultural chemistry and botany. The support of veterinary medicine by the Department of Agriculture, already closely related to the experiment stations, made important contributions to human medicine, notably in illuminating the role of secondary hosts in spreading communicable disease. Hardly less significant was the precedent set for federal support of research. The 1887 Hatch Act and the 1906 Adams Act provided government money for agricultural research, though it would be decades before this early federal interest in research made any great difference for medicine.

By the end of the nineteenth century it was not federal but private support for research that began the real transformation. Medical research was primarily in the hands of universities, but they began attracting the attention of the wealthy, particularly the most wealthy of all, notably the John D. Rockefeller family, but also Vanderbilts, Carnegies, Hopkinses, and Clarks. In 1889 Andrew Carnegie formulated the potent "Gospel of Wealth," which held that there was an obligation on the part of the wealthy to return their profits to society. If the first beneficiary of this ethic was higher education, medical research was next in line.

THE GERMAN INFLUENCE

One other factor was to make that turn to research compelling. The French were the main models in the mid nineteenth century, but the Germans made the decisive mark toward the end of that century. Their influence was set within the context of a rising dissatisfaction with the state of American medical research. In an 1873 lecture, the British scientist John Tyndall, while noting the Americans' enthusiasm for education, deplored their failure to support research and to recognize its importance.[8] Striking a similar note, other commentators saw no prospect for governmental support but began to urge a solicitation of private funds. The high standing of physicians by that time gave added force to the effort, but it was the German work that made the critical difference in giving credibility to the call for better research.

The Germans had many points in their favor. Their medical sciences had become the most advanced in the world, led by developments in cellular pathology and bacteriology. Rudolf Virchow's 1858 unveiling of a general concept of disease based on the cellular structure of the body together with Robert Koch's discovery of the tuberculosis bacillus, and the establishment of the germ theory of disease, all played their part in polishing the German research reputation. Koch, moreover, was important in encouraging the concept of devising specific therapies to cure specific diseases. If strong and historically important research was the core of German medicine, two other advantages were decisive. One of them was the generous financial support of the German government, which made a decisive commitment to the advancement of research and left the United States looking myopic by contrast. The other and related strength was the German network of universities, chairs of medicine and research, well equipped medical laboratories, advanced graduate education, and the high prestige accorded to research.

By 1890 American medical educators, inspired by the German example, aimed to teach medicine in a more scientific way and to give research a central role in the medical school mission. The number of faculty researchers steadily grew over the next two decades, and, by 1910, American medical schools had acquired as much acknowledgment for their research leadership as for their educational advances. In that year Dr. William H. Welch of Johns Hopkins was able to announce, "the recognition that has been won for American [medical] science on the other side of the water has been one of the most important developments of the last century."[9] Noting these advantages, a steady stream of American physicians traveled to Germany for postgraduate education. They brought back with them not only fine training but also a passion to promote American medical research.

Dr. Welch, himself trained in Germany, became the leader of American research. At one point, while considering an invitation to join the faculty at Johns Hopkins, he was promised $50,000 by Andrew Carnegie to establish a pathology laboratory as an inducement to keep him in New York. Hopkins won, and Welch's career thereafter was marked by an ambitious program of organizing research throughout the country as a whole. His passion for research found a perfect match among those people of wealth who wanted to make their mark on American medicine. Johns Hopkins and the University of Chicago were among the first beneficiaries of the new private largesse, but other institutions and research laboratories gained as well.

Welch's *Journal of Experimental Medicine,* established in 1896, helped move along the prestige of research by displaying its results and promise. The faculty of elite medical schools, who made their reputation as researchers, found that it attracted the best students and the wealthiest patients, a fine combination for schools that were trying to improve their shaky intellectual status. To this day academic medical centers, though under great financial pressure, remain leaders in research.

ENTER THE PHILANTHROPISTS

The philanthropists held the trump card: money. The most important and justly celebrated symbol of the enthusiasm of private supporters of research was the establishment in 1901 in New York of the nation's first independent medical research organization, the Rockefeller Institute for Medical Research. After the death of a three-year-old grandson from scarlet fever, John D. Rockefeller (an otherwise firm believer in homeopathy) made an initial contribution of $1,000,000 for the institute and then a gift of $2,620,000 in 1907 to establish its endowment. By 1920 he had increased that sum to $23,000,000 and by 1928 to $65,000,000. None of his gifts might have come about but for the influence of the remarkable Reverend Frederick T. Gates, a minister who was both a skillful adviser to Rockefeller and a savvy businessman. Moved by deaths in his own family and by a reading of William Osler's celebrated 1,000-page textbook of medicine during a family vacation in the Catskills, Gates persuaded Rockefeller to champion research. For Gates, one commentator has observed, "the mere fact of the scientist's presence in the laboratory would have been enough to satisfy Jesus."[10]

"When I laid down [Osler's] book," Gates wrote later in a memoir, "I had begun to realize how woefully neglected in all civilized countries and perhaps most of all in this country, had been the scientific study of medicine. . . . It became clear to me that medicine could hardly hope to become a science until medicine should be endowed and qualified men could give themselves to uninterrupted study and investigation, on ample salary, entirely independent of practice."[11] Gates persuaded Rockefeller that the new institute should leave its staff free of teaching and clinical responsibilities, thus setting an important precedent for grants from the Rockefeller Foundation, which stipulated that medical schools receiving research money relieve their faculty of the need to supplement their income by patient care.

By the early twentieth century, clinical research was beginning to stake out its own claim to scientific rigor. It could be, its adherents held, just as scientific as laboratory research, taken at the time to be the gold standard. Those whom Harry Marks has called the "therapeutic reformers" sought to use the science of controlled experiments to direct medical practice and to judge the results of medical practice. These therapeutic reformers were persistently suspicious of corporate-sponsored research, treated as guilty until proved innocent. "Early in the century," Marks has noted, "Progressive-era reformers warned that only an independent science of drug evaluation, securely controlled by the medical profession, could resist corporate impulses to 'debauch our medical journals' and 'taint our text books.'" The early critics of the pharmaceutical industry were not necessarily hostile to business in general. "They sought," Marks has judged, "not to eliminate business from American society, but to subordinate it to the authorized voices of medical science."[12] Suspicion about that industry lingered and has never disappeared, rising and falling over the years.

Few of those suspicions infected the Rockefeller enterprise. So rapid and great was the success of the new Rockefeller Institute that, coming full circle so to speak, the new research institute founded in Germany in 1911, the Kaiser Wilhelm Gesellschaft, modeled itself on the Rockefeller Institute. The establishment of the Rockefeller Foundation in 1913 intensified the medical research drive of the Rockefeller family. The foundation expanded its interest in international health to rural health, making a strikingly impressive effort to eliminate hookworm, a serious public health hazard, in the South.[13] In the 1930s it turned to molecular biology but kept throughout what we now think of as a holistic vision, combining experimental biomedical research, the social sciences, and even the humanities. As Raymond Fosdick, who took over the presidency of the foundation in 1936, proclaimed, "Body and mind cannot be separated for purposes of treatment, they are one and indivisible."[14] For all its influence on research in general, however, the foundation succeeded only fitfully in promoting its nonreductionistic view of research, a stream of American research more neglected than praised.

The growing private support of research slowly set the stage for the federal support of research that was to be the mark of the second half of the twentieth century. But in the early twentieth century there was little public support and few strong voices pushing for the research process. Only the highly educated seemed able to appreciate it. Sinclair Lewis's character in his 1924 novel *Arrowsmith*, Martin Arrowsmith, a driven scientist, was meant to exemplify that process, struggling against a disinterest in research, full of caution, self-doubt, an obsession with precision, and loneliness. [15] Even so, scientific medicine helped the process along, eventually captivating journalism. Sophisticated medical and science writing did not come to journalism until the late 1920s and early 1930s, but magazines such as *Scientific American* and *Popular Science Monthly* earlier provided some insight into the nature of research. Even as interest in the cause and understanding of research advanced, so did the persistent virus of sensationalism. If it often enough misled the public, it fed the growing audience with information about medicine, research, and the promise of still more, ever more, to come.

As the historian Daniel M. Fox has noted, in the 1880s and 1890s "many people in America and Britain began to believe that, for the first time in history, scientists were discovering wholly new kinds of truth about nature that would, eventually, make it possible for doctors to reduce the suffering and death caused by the most threatening diseases."[16] The public prestige of medicine fostered the conviction that an increase in the supply of medical services, focusing on individual health, was the right way to go. The period 1890 to 1924 saw the transformation of American medicine, gaining public prestige, increased professional competence, and a sounder foundation in research. Together with the reform of medical education that took hold after the turn of the century and the Flexner Report in 1910, reforms going back to the late nineteenth century and earlier, the struggle against disease was organized into an effective campaign by the early twentieth century.

To onlookers in 1910, Kenneth Ludmerer, a historian of medical education has written, "the achievements were impressive. The nineteenth-century legacy was one of havoc from illness, suffering, and premature death. Epidemics continued to ravage the land; average life expectancy in 1900 was still less than 50 years. A certain fatalism toward disease characterized the attitude of virtually every American. . . . In this context, the early achievements of scientific medicine were stunning. Disease and suffering for the first time were seen not to be inevitable features of the human condition; they could be alleviated, relieved, prevented."[17]

A physician writing in the *Journal of the American Medical Association* stated that scientific medicine "has possession of methods which ultimately will lead to a solution of most if not all of our [medical] problems."[18] Another claimed, "In fifty years science will have practically eliminated all forms of disease."[19] Even the more sober General Education Board, a Rockefeller creation, said, "Though relatively few human ills have been subjugated, the method and the techniques by means of which successive diseases may and perhaps will be ultimately conquered have been definitely established."[20] Reverend Gates referred to the Rockefeller Institute for Medical Research as a "sort of theological seminary." "Medical research," he wrote "will find out and promulgate, as an unforeseen by-product of its work, new moral laws and new social laws—new definitions of what is right and wrong in our relations with each other. Medical research will educate the human conscience in new directions and point out new duties."[21]

Such pronouncements are simply part of a tradition of exuberant optimism going straight back to Thomas Jefferson and Benjamin Franklin, but they began to deserve some credibility by the early twentieth century. By then also, the first steps toward the research imperative had been taken. Fatalism was replaced by hope and optimism, unmarked as yet by the language of a "war," much less the later rhetoric of a necessary, morally obligatory crusade. But the foundation for that shift had been laid. The turmoil of World War II and the progress made during the 1950s and 1960s would encourage those next steps.

TOWARD THE NATIONAL INSTITUTES OF HEALTH

Much as the Rockefeller Institute's founding in 1901 signaled the coming of age for American research and an important economic stimulus to its private support, the evolution of the National Institutes of Health registered its public support. Yet its progress was slow, gaining full speed only after World War II. It began as a laboratory of hygiene in the Marine Hospital Service on Staten Island in 1887, reflecting that era's public health movement. Neither the public nor politicians thought it appropriate for the federal government to involve itself in, much less take charge of, that movement. Yet the large number of immigrants coming to the country each year, many of them sick, together with the growing knowledge about infectious disease made at least a measure of governmental support seem imperative. Cholera, yellow fever, malaria, smallpox, and typhoid fever were still rampant and fearsome. Now, people believed, government could and should do something about them.

The establishment of the laboratory, at first oriented to public health and confined to a single room, was also the starting point of a long struggle between two groups. One of them, known as the "national health movement," wanted public health to be part of a larger federal department of health. The other group, victorious in the long run, wanted the Marine Hospital Service to develop into such a body within its own institutional structure. With the laboratory of hygiene providing the opening wedge, the transformation of medical research policy, which began in the Progressive era at the turn of the century, moved slowly at first but steadily. The groundbreaking work of private philanthropists, the serious establishment of research in medical schools, the model of government-supported research in Europe, and the growing public interest in research, all played their part in what Victoria Harden has called the "increasing federalization of all the sciences in the twentieth century."[22] World War I had also played its part by revealing the poor health of so many recruits as well as the more general importance of health for national defense and the general welfare.

Harden singled out yet another important feature of this era: "On an organizational plane, this meant the rise of team research and the correlation of different fields. In the laboratory it meant increased reliance on quantitative methods, the use of experimental animals, and the development of new instruments that permitted the acquisition of more accurate data." "Objective" science was pitted against the anecdotal knowledge of clinicians.[23] At the same time, and stimulated by an active and powerful American Medical Association (AMA), public health leaders began trying to develop a role for their field distinct from that of medicine.

In 1926, Louisiana senator Joseph Eugene Ransdell introduced a bill to establish a national institute of health. Its aim would be to study the "fundamental problems" of human disease, to use the German state-sponsored university system of laboratory research as its model, and—most critically—to imbed the idea of pure or basic research in American universities. It took four years for that bill to pass after a long struggle with the national health movement, its aims embodied in a competitive bill introduced about the same time. But by 1930 the National Institute of Health was a reality, though far different from its present reality. Then in 1937 the National Cancer Institute was established, the first of many institutes, but in a sense it remains the flagship institute because of the public's fear of cancer. Characteristically negative toward government, the AMA warned, "The danger of putting the government in the dominant position in relation to medical research is apparent."[24] Of course the AMA eventually backed off from that attitude. More perennial was the warning of a prominent scientist: "This solution [to cancer] will come when science is ready for it and cannot be hastened by pouring sums of money into the effort."[25] Not that the warning mattered much. The notion that research is identical to solutions was, even then, a well-ingrained belief.

Once again war, this time World War II, accelerated the pace of research. Even before the war came to an end, President Franklin D. Roosevelt had begun to think about postwar science policy. In 1945 Vannevar Bush, director of the wartime Office of Scientific Research and Development, prepared at Roosevelt's request a report, *Science: The Endless Frontier.*[26] In the strongest call yet for a peacetime role for the government, Bush proposed large-scale federal support for research, articulating an old, but always renewable, conviction: in science lies the unlimited promise of improving human welfare. Shortly thereafter, another government report attempted to define different kinds of research with correspondingly different spheres of federal responsibility.[27] Its main consequence was to assign to the National Institute of Health responsibility for basic research, and the newly created Communicable Disease Center in Atlanta responsibility for applied research (in effect epidemics and public health crises). The Committee on Medical Research, under the National Defense Research Council, awarded a number of contracts, adding its own impetus to the postwar research drive.

Thereafter, the National Institutes of Health expanded rapidly, riding the crest of a great wave of public and political support. That support can be credited, in great part, to the dedication of a series of talented NIH directors, strong bipartisan leadership in Congress, and highly skilled lay proponents. Among the latter were Mary Lasker and her friend Florence Mahoney, who used their wealth and political skills to advance the cause of research in general and of NIH in particular. While the NIH budget for 1940 and 1941 was about $700,000, by 1948 it was $29 million, by 1955 $98 million, and by 1967 $1.4 billion. By the mid-1950s, budget increases of 25 percent a year were common. It was Lasker who was most likely responsible for a passage in Vannevar Bush's 1945 report noting that a couple of lethal diseases—no doubt cancer and heart disease—killed more people than all the lives lost in World War II. It was also Lasker who said in the 1960s, "I'm really opposed to heart attacks and cancer and strokes the way I'm opposed to sin."[28]

HARD TIMES, GOOD TIMES

Lasker's imagery was to catch the flavor of that era. In January 1971 President Richard M. Nixon urged in his State of the Union message that the conquest of cancer become a national goal, an aim that—after some confusion about how such an aspiration should be organized—was taken up by Congress. That was not so hard. In 1970 Congress had passed what one commentator has aptly called "a King Canute–style resolution," calling for a total victory over cancer by 1976, the two hundredth anniversary of the Declaration of Independence.[29] This was almost fifty years after the declaration of the first war against cancer, in 1922, and close to thirty years before Al Gore made that same goal part of his presidential campaign for 2000.

Yet if cancer research was to receive a boost in 1971, the NIH was in fact going through difficult years. The strong postwar coalition, led by Mary Lasker with the more than able support of Lister Hill and John Fogarty in Congress, and James Shannon as director of NIH, began to break up in the 1960s. That disintegration was in part the victim of the budgetary pressures brought on by the Vietnam War and in part resulted from the fallout of complaints that the NIH had not produced much in the way of therapeutic results in the twenty years since World War II. That some of the complaints came from leading coalition members made the criticism all the more stinging. The involvement of science in the Vietnam War (with the technocratic Robert McNamara as a symbol), and a belief in some quarters that scientists were to blame for environmental pollution (an unfair charge), probably did not help either.[30]

Between those criticisms and the budget pressures, weakened also by Hill's and Shannon's earlier retirement, the NIH had a difficult decade. My late friend Robert Q. Marston, director of NIH from 1968 to 1973, said to me, "after 1969 Congress no longer wrote the NIH a blank check; every request had to be justified." Struggles over the appropriate NIH balance between basic and applied research, never wholly absent, raised unsettling questions about its mission. While the NIH managed to continue giving the priority to basic research, it well understood that it owed much of its public support not simply to the promise of therapeutic gains but to actual demonstrations of such gains. Unhappily for scientists focused on freedom of research, the budgetary pressures that mixed tight funds and demands for visible results were about as disconcerting as any combination could be.

Nonetheless, after a rough period in the 1970s and part of the 1980s marked by rapid change of directors, the NIH was once again on the rise in the 1990s. By then a pattern prominent in the golden years of the 1950s began to reappear: Congress regularly complained that the executive branch had not asked for enough money and then, in protest, added more than requested. By the late 1990s, with full bipartisan support, budget increases of over 10 percent a year had become a regular event. In 1998, a campaign was launched aimed at nothing less than a doubling of the budget over the next five years. Only an increase of that magnitude, so the argument went, could do justice to the great breakthroughs just over the horizon: cancer could and would soon be cured, and the Human Genome Project would set the stage for a final and full understanding of the origin and nature of disease on the brave new frontier of genomics. That argument worked.

As with earlier bursts of optimism and grandiose claims, buried in the small print of balancing qualifications were the usual notes of caution and sober recognition that time—much time—would be needed to realize the bright dreams. Such was the response of the most careful scientists. But the large claims helped gain headlines and excite the public, a public that always likes news about new medical advances. Whatever the criticisms, the NIH has made magnificent contributions to American and international health— but almost always by steady, incremental gains, not sudden breakthroughs. Save perhaps for antibiotics, there have never been the quick and clean advances that the great triumphs against infectious disease in the late nineteenth and early twentieth centuries seemed to presage for future research. That highly misleading model lingers on today in the oft-repeated promise of eventual vaccines for cancer and Alzheimer's. They may well appear, but ameliorative therapies are even more likely.

ETHICS, MONEY, AND THE RESEARCH IMPERATIVE

So far, in the briefest of terms, I have sketched the rise and triumph of medical research in the United States. It was a triumph fashioned initially out of an emulation of German medical research, helped along by a generation of patronage by wealthy philanthropists, and eventually taken up by the federal government, which built the NIH into a hugely successful engine for biomedical progress.

Strikingly absent from my outline were the serious public ethical struggles of recent decades. The earliest history of biomedical research held a few of them, in battles over the use of cadavers and autopsies for research and education, for example; or the antivivisection movement of the early twentieth century, which brought abuses of human subjects as well as mistreatment of animals into the public eye. Despite criticism, the researchers tended to prevail, though the cessation of the first polio vaccine trial in 1939 came about as a result of pressure from the American Public Health Association. It was not until the 1960s that serious, and new, kinds of fights began to break out, and researchers had to contend with stiffer opposition. I move rapidly through that era's struggles, to give readers a context for issues I take up more fully later in the book.

Underlying the emergence of a variety of ethical and social dilemmas and disputes in the latter half of the twentieth century is a combination of developments both benign and troubling. In the benign column are some of the deep ethical problems inevitably posed by efforts to combat death and to eradicate disease and disability: how far should science go in that direction and what constitutes genuine progress of human value? Then there are problems of cupidity and pride—products of biomedical research's popularity and success, brought about by the vast amounts of money and prestige at stake—that set out a range of temptations absent from classical medicine and earlier research. Are great profits and popularity compatible with serious science?

These problems slowly came into public view in the 1960s. Most can be traced, I believe, to the research imperative, from the benign to the hazardous, slowly gathering force in the postwar years, and very much in step with the growing amount of money at stake, the heightened public expectation of forthcoming medical miracles, and a quickening reluctance among some excited researchers, members of Congress, and lay advocacy groups to let their opponents' moral objections stand in the way of promising lines of research.

The first sign of the more recent public trouble came with an article in 1965 by Henry Knowles Beecher, the distinguished chairman of anesthesiology at the Harvard Medical School, in the *New England Journal of Medicine*.[31] Destroying the myth that only in Nazi Germany had human beings been used for harmful and sometimes lethal research experimentation, Beecher showed that in the United States too such research was going on at that very moment. To the indignation of many colleagues and an embarrassed research community, he provided detailed evidence of violations of the Nuremberg Code.[32] That code, promulgated in 1947 as an outcome of the Nuremberg trials and requiring consent from research subjects and a balance of benefits over harms, was meant to avoid such abuse in the future.[33] It had not worked. Uninformed patients were injected with live cancer cells at the Jewish Chronic Disease Hospital, mentally disabled children were infected with hepatitis virus at the Willowbrook institution, and, most notoriously in the later-revealed Tuskegee project, poor black men took part in a study of the natural course of syphilis without their knowledge and were then denied effective treatment with penicillin when it became available.

Was this research carried out by cold, cruel physicians? Not at all. For them the research imperative—the overriding importance of the relief of suffering or death to future victims of disease—provided a clear justification for putting present subjects at risk (and, inadvertently, usually poor and minority subjects). How else was a healthier future to be secured? That utilitarian contention did not carry the day. As a result of Beecher's revelations and others that began appearing, the National Institutes of Health established in 1966 the institutional review board system, requiring that all federal grants using human subjects adhere to specific guidelines and be approved by an institutional review committee. But the strain between the research imperative and the protection of human subjects continued to emerge from time to time, right up through the present.

By the end of the 1960s and into the 1970s, talk of a "biological revolution" was in the air and celebrated by the media. That revolution, mainly with genetics in mind, was hailed as the successor to the physics revolution—whose most striking gifts, sometimes overlooked, were nuclear weapons and nuclear energy. The new revolution would, it was said, open the way for a radical manipulation of human nature and human traits, ranging from a greatly extended life expectancy through the cure of disease to an enhanced parental power to avoid genetic defects in their children and, even more exciting, to choose specific desirable traits. The prospect of human cloning, in the wake of a successful cloning of salamanders, was put forward as a particularly striking prospect.[34]

Ethical Troubles

If the 1970s and 1980s were to be dominated by other issues, the animal rights movement should not be overlooked. While the antivivisection movement had roots going back for at least a century, the 1960s saw a fresh version of that movement. It brought to the protection of animals the language of "rights" and an uncommon, sometimes violent, zeal. The Australian philosopher Peter Singer's 1975 book *Animal Liberation* intensified a worldwide effort to restrict the use of animals for medical research and to ensure that, when animals were used for that purpose, their use would be minimized and the conditions under which they were housed would be decent.[35]

Medical researchers were alarmed, not only because of the terrorism and vandalism of some extremists in the decades that followed, but also because they said they needed animals for research. Their argument was not too different from that used by researchers anxious about a curtailment of human-subject research: good medical research depends on animal research, just as it depends on human-subject research. There is no good alternative to the use of animals, particularly if information is needed about the likely effect on humans of new drugs or medical procedures. Therefore, the research must go forward.

Pitting the research imperative against the protection of animals, the encounter led to a compromise. Congress established a set of animal welfare regulations in the 1960s, frequently amended thereafter, and eventually set up the Institutional Animal Care and Use Committee. Though carefully regulated, the use of animals for research continued. Arguments for the value, indeed the necessity of such research for human health, withstood the strong and ongoing efforts to either end such research or curtail it far more drastically.

If the Beecher revelations and the animal rights struggle were the first signs of trouble within medical research, a more public crisis soon followed. The advent of recombinant DNA (deoxyribonucleic acid) research—gene splicing as it was popularly known, allowing the construction of hybrid DNA molecules—brought it about. While its development was a great thrill for the scientific community, there were also potential harms of a serious magnitude: the recombined molecules might get out of control, infecting future generations. In July 1974 an important group of researchers led by Paul Berg of the Stanford Medical Center and with the support of the Nobel laureate James D. Watson called for a moratorium on the research, which was effectively observed internationally.[36]

Then in March 1975, at a meeting held at the California Asilomar conference center, an international gathering of scientists decided to end the moratorium. Leading that charge were Watson and Joshua Lederberg. Watson in particular came to feel that the moratorium itself had been a mistake, serving only to inflame an uninformed public and opening the research to the prospect of an outright ban. That almost happened in Cambridge, Massachusetts, when the city council, with the support of a few dissident scientists, tried to enact a moratorium on such research at Harvard and MIT (though the mayor wanted an outright ban). The Asilomar conference participants did, however, propose a set of stringent regulations for recombinant DNA research that were shortly thereafter embodied in the work of a recombinant advisory committee at the NIH, a oversight body meant to regulate and monitor the research.

In the aftermath of the moratorium, sparked by Watson's misgivings, a conviction unfortunately spread among many researchers that never again should scientists risk their research in such a naive way. An issue of the journal Daedalus in the spring of 1978 on the "Limits of Scientific Inquiry" did not in fact propose much in the way of limits, but it required a certain nerve to raise the subject at all. While researchers had a strong core of belief in the social responsibility of scientists, in practice it made them nervous, fearful of the public impact of expressed worries and of the impact on research funded by a no less nervous Congress. By the end of the 1970s bans on research seemed just about unthinkable in the United States—even if they were frequently discussed, and even if federal support for research grants on controverted scientific initiatives could be withheld. The via media of regulation and oversight proved to be the popular way to go, with moratoriums as the last resort. Research may be slowed and often hindered but not permanently stopped. With the advent of the idea of therapeutic cloning (cloning for research rather than reproductive purposes), however, the idea of bans returned to the front of the stage (see chapter 7).

The public hardly noticed another consequence of the recombinant DNA development: a new entrepreneurialism among academic researchers, eager to push along the suddenly exciting field of biotechnology and to cash in on its expected profits. Herbert Boyer and Robert Swanson founded Genentech; a rash of other small companies quickly followed. Traditionally, even after medical research had passed through the era of a dependence on private philanthropy and its early support by the postwar NIH, it remained a relatively elite, nonmonetary pursuit, at least within universities. Knowledge and prestige were the prizes, not personal enrichment, as Watson makes clear in his book *The Double Helix,* recounting the discovery of the structure of the DNA molecule with Francis Crick.[37] That ethos changed rapidly in the 1970s and 1980s, as first individual academics and then universities themselves sought to find ways to turn their research into wealth (see chapter 8). The emergent biotechnology industry and the older pharmaceutical industry were beckoning gold mines, even if it took over a decade for the start-up biotechnology companies to show any profit (and some never have).

There were earlier precedents for such an entrepreneurial move in schools of engineering and agriculture, where university-industry relationships were more common. In her book *The Business of Breeding,* Deborah Fitzgerald tells the story of the close, often compromising, ties between agricultural scientists in the early twentieth century, working in land-grant universities to develop hybrid corn, and the seed-producing companies of the day.[38] Those ties created a crisis for the universities. All went well enough when research was the only joint focus, but once the new seeds for hybrid corn became a commodity the collaboration became a new, and tense, story. Who was to gain the profits? It took years for the land-grant colleges to pull back from those early relationships. No such move appears on the horizon with the new biotechnology or closely developed, eagerly sought bonds between the pharmaceutical industry and universities that were just beginning to emerge in the 1980s.

That decade brought another eruption, fetal tissue research. Research dependent on the derivation of fetal cells from deliberately aborted fetuses rather than miscarried pregnancies was thought promising for the relief of Parkinson's disease. Becoming the prototype for a group of similar cases that came up in the 1990s, the issue aligned the pro-life lobby against the various scientists and patient-interest groups that wanted the research to go forward. The National Institutes of Health reacted quickly, appointing a special committee to make ethical and policy recommendations. The committee supported the research, but the Reagan administration ignored its recommendations and forbade federal research grants. When a host of similar battles emerged in the 1990s, together with a few new ones, some repeated the fetal-cell issues while others brought into focus questions about human-subject research and the equitable outcome of research efforts.

If fetal cells were valuable to many researchers, human embryos were no less attractive to others for many of the same reasons. Some years earlier a British commission had approved the use in research of spare human embryos at up to fourteen days of development, but approval was to prove less easy to obtain in the United States.[39] Once again the NIH appointed a committee to make recommendations, and, not surprisingly, it supported the research and the provision of federal grants for that purpose.[40] On that occasion the Bush administration pushed aside the recommendation, issuing an executive order—with no strong congressional opposition—prohibiting such research grants. However strong the research imperative was in the research community, in disease advocacy groups, and in a large portion of the politically liberal educated community, it had less influence with many members of Congress.

Opposition to embryo research and use became more vehement in 1999 when the prospect of embryonic stem-cell research appeared on the horizon. Embryonic stem cells are pluripotent, meaning they can develop into all the cells and tissues of the human body and divide many times. In principle they could be used to treat many diseases, producing new pancreatic or heart tissue, for instance. They are best harvested from embryos. The House of Representatives' Pro-Life Caucus and the National Conference of Catholic Bishops managed to gain an executive order forbidding grants for any experiments that deliberately create or destroy a human embryo, but this time Republican Senator Arlen Specter opened a new battlefront, invoking the argument that lives might be saved and suffering avoided if the research could be allowed to proceed with federal support.

The Birth of Dolly

For all the drama of those battles, they seemed minor in comparison with the 1996 cloning of a sheep, Dolly, in Scotland by Ian Wilmut. That effort, achieved as the result of years of quiet work, directly opened up the prospect of the reproductive cloning of human beings. The immediate outcry was to oppose any effort to pursue research cloning in that direction, a position firmly stated by President Clinton and seemingly supported by a majority of the public. A prohibition of federal funding for human cloning research was then quickly put into place, with the prospect of a public and private ban apparently in the immediate offing. A number of scientific societies and professional associations (including the AMA) expressed opposition to research on human cloning but rejected the calls for an outright ban.

When a bill was introduced into the Senate in 1998 to ban the research, a coalition of prominent scientists opposed it, not only attacking the very idea of a ban on scientific research but also expressing worries about limiting any form of research that might produce a gain in knowledge. Connie Morella, chair of the House subcommittee on science, recapping the scientists' viewpoint in the most vivid terms, said that "the promise of cloning technology holds tremendous agriculture and medical benefits which could substantially improve our quality of life. These include revolutionary medical treatments and life-saving cures for diseases such as cancer, hemophilia, cystic fibrosis, sickle cell anemia, and emphysema . . . [and] may one day lead to . . . the repair and regeneration of human tissues in severe burns and spinal cord injuries, and bone marrow regeneration for patients undergoing cancer chemotherapy."[41] This list of benefits, as we will see, is not much different from those earlier identified for embryo research and later for embryonic stem-cell research. The National Bioethics Advisory Commission (appointed by President Clinton in 1995), unable to agree ethically on anything other than possible safety hazards in trying to clone a child, proposed a five-year moratorium on further research in order to accumulate more evidence and allow public debate to mature.

That outcome, while hardly an endorsement of cloning—despite the imaginative efforts of some ethicists, in the name of unlimited procreative rights, to show benefits for certain parents in procreating cloned babies—helped cool the opposition. The research imperative is best fed by public support, but it has shown itself capable of surviving well enough if the opposition can be quieted and the prospects of health gains constantly underscored. It is often forgotten, moreover, that controversial biomedical research in the United States always has an available ace in the hole: fetal tissue, embryo, stem cell, and human cloning research can go forward utterly unimpeded in the private sector, and in most cases it has. That is not something the biotechnology and pharmaceutical industries care to advertise, but there is nothing to stop them. And there is one important precedent. When in vitro fertilization research encountered heavy opposition in the early 1970s, the British researchers continued in silence, neither talking with other scientists nor publishing any preliminary results. Only with the birth of Louise Brown in 1978 did the public learn that the research had never stopped (and the public, as it happened, cheered). Federal funding now seems sought as much to give the research open public legitimization as to bring additional money to those working outside an industry context.

For all the attention they gained, the range of issues just discussed hardly exhausts the outburst of ethical problems that marked the steps of research in the late 1990s and into the new millennium. In each case, the research imperative was at work, pitting research proponents against those with moral objections. The least noticed, except among medical professionals, were worries about the impact of research on privacy, particularly in gaining epidemiological information. Far more visible were nasty exchanges and policy struggles over human subject research. Though institutional review regulations and committees have been in place for over thirty years, their success has waxed and waned, the subject of a series of commission studies and reforms over the years.

By the year 2000 another cycle of reform was under way, with frequent complaints about compromised informed consent, perfunctory reviews, and poor procedures. The research imperative was leading many researchers away from a careful protection of subjects. The most strident argument turned on human subject research in developing countries, particularly in relationship to the testing of preventive treatments aimed at pregnant women, seeking to spare their babies from the transmission of the AIDS virus. Is it fair to use as subjects women who could not give real informed consent or might be put in a trial's placebo arm, and who in any case—even if the research was a success—might not be able to afford the treatment? Is it right to carry on human subject trials in poor countries under circumstances that would not for a moment be tolerable to subjects in affluent countries? Yet is it wise, in the name of ethical probity, to oppose research that might at first not be equitably available to all but might be at a further time?

That last question touches on a distinct ethical and political question that surfaced toward the end of the 1990s and remains a political open wound: the cost of pharmaceuticals and equitable access to them. The pharmaceutical industry's principal defense of those costs has been a research imperative argument: the high prices are necessary to carry on lifesaving research. In the developed countries, including most prominently the United States, it was becoming obvious that pharmaceutical costs were becoming a critical item in the return to inflationary health care costs. If the costs were hard on hospitals, HMOs, and health care insurers, they bore even more heavily on the elderly, not provided outpatient pharmaceuticals under the Medicare program, and on the uninsured or underinsured, forced to pay for drugs themselves. Proposals for price controls or for the use of governmental power to permit, for instance, drug purchasing coalitions or the import of drugs from foreign countries, even reimportation from Canada, met strong pharmaceutical industry opposition.

Complaints about the costs of drugs were hardly new in the United States, going back to the nineteenth century, but this time they signaled real trouble for the industry.[42] Its response was to invoke the high cost of discovering new drugs in the first place and to invoke a much-repeated claim: any control of costs, or governmental pressures to cut industry profits, the industry said, would harm the needed research for still more drug breakthroughs in the ongoing fight against disease and suffering.

For the developing countries, the problem is far worse. They cannot come close to affording the expensive, and even many of the inexpensive, drugs available in the developed countries. Nor do the pharmaceutical companies devote much research money to the diseases afflicting their populations, particularly the lethal tropical diseases such as malaria. Those companies focus on the development of drugs that people in affluent countries can afford, many of them of a life-enhancing kind, such as Prozac, rather than those that could make a real difference in the mortality and morbidity of those in poor countries. The final insult for many poor countries is that they offer drug companies an attractive combination—lax standards for human-subject research and lower research costs—that makes them useful venues for the conduct of clinical trials for pharmaceuticals that will mainly be sold in developed countries.

ENVIABLE SUCCESS

I have sketched, in a panoramic way, the history of what I believe we now have on our hands, a research imperative ever more optimistic about success (given the optimism that has reigned since Jefferson and Franklin, an amazing feat) but increasingly—because of its ever-growing ambition—generating more ethical dilemmas and sociopolitical problems of a kind relatively rare earlier. The debates have increased in scope and fury. Again and again the proponents of research invoke arguments for its moral necessity, its economic benefits, the importance of American research leadership, and the still endless frontier of research possibilities.

None of the debates about research have done much damage to its reputation, its public support, or its exceedingly high standing in Congress. The budget of the National Institutes of Health should reach $27 billion in 2003.

According to the *Pharmaceutical Industry Profile 2000*, some $24 billion would be spent in 1999 on pharmaceutical research and development, $20.1 billion within the United States and the remaining $3.9 billion spent abroad by U.S.-owned companies.[43] Yet while the budget of the NIH has more than doubled over the past decade, its national share of research and development expenditures has decreased from about 35 percent in the mid-1980s to about 29 percent in 1999. During that same period the private sector's share has increased from 34 to 43 percent. With a growth rate in its research expenditures now near 10 percent a year, that gap between the public and private sectors will grow.

If the drug companies have done well, so have all supporters of even more medical research. Research!America is an aggressive and effective lobby for increased research spending, as are a large number of disease-oriented activist groups such as the American Cancer Society and the American Heart Association. They have considerable public support. Some 84 percent of the public believe it important that the United States remain the world leader in medical research.[44] Support for increased federal spending is strong, with 66 percent in favor (as of 1999) in doubling national spending on medical research over the next five years, while 60 percent would favor spending part of the federal budget surplus to fund research. One poll finding that should please NIH researchers is that 81 percent believe the government should support basic research even if it brings no immediate benefit. Some 61 percent would be willing to accept a small tax increase to increase research.

Less clear are the public priorities for research. By a 46 to 23 percent majority the public favors spending a higher proportion of all health care dollars on health promotion and disease prevention, but whether it would support a research shift in that direction at the expense of medical research is less evident.[45] The important initiative of the American Heart Association, which will now devote 50 percent of its research budget to health promotion research rather than medical research, could signal an important national research shift in that direction. The National Institutes of Health has been under greater, if still relatively gentle, pressure to spell out its priorities in a more explicit fashion, both to satisfy Congress that its money is being well spent and its critics among disease-advocacy groups who complain about unfair priorities and spending patterns (see chapter 8). Complaints have been heard for years that the NIH does too little to support health promotion and disease prevention efforts, with its bias—as the Human Genome Project suggests—heavily oriented in a biomedical direction.

Understanding the Research Imperative

In sketching the history of medical research in the United States, I have tried to signal those historical moments when a research imperative emerged, an imperative either in the benign sense of the term—a heightened drive to do more research for its own sake or to relieve suffering—or in the more hazardous sense of an imperative that threatens other important values, as in the case of morally flawed human subject research. The remaining chapters of the book aim to provide many more of the details that I hope will make my case more plausible. While I cannot claim to have a full explanation of the gradual transformation that took place, producing the research imperative, I believe it is possible to identify the critical ingredients that have been part of it.

Perhaps the most important ingredient has been the success of the medical research enterprise. It has been a wonderful contributor to a reduction in mortality, to improved health, and to the relief of pain and suffering. It has thus, by most measures, been a glorious enterprise. It works, and we want more of it. But its very success has had two paradoxical features. One of them is that, as health has improved, and mortality and disability declined, the drive for research has increased, not decreased. There seems to be no such thing as enough, no level of individual or population health that leads to a reduction in research aspiration. A naive witness to discussions of American health might think that we have never been worse off, with a long and intimidating list of miseries still to be dealt with. The other feature, closely related, is the escalation of personal health standards: the healthier we are, the healthier we want to become; and what would have been a satisfactory level of health and functioning is no longer satisfactory. "Our medical efforts," Dr. Arthur Barsky has observed, "have by some perverse trick of fate left us with diminished, rather than enhanced, feelings of well-being . . . the healthier we become, the more concerned with health we become. . . . Because our dream is so alluring and our ambitions are set so high, our efforts inevitably leave us feeling disenchanted."[46] The cycle is clear: the better off we become, the worse we feel; and the worse we feel the more we demand of research; and the more research gives us, the more we ask of it; and when we get what we want we ask for still more.

Whether it be the Human Genome Project or embryonic stem cell research, the promise is now for a generic research breakthrough, one that will not just cure cancer (the old foe) but put science in a position to cure all disease. Moreover, as the success of research and those promissory notes portend, old-fashioned fatalism seems to have, so to speak, received a fatal blow. There is no reason in principle any longer—so the implicit message goes—to accept stoically any known disease or disability. The causes of death can be vanquished, aging pacified, diseases cured, disabilities eliminated. If once religion helped people find a meaning in death and suffering, seemingly fixed parts of the human condition, a more secularized, science-soaked culture has put in its place a confident and nature-defiant weapon, medical research. It is not a weapon to handle gingerly: tough nerves, risk-taking, high hopes, and broad visions are requisites to make it work.

None of those forces might have been so potent but for another, classically American, ingredient: money. The post–World War II expansion of biomedical research money, public and private, brought fresh and steadily increased funds to individual researchers, gradually transforming research from a once-elitist pursuit to a more egalitarian venture. Fellowships and money for equipment, laboratories, and research assistants became open to anyone with the talent to go after them. The influx of money also contributed mightily to the rise of academic medical centers, research laboratories and institutions, and much-strengthened professional and advocacy associations. The net result was the growth of a research establishment that needed more and more money to do what it wanted to do; and it drew encouragement to do more of what it wanted to do from the money that was there to do it—and always more of it.

All of that might be judged as splendid, save for one drawback: the research establishment depends on a steady flow of money to sustain the practices, policies, and institutions that the influx of massive funding makes possible. Here the private sector makes a great difference, supplementing the federal funds at first and then, eventually, spending even more on research than the government. Thus a new wealthy patron–dependent research relation came into being. As with the research venture as a whole, the more money that went into it the greater the expectations, and the greater the changes in those expectations, the greater the need to keep the whole venture going. The rapid increase of the NIH budget means that programs and projects will be put in place that will need continued support in the future, requiring a budget that will continue to rise or will cause economic and institutional dislocation if it does not.

The researchers, far from feeling more comfortable with increased funds, often find themselves feeling needier than ever. If nothing else, the cost of research keeps rising as new technologies emerge. Like the rest of us—apt to consider any retrenchment a disaster—medical researchers are part of an enveloping American culture that has intensified even as it has contributed to the research culture. For at least four decades, health care has served to generate jobs and income, in both the research and delivery phases of health care. In Congress, a federal investment in research has been backed as the source of valuable exports and international prestige; and, by the by, good for health also. The great success of the Manhattan Project during the war, and the sending of men to the moon in the 1960s, provided a model of how successful a highly focused and ambitious American research and technology innovation effort could be. The war against disease could and should be one more such bold effort.

The striking fact that the NIH budget has garnered overwhelming bipartisan support—in a way little else has in a budget-cutting, antigovernment era—suggests that the research imperative has a symbolic function of a high order, cutting through pluralistic discord, drawing together disparate supporters, eliciting transcendent ambitions, and remaining remarkably resistant to serious criticism or second-guessing. Precisely the combination of great ambition and great hubris, large amounts of money, university and research institution prestige, and professional competition helps explain the research imperative in its best and worst expressions.

The research imperative, then, draws on many sources, medical, economic, and political, and it is their interaction that creates its great force. It can be called a cultural force because, without the facilitating power and permeation of background American values, it would have far less momentum. No other country is so enamored of medical research as ours, gives it so much public and media attention, or accords it such an extraordinarily high place in promoting an optimistic view of the human future.

Hence we can usefully begin our examination of the research imperative by looking at the historical ideals of scientific research, at the social responsibilities of scientists, and at some of the more obvious dangers that threaten its good name. If those threats are by no means wholly new, many of them now can be traced to the combination of scientific aspiration, American individualism, the influence of money and market ideology, media interest, and sometimes utopian public hopes that is part of the research imperative tapestry.

2   Protecting the Integrity of Science

The research drive has the deepest possible roots, a defining part of what it means to be human. It helps us know ourselves, the nature of which we are a part, the ills of the body and mind. That drive now also connotes power and money and prestige, set within a network of politics, profits, and personalities that has of late brought dangerous viruses into the institution of science, joining those already present. In varying ways curiosity, ambition, hope, cupidity, and altruism motivate the scientific community that runs this institution. What are that community's obligations? What does it need for its own flourishing? What do those of us who will have our lives affected by research, and whose private purchases and public taxes pay for it, have a right to expect from it?

Biomedical research rests on a moral foundation of values common to science as a whole. These values—the professional norms and ethical commitments that scientists use to judge their own probity and that others may use to judge them—animate the scientific enterprise. Both because science holds a high, trusted place among our social institutions and because the research knowledge it generates affects our lives, it has exacting moral obligations. We need to know what research might do for us, how it might improve and change the world (and our bodies) through its technological applications, and what dangers it may put in our path.

Inevitably, the community of scientific researchers has less control over the impact of its research than over its interior life and professional standards. Scientists know one another, are familiar with the work being done by others, and have effective means of deciding who should, or should not, be considered responsible. They choose what they want to work on, how they conduct their research, and what they are prepared to tolerate among their colleagues. Even when the use made of their discovered knowledge slips out of their hands into that of others, scientists can be a strong influence on what happens. As a community, they have the political power and social prestige to influence public opinion as well as the judgment of legislators, judges, the media, industry, and public administrators. Hence the integrity of science depends on how it deploys its community of researchers and how it evaluates and shapes its results. The power of science and research are considerable. The standards of judgment and expectation should be high.

My argument moves through two stages: a review of the modern values and ideals of science in general and, in light of those values, an inventory of threats to good biomedical research. As with the leading edge of a storm, it is possible to discern the emergence over the past few decades of a cluster of problems jeopardizing the integrity of scientific research. My emphasis in this analysis is on recognized threats, not on those controverted issues where the threat is disputed (which I will take up in chapter 7).

In recent years a garden-variety level of scientific misconduct has engaged Congress and the public just as much as the scandals coming out of human-subject research. This misconduct seems to strike at the very integrity of science as a truth-privileged, socially critical discipline: the falsification of data, conflict of interest, a misuse of the media, and the intimidation of researchers. Unlike abuses of human-subject research—which are usually accounted a moral and not a scientific failure—misconduct seems to threaten science itself, cutting against its deepest values and most esteemed sources of public credibility.

A 1942 essay by the eminent sociologist of science Robert K. Merton has stood the test of time in setting forth classical values of science. Merton identified four "institutional imperatives" that comprise the "ethos of science":[1]

> universalism: any claims to truth made on behalf of science must be subjected to "preestablished impersonal criteria"; that is, they must bow to a rigorous standard of objectivity, not dependent on any standards dictated by politics, money, race, or class.

> communism (or "communalism," which might sound better to contemporary ears than "communism," since it refers to "substantive findings of science [that] are a product of social collaboration and are assigned to the community"): the findings of science constitute a "common heritage," and "property rights are whittled down to a bare minimum by the rationale of the scientific ethic."[2]

> disinterestedness: science is a self-regulating institution. "The activity of scientists is subject to rigorous policing, to a degree perhaps unparalleled

in any other field of activity . . . [and it is] effectively supported by the ultimate accountability of scientists to their compeers."[3]

organized skepticism: the temporary suspension of judgment "and the detached scrutiny of beliefs in terms of empirical and logical criteria."[4] I would put this standard in a more homely fashion: it is the demand to challenge all claims to scientific knowledge, forcing them to meet the highest standards of rigor and testing. There is no such thing as the benefit of doubt in good science.

If these are the core Mertonian values, other commentators have added to or refined them in the same vein to encompass rationality, emotional neutrality, honesty, and tolerance.[5] Merton did not include freedom of scientific inquiry, an odd omission, but it too is an "institutional imperative."

But is this the whole story of scientific values, much less those that are supposedly institutionalized in the practice of science? In subsequent years, a number of commentators denied that they were—sometimes characterizing them as the high school version of science—and Merton himself tried to account for the deviation from those norms visible in the history of science. The most interesting and decisive debate in this respect was stimulated by the carefully documented claim that science did exhibit the norms discerned by Merton, but that very strong "counter-norms" have a high institutional standing also.[6]

In fact, the counter-norms can themselves be understood as essential to the progress of science. The counter-norm to emotional neutrality is that of emotional commitment, even at times unreasonable commitment, useful in pushing forward with difficult, time-consuming, and often frustrating research. Universalism as a norm has as its mirror opposite particularism, which often amounts to following those scientists whose work is particularly reliable; they are simply worthy of greater trust than others. The value of communism (communality) has the counter-norm of secrecy, which in many respects is not a harmful value. It helps, for instance, avoid research discovery priority disputes and—because others may want to steal or otherwise appropriate a scientist's work—serves as a stimulus to a researcher to persevere in his own work. Secrecy is by no means always a valid ideal, but then neither is total openness of information. In sum, a flourishing science needs counter-norms no less than Merton's imperatives. They work together.

The debate did not end here. Still another sociologist, Michael Mulkay, argued that neither standard norms nor counter-norms have been established as the institutional norms of science.[7] Merton's norms were too heavily drawn from the writing of the greatest and rarest of scientists, while I. I. Mitroff worked selectively with the descriptive and prescriptive accounts of working scientists, culling out various "verbal formulations." But why take such formulations as institutional standards? The reward system of science, Mulkay contended, is determined by the quality of the research, not by the moral traits or behavior of scientists. The technical standards of the particular kind of research are the real norms that must be met; if so, then the scientific results will be accepted, and the researcher rewarded.

In the post–World War II era, scientists sought increased governmental support but at the same time aimed to hold on to their autonomy. An ideology of pure science in the prewar period stressed the universality and objectivity of science, but in a way such that only scientists could understand those notions, thus effectively excluding nonscientists. The aim was a science certified for its validity, rightfully to be supported by federal funds, but free of outside interference.[8] In the 1950s, a mutuality of cultural purpose and social contributions enhanced the status of science by likening it to American democracy, to the benefit of both parties. Science as a source of national progress worked hand in hand with science as the source of broader human progress: the virtues of science are the virtues of a good society and of good human beings.

The science in question was principally basic, or what was once called "pure" science. But that theme had its political counterpart in the emphasis on the practical contributions of science. A combination of basic and applied science gave it such national and human importance, looking both to the depths of things and yet no less to putting science to good use in the day-to-day world. Gerald Holton's characterization of Jeffersonian science applies equally well to the medical sciences: locating the "center of research in an area of basic scientific ignorance that lies at the heart of a social problem" (see page 11).

THE SOCIAL RESPONSIBILITIES OF SCIENCE

If Merton and others were able to glean from the history of science a list of values for the practice of science, integral to it as a discipline, a parallel list of scientists' social and ethical responsibilities was more elusive. For a time, it was common in the aftermath of World War II—and the development and use of atomic weapons—for some scientists (though not Niels Bohr or Robert Oppenheimer) to claim that they bore no moral responsibility for their discoveries or the uses to which they might be put. A famous satirical song by Tom Lehrer in the 1960s had someone—alluding to Dr. Werner Von Braun, a major designer of intercontinental rockets—say that he took responsibility only for getting the rockets in the air, not for where they came down. But many other scientists worked in the 1950s and 1960s to bring the social implications of research before the public eye, with the earliest focus on nuclear arms and energy, then on scientific and social issues that emerged during the Vietnam War, and then by the 1970s on biological and research issues, most notably a moratorium on recombinant DNA work. The Center for Science in the Public Interest, the Scientists' Institute for Public Information, and Science for the People were important leaders in the scientific responsibility movement.[9]

The biologist Bentley Glass caught as well as anyone the new standards of scientific responsibility that could be distilled from a number of debates in the 1960s and 1970s. He identified three ethical and social responsibilities of scientists:[10]

to proclaim science's benefits: while scientists can hardly predict with any certainty the outcomes of their research and its possible social implications, they are in as good a position as anyone to foresee where it might lead. And they ought to tell us that. After noting that science these days is hardly shy about the "advertisement of [its] benefits," he adds an ironic and wise comment. "Every bit of pure research is heralded as a step [toward the] elimination of cancer and heart disease. . . . The ethical problem here is merely that of keeping a check-rein on the imagination and of maintaining truthfulness. But the truth itself is so staggering that it is quite enough to bemuse the public."[11]

to warn of risks: Glass adduces the postwar effort to warn the world of the great risks of a nuclear arms race and the further development of nuclear weapons, but his point would work as well with medical research, particularly genetic research. "It is," he contends, the duty of the scientist to "state his opinion on matters of social concern, but at the same time to distinguish clearly between what he states to be fact and what opinion he holds."[12]

to discuss quandaries: "It is the social duty and function of the scientist . . . to inform and to demand of the people, and of their leaders too, a discussion and consideration of all those impending problems that grow out of scientific discovery and the amplification of human power. . . . Science has found its social basis and has eagerly grasped for social support, and it has thereby acquired social responsibilities."[13]

Glass does not take up the question of the standards for judging the risks and benefits of research. Who is to set those standards? What considerations are pertinent to fashioning them? Which standards apply to society as a whole, which rest on individual choice? Those are the subject matter of later chapters, but here I focus on obvious threats to scientific integrity that challenge the Mertonian norms or may reflect counter-norms.

RESEARCHERS' MISCONDUCT

When Robert K. Merton wrote his 1942 article on the ethos of science, he could say that the history of science had been remarkably clean. This may have been an exaggeration. Yet over the past few decades scientific misconduct has become a serious problem. The federal government established in 1989 an Office of Research Integrity (ORI) within the National Institutes of Health and then, in 1994, made it an independent entity reporting directly to the secretary of the Department of Health and Human Services. There is no reliable estimate of how much misconduct there has been. It is hard to detect in the first place and, even if detected, often difficult to distinguish from simple error. Whether intentional deception has increased or decreased in recent years is uncertain; its present prominence may reflect greater public interest in the subject, better reporting, and more legislative attention.

Misconduct is one of those issues, however, where the actual extent of the problem may be less important than the public perception of its scope and meaning. It was all too easy in the early 1990s for Congressman John Dingell—something of a grandstander and often unfair to researchers—to create a major public furor over misconduct, playing straight to the media and playing up the waste of federal money that it can cause. David Baltimore, a distinguished Nobel laureate, was one of the victims of what can only be called the hysteria Dingell helped bring about.[14] When Thereza Imanski-Kari, a junior coauthor on a paper jointly published with Baltimore, was accused of fraud, Baltimore came to her defense with a vigor that dismayed many of his colleagues, harming his own reputation at the time. In particular, many scientists criticized Baltimore for directly confronting Dingell, worried about possible harm to research funding. Imaniski-Kari was eventually exonerated, and Baltimore went on to become president of the California Institute of Technology.

Scientific misconduct is defined by the federal government as fabrication, falsification, and plagiarism in proposing, performing, or reviewing research, or in reporting research results.[15] *Fabrication* is making up results and recording or reporting them. *Falsification* is manipulating research material, equipment, or processes, or changing or omitting data or results such that the research is not accurately represented in the research record. *Plagiarism* is the appropriation of another person's ideas, processes, results, or words without giving appropriate credit, including those obtained through confidential review of others' research proposals and manuscripts. A finding of research misconduct requires, first, that there be a significant departure from accepted practices of the scientific community for maintaining the integrity of the research record; second, that the misconduct be committed intentionally, or knowingly, or in reckless disregard of accepted practices; and, third, that the allegation be proven by a preponderance of evidence.

The case against such misconduct is hardly difficult to make. It damages the reputation of the research community, wastes resources, and creates an atmosphere of suspicion.[16] Most simply, as Douglas Weed has put it, "Science, after all, is a search for truth. Misconduct, especially in the form of falsification or fabrication, is its antithesis."[17] In terms of the standards Merton discerned, it is a gross violation of the principle of disinterestedness. The self-interest of the researcher wins.

Why does it happen? Could the counter-norm of emotional commitment help explain a desperate if misguided attempt to show the validity of scientific work? That is a plausible explanation in some cases even if it hardly works as a viable defense. We might look also to the larger culture of which biomedical research is a part—to reports of greater cheating among high school and college students, for instance—suggesting a decline in ordinary moral standards. Closer at hand is a fair degree of consensus on the motives behind recent misconduct: the increased importance for professional advancement of publications and research grants, an intimidating "publish or perish" atmosphere in universities and medical schools, and the difficulty of detecting and punishing misconduct.[18] Is misconduct an instance of the old "rotten apple" problem, or can the culture of universities and laboratories play a part? A significant group of researchers believe it to be a systemic problem.[19]

As for its frequency, something (though not much) can be said. Between 1993 and 1997, the Office of Research Integrity received approximately 1,000 allegations of misconduct, of which it investigated 151 cases and made 76 findings of misconduct. The majority of the cases (81 percent) were for falsification of data.[20] Another study showed a number of misrepresentations in the bibliographies of applicants for medical school faculty positions: out of 250 applicants with a total of 2,149 reported articles, 39 applicants had 56 misrepresentations, with 11 applicants making 2 or more misrepresentations.[21]

No less serious are reports of research on drugs that have grossly exaggerated their effectiveness, with of course potential harm to patients. Three likely sources of these forms of research misrepresentation have been identified: *publication bias* presents for publication studies showing positive results rather than those showing negative results; *redundant publication of data* involves a second article based on the same study but with a different title and different authors; and a *purposely poor experimental design* compares the new drugs with those known to be ineffective, thus guaranteeing that the new drugs will look good.[22] The use of ghost authors and the listing of authors who did not substantially contribute to the research are still other forms of misrepresentation.[23]

What is being done about misconduct? The establishment of the Office of Research Integrity was surely an important step, but a severe limitation on its work is that the research institutions themselves, not the ORI, are primarily responsible for the prevention and detection of any misconduct. This can be a great burden on universities, which may have to spend a considerable amount of time and money investigating misconduct reports.[24] There is, moreover, a serious conflict of interest for universities forced to carry out investigations. Among other things, it can hurt their reputations, certainly not an incentive for aggressive investigations.[25] There has long been doubt that universities have pursued reports of misconduct with the necessary zeal. It is not hard to understand why that might happen, quite apart from the embarrassment of it all.

For many of those reasons, there has been pressure to take the burden of investigation away from universities and put the decisive power in the hands of the government. The federal Fake Claims Act, focused heavily on institutional misconduct, is a move in that direction.[26] Naturally, that act is unpopular, and a variety of proposals for scientific self-regulation have been put forward.[27] The idea behind most of the proposals is to promote scientific integrity rather than to emphasize scientific misconduct. Many other professions have had similar debates, but few have been able to manage an emphasis on virtuous practitioners without recourse to strong outside regulation. The record of clinical medicine in disciplining its practitioners, for instance, is weak to the point of being meaningless, burdened by a reluctance to blow the whistle on colleagues and a legalistic structure for dealing with charges that make it difficult for the profession to punish or eject those who behave irresponsibly.

At stake in this debate, though not sufficiently noted, is the severe threat to the scientific community that external regulation of an even more stringent kind would bring with it. As the Merton standards bring out, the great strength of science rests on the integrity of its community. Peer judgment, pressure, and oversight are at the heart of good science. The public must trust scientists, who in turn must trust one another.

"Trust" that requires outside sanctions to make it work is not trust at all; it is fear of punishment masquerading as trust. Outside regulation of too severe a character is no guarantee to curb bad behavior, but it greatly increases the possibility of harm to the scientific community. Exacerbating that possibility, the charge that misconduct represents a waste of public money sometimes gets as much political attention as threats to health brought on by bad research. The need for outside money, public or private, to pay for research is—though unavoidable—itself the source of many serious problems for the scientific community. That is less so when the money comes from the public rather than the private purse, but legalistic governmental oversight of a kind destructive to the trust necessary for good research is also harmful.

INTIMIDATION OF RESEARCHERS

When researchers take on projects that can directly affect the financial or professional interests of other specialties or specific companies, they should be ready for trouble.[28] In the mid-1990s, for example, a group of researchers brought down upon themselves the wrath of a surgical specialty group when they reported that spinal-fusion surgery had few positive scientific indications, higher costs, and more complications than other back operations. The North American Spine Society did not like that finding at all and no doubt reacted even more strongly to the study's conclusion recommending a nonsurgical approach in most cases.[29] The society then undertook a nasty campaign to discredit the research and to attack the Agency for Health Care Policy and Research that had provided the money for it. A letter-writing campaign to Congress and a lobbying organization set up by the society, the Center for Patient Advocacy, almost managed to have the agency eliminated. It did, unhappily, succeed in leading the agency to end its guideline-development work.

In another case, a study cast doubt on the immunodiagnostic tests used to support disability and liability claims for chemical sensitivity.[30] A large number of groups, with financial and legal interests at stake, undertook a harsh campaign against the researchers, claiming scientific misconduct and distributing material at scientific meetings charging the investigators with fraud and conspiracy. Preliminary investigations were carried out by no less than five different organizations, including the federal ORI. Though no basis was found for a full-scale investigation, the investigators spent over a year dealing with a barrage of complaints that diverted much of their attention from the institution where they worked. A third case was that of a research study showing that short-acting calcium-channel blockers were associated with a 60 percent increase in the risk of a myocardial infarction in comparison with diuretics and beta-blockers.[31] Outraged pharmaceutical companies undertook a campaign to discredit the results and the researchers, triggering legal challenges, phone calls from doctors and patients, and efforts prior to publication to identify the journal to which the study had been submitted. Pressure against the principal researcher was initiated through his dean, who might be expected to defend a beleaguered faculty member.

Researchers have no ready defense against attacks of this kind. As Deyo and his colleagues note, the world of law and public pressure is very different from that familiar to researchers. The former has a set of rules "more like the aggressive marketing hyperbole, entrenched positions, and relentless character attacks of political campaigns and high-profile court room battles . . . [that leave] investigators feeling relatively defenseless."[32] There is no sure way to protect researchers against campaigns of that kind. Meticulous reporting of research results to the media may help, as will a clear absence of any conflict of interest, support from the researchers' professional organizations, and institutional help in dealing with charges.

Efforts to suppress research results are clearly a threat to the research enterprise. A failure of colleagues and pertinent institutions to come to the assistance of those under assault is no less a threat. As for attacks on funding agencies, as great an insulation from politics as possible is wise, supported by a solid system of peer review to keep the reputation of the funding agency at a high level. All this is easier said than done: the agency may itself have been a creation of politics (which can do as much good as bad).

CONFLICT OF INTEREST

Does the fact that a researcher has a financial stake in the outcome of the investigation or is carrying out the research for a company with such a stake automatically skew the research and compromise its scientific value? Not necessarily, at least as a formal, abstract issue. Researchers bring all kinds of interests to their investigations, financial and otherwise: the desire for praise and prestige, the need for academic tenure, the spur of prizes and fame, or simply a fixed view of the truth that their research should (surely) reveal. Yet a serious, conscientious researcher can overcome such tendencies by designing the research well, letting the results speak for themselves, and swallowing any personal disappointment that the results might bring.

That abstract possibility does not, unfortunately, dispose of the issue. It is not simply a matter of doing good, but of looking good—in the best sense of "looking good," that of being free of self-interest (which represents a conflict of interest)—in designing the research, carrying it out, and presenting the results. At stake are the good name and credibility of the researcher, any institution of which she is a part, and the larger public reputation of science itself. For just those reasons, it is important to avoid any *appearance* of a conflict of interest. This is particularly true when money is at stake, if only because financial self-interest is seen as comparatively more reprehensible than, say, a desire for prestige, but also because it is somewhat more accessible to public inspection. In the end, only the researcher knows the extent to which a desire for fame, or a vested psychological interest in a particular research outcome, is working its influence; and in many cases, self-deception can mask such motives.

Conflict of interest can come in many forms, and it is worth noting them to understand the kinds of pressures that researchers find at work, and what might be done about them. The increased dependence of researchers on the pharmaceutical industry is part of the problem, as are the entrepreneurial interests of researchers.[33] By far the most public attention has been paid to financial conflicts: carrying out paid research for a company with a financial stake in the outcome; owning stock in a company that makes a product the researcher is investigating; failing to disclose a financial connection or interest in publishing research results; lending one's name to the discrediting of otherwise valid research because it challenges a commercial interest; and, in human subject research, being paid to recruit subjects. Money talks, as the old saying has it, and offers many incentives to behave badly.[34] For universities caught up in such problems, it may be true, but sobering, that "academia is gradually assuming an economic development function within regional and national contexts. . . . Conflict of interest disputes are not only symptomatic of a clash of values but reflect an underlying social structure."[35]

To do something about conflict of interest is never easy. The most common strategy is to require the filling out and signing of a financial disclosure form, whose scope can include various forms of conflicts of interest: consultancies, employment, stock ownership, honoraria, and paid expert testimony. Many universities forbid medical school faculty to own stock in companies providing money for their research, while others set limits on how much stock faculty can own in companies for which they do research or on what they can earn in consultancy fees.[36] The Association of American Medical Colleges has urged universities to disqualify investigators from conducting clinical trials if they hold a significant financial interest in the outcome. Since public disclosure strategies may not be very revealing, institutional limitations may be the best direction to take.[37]

While noting that the great expansion of human-subject research in recent years opened the door to many abuses, Stuart E. Lind has argued that, by taking such research out of the hands of the professional experimenters who were dominant in the 1950s and 1960s, "those changes moved research out in the open so that others, including housestaff and practicing physicians could witness, judge, and monitor research practices."[38] The combination of university controls and a greater research visibility may turn out to be more important than disclosure policies.[39] In 2001 the editors of eleven major medical journals announced they now "routinely require authors to disclose details of their own and the sponsor's role in the study."[40] That may help too but does not take full account of disclosure policies.

There is an obvious problem with disclosure, however sensible and necessary it is. Awareness of someone's financial tie to a company or other financial stake in a piece of research offers not the slightest clue to the validity of the research or the rectitude of the researcher. The research may be solid or it may be biased, but financial disclosure offers no insight into either. It is at best a caveat emptor declaration, but one that is inevitably unclear in its meaning. If research results are published in a peer-reviewed journal, that fact in itself seems to automatically establish scientific credibility. Does not the acceptance of the results by peer reviews imply that no bias or impropriety has been detected and that those results should be given the benefit of the doubt? And does not the willingness of someone to disclose a financial interest—even if required—itself seem to suggest good faith and serious science? The answer to these questions is not necessarily. As more and more researchers receive support from industry, conflict-of-interest declarations may become as common as authors' institutional identifications. They will then cease to be a meaningful indication of anything.

There is a sense also in which the whole is greater than the sum of the parts. When the number of researchers with financial connections becomes large, a miasma of suspicion envelops the entire research enterprise. The journals that publish the research are heavily dependent on advertising revenue from companies whose products may be reviewed in their pages, the editors of the journals may own considerable stock in medical and pharmaceutical companies, and the reviewers to whom they turn may have, if not a stake in a particular product under review, a stake in the well-being of the pharmaceutical industry as a whole, in which they have investments. In those circumstances, public distrust easily takes hold, requiring only a few scandals to taint the entire enterprise.

Scandals have also attended well-publicized cases where researchers who have taken commercial money to support their research have also signed confidentiality agreements about their findings. A professor at the Brown University School of Medicine conducted paid research for a textile company on an outbreak of lung disease at one of its plants.[41] When he planned to reveal at a professional meeting his finding of a higher than expected incidence of interstitial lung disease at the plant, the company threatened to sue him. He then broke off the consultancy agreement and went ahead with the public disclosure. While some individual faculty members supported him, both the medical school and the hospital at which he worked did not, instead upholding the confidentiality agreement.

In another case, it took nine years for two pharmaceutical companies to concede that they had tried to suppress a study that found three cheaper drugs were just as effective as Synthroid, a synthetic hormone used to treat thyroid disease. Again, a nondisclosure agreement signed by the researchers was the focus. Only a story about the suppression effort in the *Wall Street Journal* forced the companies to back down.[42] The president of one of the companies that had withheld data, Knoll Pharmaceuticals, apparently received a grand insight. "The company," he was quoted as saying, "had gained a better understanding of the importance of supporting academic freedom and the peer review process." That was not, it seems, equally true of the University of California, San Francisco, which upheld the nondisclosure agreement signed by its faculty members, no doubt wary about its own legal liability.

At about the same time, a survey of life science researchers found that 20 percent of 2,197 respondents reported withholding results or refusing to share data. As the authors of the study implied, nothing less than a violation of the scientific norm of communalism identified by Merton was at issue. The free exchange of scientific information is central to the healthy life of science. Another study found that 58 percent of life science companies sponsoring academic research require a six-month waiting period before publication, and nearly 20 percent of life science faculty withheld publication of research results for more than six months to protect its commercial value.[43]

Is the counter-norm of secrecy exculpatory here? Perhaps so, but only if we consider proprietary reasons sufficient to overcome the norm of communalism. That answer divides for-profit research (which needs secrecy for commercial, competitive reasons only, not scientific reasons) from nonprofit research (which does not). Any delay of publication will deprive the scientific community of potentially valuable information; it thus undercuts communalism. At the same time, to be sure, but for the profit motive to initiate the research, there might be no publications, and no research, at all.

Obvious problems with the Faustian nondisclosure agreements many faculty members are willing to enter into in order to raise—or to make—money are hardly the only pitfalls. Biomedical symposiums sponsored by the pharmaceutical industry have, as one survey gently put it, "promotional attributes" and are not peer reviewed. Nonetheless, the papers are often published in peer-reviewed journals, often with misleading titles and the use of brand names.[44] Publication of papers under those circumstances is no doubt pleasing to the authors. Corporate gifts to researchers over and above direct grant and contract support—for biomaterial, discretionary funds, research equipment, trips to meetings, and student support—are another common practice. In return, a significant proportion of the researchers are asked to allow prepublication review of articles or reports stemming from the gifts, to provide testing of a company's product, and to turn over patent ownership rights from such research.[45] Though little noticed, biotechnology and pharmaceutical companies make a strenuous effort in their advertising to develop and enhance commercial bonds with practicing scientists.[46]

THE USE AND ABUSE OF THE MEDIA

Though the media's interest in medicine and the biological sciences caught fire only in the 1920s, that fire has never ceased burning, fed by many combustible elements. At the top of the list is the public fascination with science in general and medicine in particular. It is a popular topic, and the media have responded by creating a large core of science and medical writers, television producers, traditional and Internet news services. Helping fan the interest are many university, pharmaceutical, and biotechnology publicists, fast with handouts and releases, news services of their own, and a well-used list of media contacts to promote scientific work.

As any public relations person knows, the media and their sources of information need one another. It is a classical symbiotic relationship.[47] The result is a constant and massive outpouring of biomedical information and analysis, spread from the front pages of newspapers and network TV news to the industry-centered specialty news services and publications.[48] Universities court the publicity this outpouring can bring. Venture capitalists and start-up firms need the high level of excitement the media induce to attract eager but wary investors. The National Institutes of Health is immensely helped in gaining money from Congress by steady news of possible "breakthroughs" on spine-tingling frontiers of research. Individual scientists can find the media helpful in promoting their line of research, publicizing their findings, getting their name before the public, and gaining a leg up on grants and contracts.

The principal threat to scientific integrity, and particularly the value of objectivity, comes from the occasional complicity of scientists in presenting misleading reports to the media, usually in the direction of exaggerating the value of research findings or their likely clinical benefits. It is no less the case, however, that the findings of research are misused and misconstrued despite the most careful efforts of the researchers to avoid that hazard.

The media can sow confusion, mislead the public, and do harm to science as a discipline and to the individual scientist. For well over a century, news of pending triumphs in the war against cancer has won headlines. I choose, almost at random, an example from 2000. "We are going to see a global conquering of cancer in five to ten years," Dr. Carlos Gordon-Cardo, director of molecular pathology at the Memorial Sloan-Kettering Hospital, says in a comment splashed across the front cover of *New York* magazine. The accompanying article cites him and many other equally enthusiastic prominent scientists. One of the boxes presenting lively phrases quotes Dr. Dennis Salmon, a distinguished cancer specialist at UCLA, as saying that genetic knowledge "could mean the end of disease as we know it."[49]

The full quotation, however, contains an important "if": "If we put enough . . . information together [about genes and their functions] . . . it really could mean the end of disease as we know it." The palpable flavor of excitement and possibility overwhelms other qualifications and cautions in the article. On occasion, there are more sobering reports from the front about the progress of the war on cancer, but they receive considerably less attention. At about the same time a *Wall Street Journal* article by a British physician, Anthony Daniels (writing under the pseudonym Theodore Dalrymple), attacked Vice President Gore's proposal for a reinvigorated war against cancer, this time one advertised by Gore as more or less guaranteed to be successful. Daniels noted the correlation of cancer and aging, the lack of any solid knowledge about the causes of cancer, and the fact that prevention and other public health measures are likely to be more effective against cancer than a clean cure.[50]

That viewpoint does not gain headlines (though it did get published), any more than another, similar, article at the same time did. In answer to the question posed in the article's title— "Are Increasing 5-Year Survival Rates Evidence of Success Against Cancer?"—an outcomes research group said no. "Our analysis shows," the authors wrote, "that changes in 5-year survival over time bear little relationship to changes in cancer mortality . . . they appear primarily related to changing patterns of diagnosis."[51]

It is a paradox that, while the media are generally drawn to disasters and the nastier aspects of life, when it comes to that most neglected of research virtues, its skepticism, the media are often quiet. Supposed cures that did not pan out, money lost in failed research efforts, revelations about expensive, popular brand-name drugs working no better than cheaper generics, do not sufficiently gain the attention of writers or editors. As Dorothy Nelkin once noted, science writers tend to be science enthusiasts, as excited by breaking medical news as anyone else. Many, moreover, see themselves as allies of the scientific enterprise. They want it to succeed.[52] They are not particularly drawn to write about the failures of research or the personal sins of researchers (even if that attracts some editors). Who is eager to hear about the doctoring of data to produce a good outcome, or to hear stories about the continuing high death rates from lung or pancreatic cancer, or failures of new drugs, or of researchers whose "promising" work has come to nothing?

Yet it is precisely information of that kind, a vital part of the work of scientists, that is necessary for research vitality. Most scientists are cautious and responsible, willing to admit skepticism about touted breakthroughs. But not always or strongly enough. As *New York Times* science writer Gina Kolata noted in a review of the stem cell debate, the research is difficult, will take many years, and will almost certainly disappoint those looking for quick cures. Scientists know that. "But," she wrote, "as the exaggerations and talk of revolutionary treatments continued, few made concerted efforts to set the record straight. And some small biotechnology companies continue to promise quick cures."[53]

It is all too easy, but not always fair, to blame the media for failure to report on biomedical research carefully, soberly, delicately, and candidly. That's not what editors are necessarily looking for, what writers are most attracted to, or what will draw the public to medical and science writing. There is something less noticed: whatever the media do, good or bad, they do in collusion with researchers. If many researchers are hostile to, or at least highly ambivalent about, the media, many others recognize, even if ruefully, the value for them. They know that favorable publicity fuels popular interest and financial support. It will not hurt their careers, their institutions, or the annual budget of the NIH. They know that they may well be misquoted by the media, that their hesitations and qualifications and skepticism will probably not appear at all, or be buried deep in a story—but that, like many other fields in the public eye, they (almost) must live or die by the media. They may hate publicity, but they need it. The media are an unavoidable part of contemporary life, ignored at researchers' peril, and all the more so the higher they move up the ladder of public prominence.

The headline news came just as I began this book: the Human Genome Project had (all but) been completed. Even the normally sober journal *Science* could not resist a grandiose description of the event. "Finally," it said in 16-point type, "The Book of Life and Instructions for Navigating It."[54] A skeptic could well ask whether a mapping of the genome amounts to the "book of life" and how gene sequencing provides a navigation plan.

But at that moment, who cared about finely calibrated claims? Pride of accomplishment, hyperbolic language, and projections of a transformed human future were the prevailing spirit. No mention was made of the increase in costs that might come about in the transformation of theoretical knowledge into clinical application—assuming its completion—or of the information's possible misuse. Many, though not all, of the stories reported cautions about expecting too much, too soon. It could take decades, perhaps a century, to realize many of the mapped genome's benefits. But that was not a prominent theme. Nor were the media, or the scientists, wholly to blame for the perhaps excessive enthusiasm. As the *New York Times* columnist Gail Collins noted just after the announcement of the completion of the genome project, "For those of us who are scientifically illiterate, the precise meaning of the genome research project is a tad murky. But the verbiage floating around— 'eradicate once incurable disease' (Bill Clinton) or a 'limitless progression of new medical breakthroughs' (Mr. Gore)— seems to suggest that our biotech guys are six months away from curing death."[55]

The cautious view of Steve Jones, professor of genetics at the Galton Laboratory of University College, London, well caught in the title of his *Genetics in Medicine: Real Promises, Unreal Expectations*, was not the kind of mixed message to spread about.[56] Even the high reputation of Richard Lewontin, professor of biology at Harvard, was not likely to draw reporters to his door for writing, in the best tradition of skepticism, that he agreed with the view of a colleague that it was "complete trash" to think that with a complete sequencing of the human genome "we will know what it is to be human."[57] The news, not too long after the end of the genome project, that the number of genes may be closer to 35,000 or 40,000, not well over 100,000 as earlier speculated, and the recognition that those fewer genes must each control a larger number of proteins, made it clear that the therapeutic translations would be much harder than anticipated, was reported— but not on the first page above the fold.

Science and Social Responsibilities

Some of the problems and practices I described above pertain to research and the private sector, which chapter 8 explores. But even milder and moderately hazardous expressions of the research imperative—particularly the combination of money, ambition, and excessive hype—are at work, putting strong economic temptations directly in the path of many researchers, on occasion casting doubt on the validity of biomedical research, and infecting the institutions of which they are a part. From every indication, these problems may be on the increase if only because there are larger numbers of researchers.

Apart from a passing reference here and there, earlier studies of medical research did not mention scandals and bad behavior. Scientific misconduct, the suppression of research results for economic reasons, reprisals against researchers for telling the truth, and the lure of money to carry out and then distort or suppress research for commercial ends were simply not prominent issues. For the steadily strengthening pressures on medical researchers to do well, to look good, to gain tenure or money or prestige—all of them a testimony to the high social place accorded research—also, ironically, stem from the research imperative in its most benign sense. It too has gained strength. In great part because of its past benefits and future promise, the research imperative is increasingly subject to forces that subvert the ethic that has always sustained it and burnished its high reputation.

Since good science emerged from those earlier eras with its reputation intact, nothing in the nature of science as such invites abuse. That abuse comes from the external pressures on science: a mix of the money to be made in selling the products of research, the reputations (and money also) to be had in scientific distinction, the intense pressures of the American university where jobs are scarce and tenure a hard prize to win, and high public expectations. Those expectations blossom in a climate of taken-for-granted progress of science in improving life, where more is always expected, and where the media exaggerate our hopes of conquering suffering and death.

In light of such pressures, what is to be the fate of the standards of social responsibility Bentley Glass proposed? As my friend and longtime colleague Willard Gaylin, a physician and psychoanalyst, discovered some years ago, there are no ritual congratulations for bringing the ethical problems of science into the open, particularly if the writer wonders openly whether certain lines of research are conducive to the human good. Gaylin published an article in the *New York Times Magazine* on the moral challenges raised by the possibility of human cloning, still far in the distance but actively discussed as a paradigm case of what was then called the "new biology."[58] His enraged dean at the Columbia University College of Physicians and Surgeons lambasted him for writing an article on such a futuristic kind of problem and, in the process, for sensationalizing important new scientific developments (which they were not). Nor was that all. The real danger of articles of that kind, he was told, was to alarm the public and endanger the flow of grant money. Gaylin was then a senior and prominent member of the medical school faculty, and he could get away with incensing the dean. It was then, and is probably now, unlikely that untenured younger faculty members would dare to outrage their dean.

I have not been able to determine the extent of intimidation researchers encounter to raising, and seriously pursuing, the responsibility Glass identified "to warn of risks." Paul Berg did raise questions about recombinant DNA research, though his career was vulnerable (and he later won a Nobel Prize), but it is not easy to find contemporary examples of scientists warning about the risks of research, much less leading a campaign to have those risks taken seriously. Perhaps the most effective science group in the 1970s in addressing research risks was Science for the People (mentioned above). It gradually declined and went out of existence in 1991.[59] The Council for Responsible Genetics is an exception, but it is small and almost unknown among scientists and the public. Many scientists have spoken out in a number of recent debates but almost always on the side of supporting research initiatives, working hard to minimize the hazards and dampen ethical worries (as we will see with efforts to promote embryonic stem cell research).

The 1970s recombinant DNA debate may have left its mark, but not in a healthy way. A good example of how to discourage scientists from openly warning about risk can be found in a 1980 article analyzing the outcome of the earlier debate on the possible risks of recombinant DNA research. In light of the scientific evidence as of the end of the late 1970s, Vincent Franco concluded that a "wealth" of research "supports the conclusion that the recombinant DNA technique poses no real hazard to public health, laboratory workers, or the environment." Franco made a good case, and no serious evidence (though there is some evidence) has turned up since then to give substance to the earlier fears. He then drew the wrong conclusion: the debate had been a mistake from the beginning: "Debate has been so insufferably protracted because the scientific community six years ago did a reckless job of exercising its responsibility for transmitting conjectural information to an easily alarmed public." He approvingly quoted a statement of Philip Handler, then president of the National Academy of Sciences: "Those who have inflamed the public imagination [over recombinant DNA] have raised fears that rest on no factual basis but their own science fiction." Dr. Franco piously concluded that scientists should "develop mechanisms of communicating the collective judgment of their peers in a manner that helps the public distinguish between rational and irrational views."[60]

He utterly missed the point, in a way that could only discourage those who might feel compelled to voice their anxieties and risk the wrath or condescension of their colleagues for doing so. First, the scientists in question, accused of irrationality after the fact, were a distinguished group, none of whom would ordinarily be accused of irrationality. Their credentials and reputation were as solid as any of those scientists who imagined no harms. If the public subsequently had fears about the research, it did so because— and only because—many reputable scientists said anxiety was the most reasonable response. Second, that their fears turned out to be unfounded does not speak to the question of whether, whatever scientists knew at the time— that is, knowing as little as they did—they were foolish to voice their concern. If they believed what they said, then—taking Glass's duty "to warn of risks" seriously—they had a duty to speak out. At worst, recombinant DNA research lost a couple of years, a small price to pay for an important exercise of scientific responsibility. Third, they did indeed use their imaginations but—in the face of little or no solid evidence in dealing with a technology just invented—they did what any rational person should have done. There was no objection to other scientists' imaginative rhapsodies about the potential benefits of the research, no charges of irrationality against them. There should have been none, none at all, to projections of possible danger. The same standard applies to both cases.

Science itself is heavily dependent on imagination to project possibly fruitful lines of theoretical inquiry or potentially valuable therapies. Occasionally projections must turn out to be wrong. If an institution attacks any of its researchers who sound an alarm—rightly or wrongly as later data may reveal—then it deals a major blow to the very idea of speaking out in public and thus to the idea of responsibility itself. Worse still, nothing but the most destructive kind of myopic self-interest would permit science to tolerate only the upbeat and the optimistic, much less to pander to the media in doing so. To repress or scoff at those who believe that science is about uncovering the truth, and only that, and not about engaging in the kind of spin control that gains money and generates popular (and congressional) excitement, is to drive a dagger through the heart of its deepest historical commitment.

That commitment is to uncovering the truth about the empirical world—the way it is. Medical research in particular works toward improving the human condition, both to acquire biological knowledge for its own sake and to use that knowledge to help us deal with our bodily and psychological miseries. Despite the shadows I have been highlighting, commitment is only part of the story. Far more important are the goals of medicine and medical research. What is it we—as individuals, or as a society—want from research? Just how imperative is the research imperative as a struggle against sickness, death, and aging? Sometimes an excessive pursuit of those goals, in the name of a morality aiming to reduce pain, suffering, and death, causes harm. Or if that is too strong—none of us embraces those evils—then the single-minded pursuit of them is a mistake.

3 Is Research a Moral Obligation?

In 1959 Congress passed a "health for peace" bill, behind which was a view of disease and disability as "the common enemy of all nations and peoples."[1] In 1970 President Nixon declared a "war" against cancer. Speaking of a proposal in Great Britain in 2000 to allow stem cell research to go forward, Science Minister Lord Sainsbury said, "The important benefits which can come from this research outweigh any other considerations," a statement that one newspaper paraphrased as outweighing "ethical concerns."[2] Arguing for the pursuit of potentially hazardous germ-line therapy, Dr. W. French Anderson, editor in chief of *Human Gene Therapy*, declared that "we as caring human beings have a moral mandate to cure disease and prevent suffering."[3] A similar note was struck in an article by two ethicists who held that there is a "prima facie moral obligation" to carry out research on germ-cell gene therapy.[4]

As if that was not enough, in 1999 a distinguished group of scientists, including many Nobel laureates, issued a statement urging federal support of stem-cell research. The scientists said that because of its "enormous potential for the effective treatment of human disease, there is a moral imperative to pursue it."[5] Two other ethicists said much the same, speaking of "the moral imperative of compassion that compels stem cell research," and adding that at stake are the "criteria for moral sacrifices of human life," a possibility not unacceptable to them.[6] The Human Embryo Research Panel, created by the National Institutes of Health, contended in 1994 that federal funding to create embryos for research purposes should be allowed to go forward "when the research by its very nature cannot otherwise be validly conducted," and "when the fertilization of oocytes is necessary for the validity of a study that is potentially of outstanding scientific and therapeutic value."[7]

The tenor of these various quotations is clear. The proper stance toward disease is that of warfare, with unconditional surrender the goal. Ethical objections, when they arise, should give way to the likely benefits of research, even if the benefits are still speculative (as with stem cell and germ line research). The argument for setting aside ethical considerations when research could not otherwise be "validly conducted" is particularly striking. It echoes an objection many researchers made during the 1960s to the imminent regulation of human subject research: regulations would cripple research. That kind of reasoning is the research imperative in its most naked—and hazardous—form, the end unapologetically justifying the means. I am by no means claiming that most researchers or ethicists hold such views. But that reasoning is one of the "shadows" this book is about.

What should be made of this way of thinking about the claims of research? How appropriate is the language of warfare, and how extensive and demanding is the so-called moral imperative of research? I begin by exploring those questions and then move on to the wars against death and aging, two fundamental, inescapable biological realities so far—and two notorious and clever foes.

THE METAPHOR OF "WAR"

Since at least the 1880s—with the identification of bacteria as agents of disease—the metaphor of a "war" against illness and suffering has been popular and widely deployed. Cancer cells "invade" the body, "war stories" are a feature of life "in the trenches" of medicine, and the constant hope is for a "magic bullet" that will cure disease in an instant.[8] Since there are surely many features of medicine that may be likened to war, the metaphor is hardly far-fetched, and it has proved highly serviceable time and again in the political effort to gain money for research.

Less noticed are the metaphor's liabilities, inviting excessive zeal and a cutting of moral corners. The legal scholar George Annas has likened the quest for a cure of disease to that of the ancient search for the Holy Grail: "Like the knights of old, a medical researcher's quest of the good, whether that be progress in general or a cure for AIDS or cancer specifically, can lead to the destruction of human values we hold central to a civilized life, such as dignity and liberty."[9] "Military thinking," he has also written, "concentrates on the physical, sees control as central, and encourages the expenditure of massive resources to achieve dominance."[10] The literary critic Susan Sontag, herself a survivor of cancer, has written, "We are not being invaded. The body is not a battlefield. . . . We—medicine, society—are not authorized to fight back by any means possible. . . . About that metaphor, the military one, I would say, if I may paraphrase Lucretius: Give it back to the warmakers."[11]

While some authors have tried to soften the metaphor by applying a just-war theory to the war against disease (a sensible enough effort), the reality of warfare does not readily lend itself to a respect for nuanced moral theory. Warriors get carried away with the fight, trading nasty blow for nasty blow, single-mindedly considering their cause self-evidently valid, shrugging aside moral sensitivities and principles as eminently dispensable when so much else of greater value is thought to be at stake. It is a dangerous way of thinking, all the more so when—as is the case with so much recent research enthusiasm—both the therapeutic benefits and the social implications are uncertain.

Is Research a Moral Obligation?

Yet if the metaphor of war is harmful, lying behind it is the notion of an insistent, supposedly undeniable moral obligation. Nations go to war, at least in just wars, to defend their territory, their values, their way of life. They can hardly do otherwise than consider the right to self-defense to be powerful, a demanding and justifiable moral obligation to protect and defend themselves against invaders. To what extent, and in what ways, do we have an analogous moral obligation to carry out research aiming to cure or reduce suffering and disease, which invade our minds and bodies?[12]

Historically, there can be little doubt that an abiding goal of medicine has been the relief of pain and suffering; it has always been considered a worthy and highly defensible goal. The same can be said of medical research that aims to implement that goal. It is a valid and valuable good, well deserving of public support. As a moral proposition it is hard to argue with the idea that, as human beings, we should do what we can to relieve the human condition of avoidable disease and disability. Research has proved to be a splendid way of doing that.

So the question is not whether research is a good. Yes, surely. But we need to ask how high and demanding a good it is. Is it a moral imperative? Do any circumstances justify setting aside ethical safeguards and principles if they stand in the way of worthy research? And how does the need for research rank with other social needs?

The long-honored moral principle of beneficence comes into play here, as a general obligation to help those in need when we can do so. Philosophically, it has long been held that there are *perfect* and *imperfect* obligations. The former entail obligations with corresponding rights: I am obliged to do something because others have rights to it, either because of contractual agreements or because my actions or social role generate rights that others can claim against me. Obligations in the latter category are imperfect because they are nonspecific: no one can make a claim that we owe to them a special duty to carry out a particular action on their behalf.[13]

Medical research has historically fallen into that latter category. There has long been a sense that beneficence requires that we work to relieve the medical suffering of our fellow human beings, as well as a felt obligation to pursue medical knowledge to that end. But it is inevitably a general, imperfect obligation rather than a specific, perfect obligation: no one can claim a right to insist that I support research that might cure him of his present disease at some point in the future. Even less can it be said that there is a right on the part of those not yet sick who someday might be (e.g., those at risk of cancer) to demand that I back research that might help them avoid getting sick. Nor can a demand be made on a researcher that it is his or her duty to carry out a specific kind of research that will benefit a specific category of sick people.

This is not to say that a person who takes on the role of researcher and has particular knowledge and skills to combat disease has no obligation to do so. On the contrary, the choice of becoming a researcher (or doctor, or firefighter, or lawyer) creates role obligations, and it would be legitimate to insist that medical researchers have a special duty to make good use of their skills toward the cure of the sick. But it is an imperfect obligation because no individuals can claim the right to demand that a particular researcher work on their specific disease. At most, there is an obligation to discharge a moral role by using research skills and training responsibly to work on some disease or another. Even here, however, we probably would not call a researcher who chose to carry out basic research but had no particular clinical application in mind an irresponsible researcher.

These are no mere ethical quibbles or hair-splitting. If the language of an "imperative" applies, we can reasonably ask who exactly has the duty to carry out that imperative and who has the right to demand that someone do so. If we cannot give a good answer to those questions, we might still want to argue that it would be good (for someone) to do such research and that it would be virtuous of society to support it. But we cannot then meaningfully use the language of a "moral imperative." We ought to act in a beneficent way toward our fellow citizens, but there are many ways of doing that, and medical research can claim no more of us than many other worthy ways of spending our time and resources. We can be blamed if we spent a life doing nothing for others, but it would be unfair to blame us if we chose to do other good works than support, much less personally pursue, medical research. Hence a claim that there is any kind of research—such as medical research—that carries a prima facie imperative to support and advance it distorts a main line of Western moral philosophy.

The late philosopher Hans Jonas put the matter as succinctly as anyone:

Let us not forget that progress is an optional goal, not an unconditional commitment, and that its tempo in particular, compulsive as it may become, has nothing sacred about it. Let us also remember that a slower progress in the conquest of disease would not threaten society, grievous as it is to those who have to deplore that their particular disease be not conquered, but that society would indeed be threatened by the erosion of those moral values whose loss, possibly caused by too ruthless a pursuit of scientific progress, would make its most dazzling triumphs not worth having.[14]

In another place Jonas wrote, "The destination of research is essentially melioristic. It does not serve the preservation of the existing good from which I profit myself and to which I am obligated. Unless the present state is intolerable, the melioristic goal is in a sense gratuitous, and this not only from the vantage point of the present. Our descendants have a right to be left an unplundered planet; they do not have a right to new miracle cures."[15]

In the category of "intolerable" states would surely be rapidly spreading epidemics, taking thousands of young lives and breaking down the social life and viability of many societies. AIDS in poor countries, and some classic earlier plagues, assaults society as a whole, damaging and destroying social infrastructures. But though they bring terrible individual suffering, few other diseases—including cancer and heart disease—can be said now to threaten the well-being and future viability of any developed society as a society. They do not require an obsession with victory that ignores moral niceties and surfaces at times in the present war against disease, where, to paraphrase Lord Sainsbury's words, its benefits outweigh ethical concerns.

Jonas was by no means an enemy of research. Writing in the context of the 1960s debate on human subject research, he insisted that the cost in time lost because of regulatory safeguards to protect the welfare of research subjects was a small, but necessary, price to pay to preserve important moral values and to protect the good name of research itself. But he was also making a larger point about absolutizing disease, as if no greater evil existed, in order to legitimize an unbounded assault. Not everything that is good and worthy of doing, as is research, ought to be absolutized. That view distorts a prudent assessment of human need, inviting linguistic hyperbole and excessive rationalization of dubious or indefensible conduct.[16] Moreover, as well as any other social good, medical research has its own opportunity costs (as an economist could put it); that is, the money that could be spent on medical research to improve the human condition could also be spent on something else that would bring great benefits as well, whether public health, education, job-creating research, or other forms of scientific research, such as astronomy, physics, and chemistry.

Health may indeed be called special among human needs. It is a necessary precondition to life. But at least in developed countries, with high general levels of health for most people for most of their lives, that precondition is now largely met at the societal, if not the individual, level; other social goods may legitimately compete with it. With the exception of plagues, no disease or medical condition can claim a place as an evil that *must* be erased, as a necessary precondition for civilization, though many would surely be good to erase.

Hardly anyone in medical research is likely to deny the truth of those assertions, but no one is eager to introduce them to public debate. One way to absolutize, and then abuse, medical research is to turn the evils it aims to erase into nasty devils, evil incarnate. In this way good and just wars often descend to nasty and immoral wars. The weapons of war, including those brought to bear against disease, then easily become indispensable, for no other choice is available. The language of war, or moral imperative, can thus be hazardous to use, giving too high a moral and social place to overcoming death, suffering, and disease. It becomes "too high" when it begins to encroach upon, or tempt us to put aside, other important values, obligations, and social needs.

Nonetheless, there is a way of expressing a reasonable moral obligation that need not run those dangers. It is to build on and incorporate into thinking about research the most common arguments in favor of universal health care, that is, the provision of health care to all citizens regardless of their ability to pay for that care. There are different ways of expressing the underlying moral claim: as a right to health care, which citizens can claim against the state; as an obligation on the part of the state to provide health care; and as a commitment to social solidarity. The idea of a "right" to health care has not fared well in the United States, which is one reason the President's Commission for the Study of Ethical Problems in Medicine and Biomedical and Behavioral Research used the language of a governmental obligation to provide health care in 1984.[17] A characteristic way of putting the rights or obligations is in terms of justice. As one of the prominent proponents of a just and universal care system, Norman Daniels, has put it, "by keeping people close to normal functioning, healthcare preserves for people the ability to participate in the political, social, and economic life of their society."[18] To this I add the ability to participate in the family and private life of communities. The aim in Daniels's view is that of a "fair equality of opportunity."

The concept of "solidarity," rarely a part of American political thought, is strong in Canada and Western Europe. It focuses on the need of those living together to support and help one another, to make of themselves a community by putting in place those health and social resources necessary for people to function as a community.[19] The language of rights and obligations characteristically focuses on the needs of the community. The language of solidarity is meant to locate the individual within a community and, with health care, to seek a communal and not just an individual good.

It is beyond the scope of this book to take up in any further detail those various approaches to the provision of health care. It is possible, however, to translate that language and those approaches into the realm of medical research. We can ask whether, if there is a social obligation to provide health care—meaning those diagnostic, therapeutic, and rehabilitative capabilities that are presently available—there is a like obligation to carry out research to deal with those diseases and medical conditions that at present are not amenable to treatment. "Fair equality of opportunity," we might argue, should reach beyond those whose medical needs can be met with available therapies to encompass others who are not in this lucky circle. Justice requires, we might add, that they be given a chance as well and that research is necessary to realize it.

Three important provisos are necessary. First, rationing must be a part of any universal health care system: no government can afford to make available to everyone everything that might meet their health care needs. Resource limitations of necessity require the setting of priorities—for the availability of research funds and health-care-delivery funds alike. Second, no government can justify investments in research that would knowingly end in treatments or therapies it could not afford to extend to all citizens or ones available only privately to those with the money to pay for them (chapters 9 and 10 pursue these two points). Third, neither medical research nor health care delivery is the only determinant of health: social and economic and environmental factors have a powerful role as well.

Instead of positioning medical research as a moral imperative we can understand it as a key part of a vision of a good society. A good society is one interested in the full welfare of its citizens, supportive of all those conditions conducive to individual and communal well-being. Health would be an obviously important component of such a vision, but only if well integrated with other components: jobs, social security, family welfare, social peace, and environmental protection. No one of those conditions, or any others we could plausibly posit, is both necessary and sufficient; each is necessary but none is sufficient. It is the combination that does the work, not the individual pieces in isolation. Research to improve health would be a part of the effort to achieve an integrated system of human well-being. But neither perfect health nor the elimination of all disease is a prerequisite for a good twenty-first-century society—it is a prerequisite only to the extent that it is a major obstacle to pursuing other goods. Medical researchers and the public can be grateful that the budget of the NIH has usually outstripped other science and welfare budgets in its annual increases. But the NIH budget does not cover the full range of our social needs, which might benefit from comparable increases in programs devoted to them.

In the remainder of this chapter, I turn to death and aging, both fine case studies to begin my closer look at the research imperative. Long viewed as evils of a high order, they now often serve as stark examples of evil that research should aim to overcome. Two of my closest friends died of cancer and another of a stroke during the year in which I wrote this book, so I do not separate what I write here from my own reflections. I wish they were still alive and I have mixed feelings about getting old, not all of them optimistic.

I choose death and aging as my starting point in part because, though fixed inevitabilities, they are unlike. Death is an evil in and of itself with no redeeming features (unless, now and then, as surcease from pain). With aging, by contrast, the evil is there—who wants it and who needs it?—but the flavor is one of annoyed resignation, of an evil we (probably) can't avoid but, if we let our imaginations roam, we might understand differently or even forestall.[20] Hence the fight against death is imperative, and the fight against the diseases of aging worthy and desirable, even if it does not quite make the heavyweight class of death.

THE WAR AGAINST DEATH

By far the most important opponent in modern medical warfare is death. The announcement of a decline in mortality rates from various diseases is celebrated as the greatest of medical victories, and it is no accident that the NIH has provided the most research money over the years to those diseases that kill the most people, notably cancer, strokes, and heart disease. Oddly enough, however, the place of death in human life, or the stance that medicine ought, ideally or theoretically, to take toward death has received remarkably little discussion. The leading medical textbooks hardly touch the topic at all other than (and only recently) the care of the terminally ill.[21] While death is no longer the subject no one talks about, Susan Sontag was right to note that it is treated, if at all, as an "offensively meaningless event"—and, I would add, fit only to be fought.[22]

Of course this attitude is hardly difficult to understand. Few of us look forward to our death, most of us fear it, and almost all of us do not know how to give it plausible meaning, whether philosophical or religious. Death is the end of individual consciousness, of any worldly hopes and relationship with other people. Unless we are overburdened with pain and suffering, there is not much good that can be said about death for individual human beings, and most people are actually willing to put up with much suffering rather than give up life altogether. Death has been feared and resisted and fought, and that seems a perfectly sensible response.

Yet medicine does more than resist death or fight it. Death is, after all, a fact of biological existence and, since humans are at least organic, biological creatures, we have to accept it. Death is just there, built into us, waiting only for the necessary conditions to express itself. Why, then, should medicine treat it as an enemy, particularly a medicine that works so hard to understand how the body works and how it relates to the rest of nature? The late physician-essayist Lewis Thomas had an articulate biological sense of death as "a natural marvel. All of the life of the earth dies, all of the time, in the same volume as the new life that dazzles us each morning, each spring. . . . In our way, we conform as best we can to the rest of nature. The obituary pages tell us of the news that we are dying away, while the birth announcements in finer print, off at the side of the page, inform us of our replacements."[23]

Many biologists and others have pointed out the importance of death as a means of constantly replenishing the vitality and freshness of human life as a species. New people come into the world and thereby open the way for change and development; others die and thus facilitate the new and the novel. Moreover, does our recognition of the finiteness of our lives, the brute fact that they come to an end, not itself sharpen our appreciation of what we have and what we might do to make the most of it? If we had bodily immortality in this world, would not the danger of boredom and tedium be a real possibility? "Nothing less will do for eternity," Bernard Williams has written, "than something that makes boredom *unthinkable.*" And Williams believes it exceedingly difficult to imagine an unendingly satisfying model of immortality.[24]

Jonas caught what seems to me the essence of the ambivalence about death when he wrote of mortality as, in some inextricable way, both a burden and a blessing: "the gift of subjectivity only sharpens the yes-no polar-ity of all life, each side feeding on the strength of the other. Is it, in the bal-ance, still a gain, vindicating the bitter burden of mortality to which the gift is tied, which it makes even more onerous to bear?"[25] His answer was yes, in part because of the witness of history to the renewal that new lives bring and the passing of the generations makes possible, and in part because it is hard to imagine that a world without death would be a richer biological and cul-tural world, more open in its possibilities than the world we now have.

Part of the problem is simply that we know nothing beyond the bounds of our own existence: we know that life, when it is good, is good. Only a re-ligious vision of immortality holds out hope of something better. Hence, we hold tight to what we know. Even so, simply extending life is no guarantee that the good we now find in life, at younger ages, would continue indefi-nitely into the future; boredom, ennui, the tedium of repetition may well weigh us down. Nor is there any guarantee that our bodies would remain free of frailty, late-late-onset dementia, failing organs. Even under the best prospects, there would be hazards, physical and mental, to negotiate for a prize that might hardly be worth winning.

My own conclusion is this: while it makes sense for medicine to combat some causes and forms of death, it makes no sense to consider death *as such* the enemy. To give it a permanent priority distorts the goals of medicine, taking money from research that could improve the quality of life. And so far in human history, however much we spend to combat death, it always wins in the long run. There will always be what I called elsewhere the "ragged edge of progress"—that point where our present knowledge and technology run out, with illness and death returning; and however much progress is made, there will always be such a point.[26] No matter how far we go, and how successful we are in the war on death, people will continue to die, and they will die of some lethal disease or other that disease research has yet to master. The most serious questions we need to consider are how *much* emphasis research should place on the forestalling of death, and just which *kinds* of death it should tackle.

Medicine's Schism about Death

One obstacle delays any attempt to answer those questions. At the heart of modern medicine is a schism over the place and meaning of death in human life. On one side is the research imperative to overcome death; on the other, the newly emergent (even if historically ancient) clinical imperative to ac-cept death as a part of life in order to help make dying as tolerable as pos-sible. Reflecting medicine's fundamental ambivalence about how to interpret and deal with death, the schism has untoward consequences for setting medical research priorities and for understanding medicine's appropriate stance toward death in the care of patients. My question is this: if this schism is truly present, and if it creates research pressure that generates serious clinical problems, are there ways to soften its impact, to lessen the friction, and to find a more coherent understanding of death?

In the classical world death was not medicine's enemy. It could not be helped. Only with the modern era, and the writings of René Descartes and Francis Bacon in the sixteenth and seventeenth centuries, did the goal of a medical struggle against death emerge.[27] The earlier cultural and religious focus was on finding a meaning for death, giving it a comprehensible place in human experience, and making the passage from life to death as comfortable as possible.[28] The post-Baconian medicine put aside that search. It declared death the enemy. Karl Marx once said that the task of philosophy is not to understand the world but to change it. Modern medicine, to paraphrase Marx, has seemed in effect to say that its task is not to understand death but to eliminate it. The various "wars" against cancer and other diseases in recent decades reflect that mission. For what is the logic of an unrelenting war against all lethal disease other than trench warfare against death itself?

The tacit message behind the research imperative is that, if death itself cannot be eliminated—no one is so bold as to claim that—then at least all the diseases that cause death can be done away with; and that amounts to the same thing. As William Haseltine, chairman and chief executive officer of Human Genome Sciences, breathtakingly put it, "Death is a series of preventable diseases."[29] From this perspective, the researcher is like a fine sharpshooter who will pick off enemies one by one: cancer, then heart disease, then diabetes, then Alzheimer's, and so on. The human genome effort, the latest contender offering eventual cures for death, will supposedly get to the genetic bottom of things, radically improving the sharpshooter's aim.[30]

I chose the word "logic" for the research enterprise that aims to eliminate all the known causes of death, in order to point out that its ultimate enemy must be death itself, the final outcome of that effort. But most researchers and physicians, in my experience, do not see themselves as trying to stamp out death itself, even if they would like to understand and overcome its causes. They know that death is now, and will remain, part of the human condition; medicine is not in hot pursuit of immortality. Even so, the struggle against the causes of death continues, as if researchers must and will continue until they eliminate those causes. Perhaps this tension, or contradiction, is best understood as an expression of an ideal of research confronting a biological reality: the spirit of the research enterprise is to eliminate the causes of death, even as it is understood that death itself will not be eliminated. We might, then, think of the struggle against death as a goal we may never achieve, a dream we may never realize. However we understand this phenomenon, it has its effect at the clinical level.

But why should this dream affect the care of those who are dying, having passed beyond the limits of effective help? For one thing, as already mentioned, it has turned out to be very difficult, medically and psychologically, to trace a bright line (as a lawyer might put it) between living and dying. The increased technological possibility of doing just a little bit more, and then just a little bit more again, to sustain life means that it's getting harder and harder to tell just where that line is. Moreover, the thrust of the research drive is to turn death itself into a contingent, accidental event. Why do people keep dying? Listen to the now-common explanations: they die because they did not take care of their health, or because they had genetically unhealthy parents, or because their care was of a low quality, or because the available care is inequitably distributed, or because this year's technologies don't sufficiently sustain life (but not necessarily next year's), or because research has not yet (but will eventually) find cures for those diseases currently killing us. No one just dies anymore, and certainly not from something as vague as "old age." Everyone dies from specific causes, and we can cure them. Death, in that sense, has been rendered contingent and accidental.

The Clinical Spillover

What difference does this drive or dream make for the clinician at the bedside? Such is the pervasive power of the research imperative (even of a benign kind)—rooted in a vision of endless progress and permeating modern (and particularly American) medicine—that it can easily lead clinicians to think and act as if the death of *this* patient at *this* time is accidental or a failure, not inevitable. Even if they have done everything possible to keep the patient alive, guilt is perhaps one spillover effect of the research stance toward death: maybe we could have, even should have, done more—if we had only known what it was. Understood narrowly, the technological imperative is still another spillover effect, indicating a belief that if we use technology well, this patient need not die at this time and, understood broadly, that technological innovation is the royal road to cure.

In the United States, the research imperative to fight death stands foursquare against fatalism, against giving up hope, and against thinking we cannot tame nature. Should we be surprised that its mode of thinking influences clinical medicine as well, introducing profound uncertainties about the appropriate stance toward death? Can we really expect the various reform efforts in clinical care to be as successful as they might so long as the research-induced uncertainty about the inevitability of death is so powerful?

At this point two skeptical thoughts are sure to arise. One of them is a point of logic: the biological inevitability of death does not entail its inevitable occurrence at any given point in life. We will die, but just how and when is not at all determined. Death is possible at any time by any means, coming faster or slower, brought about by one disease rather than another. In that sense death is, then, contingent. It has no predetermined, fixed time in a person's life. Since this is true, is progress possible simply by substituting later for earlier death, faster for slower, peaceful for painful? Not quite. If "later" is always assumed to be better, then the war against death admits of no victory and the research imperative against it admits of no limits. If, however, the wiser goal is a faster and more peaceful death—admitting of potential success in a way that an all-out struggle against death does not— then a more useful research agenda is possible.

The second skeptical thought is more fundamental. Perhaps the research imperative (eliminate death, disease by disease) and the clinical imperative (accept death as an unavoidable biological reality) are inescapably at odds. Perhaps they represent one of the many instances of incompatible goods that admit of no happy reconciliation. We may just have to live with the contradiction, conceding its force but remaining helpless to get beyond it. Though most of us can think of elderly people who have found an equilibrium—working to stay alive, yet ready at any moment to die—not everyone, and particularly a younger person, can, especially if they face a premature death. We want to live but know we must die, an ancient and wrenching clash.

There is no easy way beyond this clash. I find a quotation of the theologian Gilbert Meilaender (though not, I think, a theological statement) to be helpful: "We can say death is no enemy at all, or we can say that death is the ultimate enemy. Neither of these does justice to what I take to be the truth: that death is an enemy because human life is a great good, but that since continued life is not the highest good, death cannot be the greatest evil."[31]

Is a longer life necessarily a better life? A shorter life holds fewer possibilities of experiencing the goods of life than a longer life might afford. But on that view (assuming continued good health) nothing less than an indefinitely continued life will do, as goal after goal appears on the horizon. But in general, the fact that good things—poems, music, pleasant vacations, glorious sunsets—end does not subvert their value. If finitude is not inherently evil, then neither is a finite life span.

The Mixed Record of Reform

Given that background of debate, the fitful success of various efforts over recent decades to improve care at the end of life and promote a different outlook on death is easy to understand. During the early to mid-1970s, there were three major reform efforts. The first was the effort to introduce advance directives into patient care, a strategy designed to give patients choices about the kind of care they receive when dying. The second was the hospice movement, pioneered by Cicely Saunders in Great Britain and introduced at the Yale–New Haven Hospital in 1974. The third effort was to improve the education of medical students and residents on care at the end of life.

Of the three, hospice is probably the most successful, caring for over 500,000 patients a year (their deaths represent about 20 percent of the 2.3 million annual deaths). But hospice services have been mainly effective with cancer patients, even though there have been recent efforts to extend them to other lethal conditions, heart disease and Alzheimer's in particular. There is general agreement, moreover, that many terminally ill patients come to hospice much too late, sometimes just a few days before their deaths. Neither families nor physicians are always ready to accept death. Advance directives have had at best a mixed record. Despite considerable publicity for twenty-five years, probably no more than 15 percent of the population have such directives. Even worse, as a number of studies have shown, having them by no means guarantees patients of getting what they want.[32]

Death is still denied, evaded, and in the case of many clinicians fought to the end, bitter or otherwise for patients. As for the educational efforts, they have surely given the issues more salience in medical schools, but what students learn in didactic courses or seminars is often at odds with their experience during their clinical years, where the technological imperative—to aggressively use the available life-sustaining technologies—may still reign supreme. A recent survey of medical textbooks found the subject of death strikingly absent and little guidance for physicians in the care of dying patients.[33]

An important thread running through each of the struggling reform efforts has been medicine's characteristic ambivalence toward death: patients' and physicians' confusion about how best to understand and situate death in human life; an unwillingness to accept the coming of death; and the persistence of the turn to intensified technology in response to uncertainty about death. The great improvement in, and the new prominence of, palliative care is a powerful antidote to that pattern, representing both a return to older traditions of care and a fresh, less troubled response to death.

This record of mixed success has of late been met with a renewed effort at analysis and education. The Project on Death in America program of the Soros Foundation and the Last Acts Campaign of the Robert Wood Johnson Foundation have contributed generously to that work. It is too early to tell what this new round of initiatives, though most welcome, will achieve. If the schism persists, their success is likely to remain limited.

The conventional model of treatment, even if rarely articulated in any precise way, is to undertake every effort possible to save life, until that moment when treatment becomes futile, and a palliative mode replaces the therapeutic. What's wrong with that model? For all its seeming reasonableness it is beset by two confounding elements. One is the difficulty of determining when treatment is truly futile.[34] Constant technological advances mean that there is almost always *something* more that can be done for even the sickest patient, one more last, desperate intervention. The other lies in assuming that physicians—not to mention patients and their families—can suddenly and at just the exactly right moment switch from an interventionist to a palliative mode; it betrays its psychological naïveté.[35] It is often much more like an attempt to stop a large train, which goes a long distance down the track before the brakes take hold.

A Modest Proposal

Inescapably, the research imperative complicates and even undermines medicine's clinical mission, which works for better end-of-life care. How might we proceed, to bring the two sides closer? After nearly thirty years of analysis and reform efforts, the clinical side has determined that a peaceful death requires an acceptance of death by both physician and patient. The acceptance may be affirming or grudging or simply acquiescent, but it is essential. Death just is and must be given its due. The research drive, which seems to treat death as a biological accident, possible to overcome, must somehow be reconciled with the clinical perspective. To cooperate in the clinical mission, I propose several strategies.

Focus research on premature death. Not only is eradication of death an unattainable goal, it also promotes the idea among the public and physicians that death represents a failure of medicine, one that research will eventually overcome. It is, however, reasonable for medicine to seek to reduce premature death. The federal government now defines a "premature death" as one that occurs before the age of sixty-five. That standard should probably be raised a few years, but what should not be changed is the concept of a premature death. An implication of this strategy is that, when the average age of death from a disease comes later than the prematurity standard, there should be a reduction of (*not* an elimination of) research funds to combat it; the money saved should be switched to diseases where most deaths come before the prematurity line. By this standard, and in light of the fact that cancer is increasingly a disease of the elderly, the NIH cancer budget could be reduced, not constantly expanded. Understood this way, cancer remains an important research target, but one whose priority would gradually lower over time, giving way to more pressing needs.

Give "compressing morbidity" a research status equivalent to that of saving and lengthening life. The notion of compressing morbidity—shortening the period of poor health before death—has been around at least since the time of the French philosophe Condorcet two hundred years ago. It seemed only a pipe dream. But in recent years evidence has begun to accumulate that to some extent we can falsify the common adage of "longer life, worse health." For those who have good health habits and an adequate socioeconomic foundation to their lives, there can be a significantly lessened chance of a premature death and an old age burdened by illness and disability.[36] Death is not the enemy, but a painful, impaired, and unhealthy life before death. Research on health promotion and disease prevention requires much greater financial support, as does research designed to improve the quality of life within a finite life span.

Persuade clinicians that the ideal of helping a patient achieve a peaceful death is as important as that of averting a patient's death. I contended above that one clinical spillover effect of the research war against death is an implicit purveying of the notion that death is an accidental, contingent biological phenomenon. For the clinician that message has meant that the highest duty is to struggle against death and that (with the help of research) such a struggle need not be in vain. In that context, helping patients achieve a peaceful death will always be seen as the lesser ideal, what is to be done when the highest ideal—continuing life—cannot be achieved.

The two goals should have equal value. In practice, this would mean, in a patient's critical illness and with death on its way, that the physician's struggle against a poor death would equal the struggle against death itself. The two ideals, of course, rarely admit a wholly comfortable resolution. Nonetheless, a serious and meaningful tension between them would help weaken the influence of the values inherent in the research imperative against death, by giving it a meaningful competitor; and it would also help improve palliative-care medicine and good patient care at the end of life. Because we will all die, palliative care should apply to everyone and not just to the losers, those whom medicine could not save. And of course research on improving palliative care should be given an increased budget.

Redefine medical "progress." We now commonly understand the crown jewel of medical progress to be the conquest of lethal disease. And we celebrate the triumph of a declining mortality rate, whether from heart disease, cancer, or AIDS. No doubt that celebration will continue and, with premature deaths, it should. But medical progress should increasingly refer to the avoidance of illness and disability, to rehabilitating those who have succumbed to disability, to tackling conditions that do not kill but otherwise ruin lives (such as serious mental illness), and to helping people understand how to take care of their own health. Death remains an enemy, but it is only one item in a list of many enemies of life—and not in the long run the most important.

Modern medicine, at least in its research aspiration, made death Public Enemy Number One. It is so no longer, at least in developed countries, when average life expectancies are approaching eighty. The enemy now ought to be lives blighted by chronic illness and the inability to function successfully. Death will always be with us, pushed around a bit to be sure, with death from one disease being superseded by death from another disease. That cannot and will not be changed. But we can change the way people are cared for at the end of life, and we can significantly reduce the burden of illness. It is not, after all, death but a life poorly lived that people fear most, particularly when they are old. Something can be done about that, and research has much to contribute.

AGING AND DEATH

Though not death's identical twin, aging too is feared and marked by decline. Less terrible than death, it has nonetheless been considered bad enough to merit the laments of poets, writers, ordinary people, and the medically inclined, just about everyone. For centuries, the notion of conquering aging, or rendering its burdens less harsh, has been a part of every culture's reflection on human fate, joining the struggle against aging with that of the struggle against death. There is another linking characteristic: unless someone dies a premature or accidental death, aging is now more than ever understood to be the main biological gateway to death. With the decline in infant and child mortality—and with life expectancy far beyond sixty-five for a majority of people in developed countries—we cannot think about eliminating or ameliorating death without also thinking about aging, or think about improving old age without doing something also about death.

The ancient world took death to be a harsh but unavoidable reality, old age as simply a burden to endure. The modern world has been more hopeful. A softer view, going back to the Italian Renaissance, envisions an old age marked by wisdom and delight in the simple pleasures of life. Still another picture, even more common, was suggested some years ago by Gerald J. Gruman, one that joins the Enlightenment optimism of Condorcet to that of modern individualism. It counsels the elderly to reject what Gruman called "medical mortalism" in favor of a scientific attack on aging and death. No less important is a kind of living for oneself, a rejection of communal notions of a self-sacrificial life in favor of personal creativity and self-assertion. Specifically rejected are idle musings about "central questions of meaning and value," which are endlessly "open for future resolution."[37] This is not far from another look into the future, one that sees the scientific conquest of aging and added years of youth as bringing "the transformation of our society from a pattern of war and struggle to an era of utopian peace . . . [allowing] adequate time to uncover the secrets of the natural universe . . . that could serve as the foundation for a civilization of never-ending progress."[38]

Aging as "Disease"

But where does aging stand as an object of scientific research? Is it a disease like other physical pathologies or is it, like death, a "natural" biological inevitability? The strongest case for its inevitability is that, unlike other pathologies, it occurs in every human being and in every other organic creature. In a way that nothing else ordinarily classified as a disease is, aging is predictable. We may or may not get cancer or heart disease or diabetes, but we will surely get old and die. Yet much of the decline associated with age, particularly the increase in chronic disease and disability, is accessible to cure or relief. Even many of the other biological indices of aging—decline of hearing, rise of blood pressure, bone mineral loss, reduced muscle mass, failing eyesight, decreased lung function—are open to compensatory intervention though not at present to complete reversal.

In short, if aging is in many respects something other than disease, it has enough of the characteristics of disease to invite, and respond to, medical tinkering and improvement. Certainly there is no reason to classify it as "natural," if by that we mean that nothing should be done about it. On the contrary, it can be—and has in fact been—treated effectively *as if* it were a disease, not by combating old age as such but treating the undesirable conditions associated with it.[39] That route is one possibility, while the other is to take on the biological process of aging itself as a research target. Timothy Murphy has suggested two pertinent questions here. Instead of asking "is aging a disease?" we should ask, first, is "aging objectionable such that its prevention and cure ought to be sought?" Second, can a convincing argument be developed in favor of a "cure" for aging to show that "human significance warrants [it] and possibly seeks such a cure and that the social costs of curing aging are morally acceptable"?[40]

Is aging "objectionable"? Well, it is hard to find many people who welcome it, at least in its advanced phases, where the decline is steep and the disabilities crippling. But does the fact that we don't like it show that it is inherently objectionable, an offense against human dignity? That is a harder case to make, especially since various cultures have found ways to treat the aged with dignity and allow the aged to accept their aging. To make the idea of dignity dependent on the state of our bodies or minds trivializes it. If we do so, then dignity becomes nothing but an accident of biology, with some people lucky to have it and others not. That is a corruption of the idea of human dignity, the essence of which is not to reduce value of people to a set of acceptable characteristics, such as the proper race or sex, social class or bodily traits, but to ascribe dignity to them simply as human beings apart from their individual characteristics.

There is another way to look at aging. While it is possible to situate the place of death within evolution and see its value in endlessly renewing human vigor and possibility, that is not so easy to do with aging. It seems to serve no useful biological function other than as a prelude to death; and for just that reason might itself be understood as part of the same biological process. But if we can distinguish aging from the decline that brings death, perhaps we can sensibly resist the former while not equally resisting death. We might then agree that, while aging is not incompatible with human dignity, it is objectionable enough to merit serious scientific attention. The collective "we" of evolution may need it together with its twin, death, but the "we" of living cultures could do with considerably fewer of its burdens and downward slopes.

Aging and Its Longevity

Does that mean we need to find a "cure" for its burdens? An immediate difficulty here is that it is not clear what a "cure" of aging might look like. If death is the final outcome of aging for all biological creatures, does it begin at birth or in adulthood? A scientific answer to that question might then lead us to ask whether a cure would look to a perpetual youth or a perpetual adulthood (and then young or old adulthood). Or we might envision a slowing of the aging process to a snail's pace, not exactly a clean cure but an indefinite forestalling of the worst of the present consequences of aging and its final outcome, death.

I set out three meaningful possibilities for the cure or amelioration of aging (and use them also in the next chapter in another context).

Normalizing life expectancy. The aim here is to bring everyone up beyond what would be considered a premature death to what is now the average life expectancy in the most developed countries of the world (in Japan, for example, it is eighty-five for women) and bring men up a few years to a life expectancy equal to females. This trend is already under way (though not in all poor countries), driven by improved public health standards, better education, housing, diets, and economic status. Normalization must, however, be accompanied by improved standards in the quality of life, and much of that can be accomplished through research and technological innovation. The cure or amelioration of osteoporosis, arthritis, Alzheimer's disease and other dementias, and improved methods of dealing with loss of hearing and sight, would be high on any list of valuable research goals.

My characterization of normalization retains the idea of a premature death. There are at least four ways of defining a premature death, each of them arbitrary to a considerable degree. There is a death that comes earlier than the average life expectancy in a population; that might be called the statistical definition. There is the cultural definition that classifies people as young or old for various social or political purposes. Since the Bismarckian welfare programs of the late nineteenth century in Germany, the age of sixty-five has been widely used as the dividing line. Then there is what I think of as the psychological meaning of a premature death, the age at which people begin thinking of themselves as old. Finally, there is a biographical definition, that stage when people have accomplished the main tasks and goals of their lives: education, work, parenthood, travel, and whatever else their individual talents allowed.

Each of these definitions is arbitrary in the sense that each is, and always will be, variable and moving. The statistical definition will change as average life expectancy increases (most places) or decreases (Russia and many sub-Saharan countries). The cultural definition will move as more people go into old age in good health, are capable of remaining active even if not employed, and are seen as still part of the productive, nondependent segment of society. The psychological definition will reflect the cultural of course, but not entirely; people do vary in their own sense of age and aging. And the biographical definition will depend on idiosyncratic life goals.

Despite the variables in each of the definitions, they remain useful for establishing social programs, for creating conventions and expectations of behavior at different ages—many are grateful when old age relieves them of earlier responsibilities—and for helping set targets for biomedical research. Death at sixty-five now seems to require the label "premature," while at seventy it has become increasingly plausible; and the cutoff age may go up further in the future. There can well be a legitimate gap between what is culturally thought of as a premature death and the aim of bringing everyone up to the statistical average of eighty-five. My rationale for the distinction is that most people may well have lived a full and fruitful biographical life before age seventy, and thus we mourn their loss less than that of a much younger person. We may also have different reasons for setting the age of various social programs (e.g., employment possibilities) lower than average life expectancy (such as Medicare or eligibility for special housing).

Much of the research agenda is already in place for the normalizing of aging, consisting of what is already known to improve health and to avoid premature death. It is a mixture of improved public health programs, decent medical care (with an orientation to health promotion programs designed to change behavior, and primary care), healthy lifestyles, good education, jobs, housing, and a welfare safety net. Beyond that, research on chronic diseases that lead to premature death, create disability in old age, and ruin or significantly diminish the quality of life is appropriate. Equally appropriate is governmental support for such research, which contributes to the overall health and well-being of the population as a whole. This will not be true of the next category.

Maximizing life expectancy. The purpose of research efforts to maximize life expectancy would be to bring everyone up to what are now the historically longest known human life spans, between 110 and 122 years. If some few people can live that long (and want to), why not make it theoretically possible for everyone to get there? There is a certain plausibility to that idea, if only because the course of evolution has shown that species have acquired very different life spans; life spans are biologically malleable. Recent research has, moreover, begun to suggest that there may be no fixed maximum life expectancy.[41] Earlier estimates at the least have again and again been proved wrong in recent years, often because of extrapolations from past trends of causes of death or age of death, both of which have been changing.

The death of a Frenchwoman at 122 in the late 1990s and the regularity with which people living between 105 and 110 are now being reported cannot fail to catch the eye. Before 1950 centenarians were rare, and there may never have been any before 1800. Since 1950, however, their numbers have doubled every ten years in Western Europe and Japan (with women outnumbering men by four to one and even more so with higher ages); and those centenarians now alive live two years longer on average than those a few decades ago did.[42]

Nonetheless, while the trend is strongly in the direction of more people who are very old, S. J. Olshansky has presented strong data indicating how hard it will be to move everyone far along in that direction. Working with mortality trends in France and the United States, he shows that it would take huge reductions in mortality rates at every age from present levels. To move, for instance, from an average life expectancy of seventy-seven in France (combining male and female) to eighty would require an overall mortality decline of 23 percent; and it would take a decline of 52 percent for all ages to move the average to age eighty-five, and 74 percent for the average to move up to age ninety. Since mortality rates are already low for younger ages, most of the mortality decline would have to take place among those over age fifty.[43] That decline is not theoretically impossible but is in practice implausible.

To get an idea of the enormity of the task, recall that a cure for cancer, the second greatest killer in the United States, would only bring about a 1.5 percent overall decline in mortality. In response to the contention that lifestyle modifications could bring about changes of the necessary magnitude, a number of studies have suggested that mortality would not significantly change if the entire population lived in an ideally healthy way.[44] J. W. Vaupel (never citing Olshansky and admitting that his own calculations are rough) is more optimistic. He holds that a decline in mortality rates in France at the pace that has prevailed for the past means that most people can expect to live to ninety in the not too distant future.[45] Whatever the final truth here—which will take decades to appear—there is considerable good sense in Kirkwood's conclusion that "the record breakers [for individual life span] are important . . . [but] the major focus for research must be to address the main body of the life span distribution, i.e., the general population, and to improve knowledge of the causes of age-associated morbidity and impaired quality of life."[46]

Optimizing life expectancy. The most ancient version of optimization is bodily immortality, and since no clear scientific theory of how to achieve it exists, I put it aside here. The other is to move the average life expectancy to, say, more than 150 years. As the previous analysis of maximizing life expectancy suggested, it will be very hard, even if not theoretically impossible, to get average life expectancy to eighty-five, much less one hundred. Most commentators seem able to envision incremental gains within the limits of present biological and medical knowledge but agree as well that only striking genetic breakthroughs could get us to and beyond 150. The principal obstacle appears to be the multifactorial nature of the aging process; no single magic bullet is likely to do the job. All of the human organs, including the brain, would have to benefit simultaneously from the breakthrough for the results to be anywhere near desirable.

As someone who has been following the scientific developments in understanding aging for over thirty years, I am aware how remarkably little practical progress seems to have been made, even though there has been a gain in knowledge about the aging process. Among the earlier theories that have been rejected or called into question are notions of a fixed limit to the replication of cells over a life span (once thought to be fifty times), of cells' aging, or of the evolutionary necessity of unalterable programmed death. At the same time, recent research on telomeres—stretches of DNA and the proteins that bind them and protect the ends of chromosomes—has shown that they become shorter over time as a cell divides, eventually dying. It reconfirms the notion of a division limit to cells that, if better understood, could hold off the accumulated, progressive decline of the cells. It is an extension of the long-held view that the aging process is one that sees a gradual breakdown of the genetic mechanisms that preserve life; the trick is to find a way to stop or slow their decline. In this view, aging is a failure of biological adaptation, which Michael Rose says is a case of "natural selection abandoning you."[47] Research on telomeres, nutrition, free radicals, antioxidants, apoptosis (cell breakdown), hormonal regulation, cell rejuvenation, and ways of repairing DNA is well under way. Alternatively, the search is on for those positive genetic factors that protect life, have helped individuals flourish in earlier years of life, and might be enhanced to continue doing so.[48]

In sum, the genetic approach to life-span extension aims to find the basic underlying mechanisms of aging, still poorly understood, and then to discover ways of changing and manipulating them. If there is to be a radical change in life expectancy, this approach is currently the only seriously envisaged way of getting there.[49] A medical approach, by contrast, focuses on the various disabilities and diseases that bring poor health, and eventually death, to the elderly and has been (as noted above) the main approach to the incrementalism of the maximizing strategy, far more limited in its ultimate possibilities.

DO WE NEED A MUCH LONGER LIFE? CAN WE STAND IT?

Whether a form of rationalization or a higher insight, most of the imaginative literature on life extension reached a negative conclusion. Citing boredom or debility, it debunked the idea of superextending existence in its youthful or riper guise. Even so, the vision of a fountain of youth or a more up-to-date iteration of long life in good, vigorous health, hangs on. There are many people—and all of us know a few—who would like to live indefinitely; and almost everyone, if not in utter misery and given a choice, would want to live at least one more day, and one more after that. Even if I see some point in the evolutionary benefits of death and a change of the generations, that is a terribly abstract way of looking at my own life: it is doing well and not too interested in making its evolutionary contribution. A longer life beckons.

I am not alone. The National Alliance for Aging Research reported in 2000 that it had discovered twenty-five firms it labeled "gero-techs" because of their focus on applied aging research. The alliance itself sees gerotechnology as a viable market possibility that can help find ways—through improved health—to avoid rationing health care to the elderly in the future. Its director, Daniel Perry, anticipates that through gerotechnology in the twenty-first century, "the drive to discover the means to produce youthful health and vitality [will be] no less than a matter of national necessity."[50] Gerotechnology, then, would hope to assure longer and healthy lives and thus avoid the economic and other problems of aging societies.

The language of "national necessity" seems to me a variant way of speaking of a research imperative. An immediate problem comes to mind. Is the aim to improve the health of the elderly within the normalization model, that is, to get everyone up to the present average life expectancy? If so, it is, consistent with a goal of compressing morbidity, increasingly feasible. Or is the aim (of some of those gero-tech firms, for instance) to push forward the length of life into the maximizing or optimizing range? In that case, it may make geriatricians' efforts to compress morbidity that much harder. Most (though not all) of those who reach the age of 100 require significant help with what geriatricians call activities of daily living, suffer from various chronic conditions, are usually frail, and will have some degree of dementia; and it all gets worse after 105. It may well be the case that a reduction in morbidity can keep pace with a reduction in mortality, but most likely only if the net result for life expectancy gains more slowly.

Yet the health problems and uncertainties connected with increased longevity are hardly the only ones we need to think about. What are the other social consequences of efforts in that direction? That is a difficult question to answer, if only because there are different possible directions (and mixtures of directions) in which future developments could go. We are already on one path, that of normalization, aiming to improve the quality of life of the elderly, not directly trying to lengthen the average life expectancy but getting, without trying, a gradual movement in that direction.

There is already considerable knowledge about that trend. Within twenty to thirty years, when the United States' baby boom generation retires in large numbers and the proportion of elderly moves from 13 to 18 percent, there will be serious problems sustaining the present Medicare program at its present level.[51] Comparable, and perhaps even worse, problems will face officials in other countries (Germany, for example, expects to have nearly 24 percent of its population over age sixty-five). The correlative decline in the number of young people to pay for the health care of the old (the so-called dependency ratio issue) will only exacerbate the situation, as will the continued introduction of new, often beneficial, but usually more expensive technologies; public demand for ever-better medicine will not be much help either.

Something will have to give here, and there is already the expectation of moving forward the age of eligibility for Medicare, from sixty-five to sixty-seven, and further moves in that direction will occur. The promise of reduced disability for the aged in the years to come will be of great help here, but even so various unpleasant policies will probably accompany it: means-testing for the elderly rather than full and free coverage; rationing of health care, overt or hidden; constraints on health care providers and hospitals; and constant efforts to wring greater efficiency out of the system. A universal system of health care (which I support, but which is not yet on the horizon) might lead to a generally more rational and equitable system, but it would increase the governmental cost of health care and might not directly help solve the elderly health care problem. There are optimistic voices to be found, but not too many. The group on research into aging, noted above, believes that salvation lies in improved technologies to bring better health to the elderly. Others believe that some combination of greater efficiency, more choice on the part of people, and savings accounts will make it possible to weather the baby boom era—an era that will eventually end anyway, somewhere in the vicinity of 2050 or so, bringing a more affordable situation.

Once a move is made toward maximization and beyond, then a larger range of problems begins to emerge, and much would depend on the kind of age extension that research might produce. A longer life with a concomitant gain in vigor would be one possibility. Another would be a longer life but at present levels of vigor. Still another would be a longer life that simply stretched the length of the decline. And still another would be a longer life with mixed effects, mental and physical, some good and some bad.

Each of these possibilities would raise its own set of problems, and I will not try to imagine what they might be. Whatever they might be, even small changes toward any of them would have strong general effects. Included would be the impact on younger generations jockeying for jobs and promotion and positions of leadership. In the struggle to pay for the extended years without wiping out retirement and social security, would the elderly too be forced to work more years than they might like? There would also be a great impact on childbearing and child rearing, as different definitions of youth and middle age emerged and as the job market for women of childbearing age changed (and what would that age come to be?); and an impact on social status and community respect, as a larger and larger portion of the elderly emerged (and with that emergence the possibility of intergenerational conflict). Everything, in a word, would change.

Suffice it to say that a society with a much larger proportion of elderly would be a different kind of society, perhaps good, perhaps bad; much would depend on the strategies employed to cope with all the needed changes and how much time was necessary to put them in place. If by chance a striking genetic breakthrough should allow lives of 150 years, the impact would be all the more dramatic, and the necessary changes in social policy all the more radical.

Do We Need to Increase Average Life Expectancy?

Do societies worldwide need a breakthrough to the possibilities of maximizing and optimizing average life expectancy—and can any afford a research drive to achieve it? It is very hard to find any serious argument to support that development, as if future societies will be inadequate and defective unless we all have longer lives. None of our current social problems—in education, jobs, national defense, environmental protection, or other urgent issues—stem from a low average life expectancy, and none would vanish with a higher average life expectancy. Many problems would grow exponentially. At most, many individuals have said they would like to try a longer life and would probably be willing to pay for it. But for how much of the total direct and indirect costs of living out extended life spans? Ought we to want it for ourselves?

I say "ought" to force myself and my readers to ask just exactly what we think we would gain beyond a life that ended on average at, say, eighty? This question should give everyone pause since no one could know whether they would in fact fare well, whether the kind of extended life span would be one they found acceptable, and what they would do if it did not turn out as planned. We might agree that there are many unfortunate features of the present situation, and most of us can think of reasons why we would like more years. But no clear correlation between a satisfying life (assuming good health and the avoidance of a premature death) and length of life has ever been demonstrated. How many people have any of us known who died at age eighty or ninety, but for whom we felt sorrow because of all the possibilities that lay before them? I have been to many funerals of very old people and have yet to hear anyone lament a loss of future possibilities, however much they grieved to lose a friend or relative.

Some of us may be prepared to take our chances. As a policy matter, what stance should we take toward deliberate research efforts to extend average life expectancy and individual life spans? There are three possibilities: to support such research at the public, governmental level and encourage the private sector to pursue it; to refuse public grants for such research but permit it in the private sector; to refuse public grants and to use considerable social and economic pressure to discourage it at the private level (I ignore here the possibility of banning such research, which is neither likely nor easy to do).

Unless someone can come up with a plausible case that the nation needs everyone to live much longer, and longer than the present steady gain of normalization will bring, there is no reason whatever for government-supported research aimed at maximizing or optimizing life spans. Longer lives may in any case come about as an accidental by-product of efforts to improve the quality of life for elderly people; but there is no reason to court that possibility directly with targeted research. Nor is there any reason to encourage the private sector to pursue it either, and for the same reasons.

Yet that sector will undoubtedly do so if promising leads open up, and if it believes a profit can be made. Should that happen, there would be every reason to put moral, political, and social pressure on the private sector not to move on in the research unless it took part in a major national effort to work through *in advance* the likely problems that success might bring everyone. The matter would be important enough, the implications grave enough, that it would be folly to wander in with no forethought or strategies in place to deal with the economic and social consequences, many of which can be realistically imagined. To drop a new and far-reaching technology on our society, or any society, simply because people will buy it would be irresponsible. It would instead require the fullest airing over a decent period of time and in a systematically organized fashion. The public could then decide what it would like to see happen and be in a position to make a considered judgment about a collective response.

There is no doubt also that a private-sector, age-extending, antiaging product would be expensive (most new pharmaceuticals are and would not otherwise be worth developing) and probably unavailable to everyone at first (and perhaps not ever). As with many expensive new technologies, no public-sector body could reasonably deny the pharmaceutical to everyone simply because not everyone could afford it.[52] But since there will undoubtedly be disagreement on the matter, research efforts to extend life expectancy to some optimizing level should attempt to reach community consensus on the technology's merits rather than simply go by default to the market and private choice. However difficult a collective consensus may be to achieve, the numerous problems that would arise for everyone if some had the technology but others did not (of which inequity might be the least of them) are easy to imagine. Would governments have to devise different social security, retirement, and job arrangements for the former to live side by side with those who did not choose (or could not afford) to take the product? What responsibility would the former bear for the consequences of their choice—total personal responsibility, for better or worse, or would a social safety net be available to help them (paid for by those who did not choose to go that way)? Those are questions a pure market approach cannot answer, but a failure to raise and resolve them would put not only those who chose to live longer lives at risk, but the rest of us as well.

The question of research deliberately aimed at extending average life expectancy, at changing the course of aging, bears directly on the goals of medicine. I argue that death itself is not an appropriate medical target, and that there is no social need to greatly extend life expectancy. But how might we think more broadly about medical research that expands its traditional goal of preserving and restoring health to enhance human nature and human characteristics?

4 Curing the Sick, Helping the Suffering, Enhancing the Well

The knowledge that biomedical research can bring, and the translation of that knowledge into clinical application, offers a proven way of making progress against the waywardness of the body and mind, assaulted from the inside and the outside by hostile agents of death, pain, and disability. Of late, the tantalizing possibility has been raised that research may also enhance our various human traits.

We are all subject to our wayward bodies, though some are luckier than others or more blessed by access to good health care. But none of us gets a free pass from the body's vulnerability to illness and accidents. We don't like them. So when someone promises to relieve our pain and suffering with the use of old knowledge, or the creation of new knowledge, we pay attention. That is something we want, sometimes mildly and sometimes desperately, but never disinterestedly.

In chapter 3 I tried to lighten the biological reputation of two of the greatest scourges, aging and death. Not death itself but only a premature death (conceding the flexibility of that concept) should be the highest target of research. A life without aging, or a life twice as long as we now typically have, might well hold considerably less than we bargained for. But it is much harder to find a good word for the pain and suffering that can mar, and sometimes all but destroy, the time of our life before we die. The appropriate motive for medical research is that it can bring good into the world, that it can make our individual lives better, and that it can provide our collective lives with helpful relief. It is not an overriding moral imperative because it may compete with other valuable human goods. Research is just one such good, comparable to food, jobs, housing, and education. All of them together support human welfare, none is dispensable, and all of them benefit from various kinds of research, whether biological, social, or economic. Medical research speaks to the basic needs of our bodies and minds; and when they do not function well the result can be misery, the absence of health. But the absence of other basic goods can be a misery as well.

That much said, it is not instantly clear how best to pursue good health. The metaphor of a "war" against evil will not do; it invites abuse. Yet health is not a kind of luxury item, nice if you have it but otherwise dispensable. How might the struggle best be envisioned, not only that a sensible perspective can be found, but also to encourage the most useful research? Where might we best start?

Why not at the beginning, trying to make sure that we know what we are about, where the research enterprise should be pointing? To do that, I suggest, means addressing three basic issues. What is health, and what is its relationship to the limits of the body? What is the nature of medicine and public health, two indispensable means for pursuing health? And what is the relationship between health and our satisfaction with life? Or to put it more expansively, ought we in the pursuit of better health and a more satisfying life to consider enhancing body and mind, chasing our utopian dreams?

THE MEANING OF HEALTH

Good health is the goal of research, but health has peculiar traits. Without an ache or pain or worry, a person in good health doesn't even notice it: everything works as it should, hardly worth remarking on. Sickness is a different story. As I was outlining this chapter, ready to begin writing, I came down with a constant, tiring cough and a debilitating fever. I felt lousy. This chapter became irrelevant, the book beside the point. I just wanted to go to bed, and I did. It was only a severe case of bronchitis, but a diagnosis of lung cancer (not implausible as an ex-smoker) would doubtless have caught my attention even more.

For many ancient cultures, health was often seen as a sign of grace, and ill health as a disgrace, associated with sin. The Greeks thought of it as bodily integrity and harmony, order as opposed to disorder.[1] But because that notion of order is so quiet and unobtrusive, invisible when all is going well, nothing betrays its intimate link with disorder, those threats to our bodily order that make us sit up and take notice. If we did not find ourselves the victims of things going wrong, we might not care about health at all. Its reversal leads us to look toward the ideal, good health, and to seek remedies for whatever undermines it.

The attempt to characterize health by its positive features (the presence of bodily and psychological harmony) and their negative kin (whatever interferes with health) has of course led to long-standing arguments.[2] Some have objected that health is a value-laden term, subject to the vagaries of culture, the variable human responses to its absence, and its resistance to definition.[3] I think I am in good health despite a variety of minor ailments (some emphysema, a tennis wrist and elbow, inability to jog much any more, and so on). Yet I function well on most important matters: I work, I enjoy life, I interact with the world. Those few glitches don't much matter, though for others with similar problems, the reaction may be more negative (which is why people vary considerably in appraising their health). For someone subject to more serious problems—depression, or emphysema, or severe arthritis—life will be more disturbed, perhaps intolerably so (even if others with those conditions act as if nothing was wrong with them).

Health is hard to define in clear scientific concepts devoid of evaluative judgments.[4] Empirically, we can characterize it by the presence of typical capacities—to walk or see or breathe well—and measure and compare a person's health against statistical averages. But it is broadly understood as something good to have, its absence disliked. It is thus also a normative standard of judgment, subject to varying interpretations about disabling severity and wide-ranging evaluations of its subjective burden. My pain from jogging means something different to me than my aching tooth. Elderly people on dialysis, free from the pressures of a job, frequently tolerate kidney dialysis better than younger people.

My objective here is to convey the flavor of those arguments, interesting and important, not to resolve them. I settle instead on definitions that, while contestable, are not out of line with common usage. By health I mean a person's experience of well-being and an integrity of mind and body, the ability to pursue his or her vital goals, and to function in ordinary social and work contexts. That is its positive side. Health is no less characterized by the absence of significant pain, suffering, and harmful disease. By "disease," the main cause of pain and disability, I mean a physiological or mental malfunction reflecting a deviation from statistically standard norms and likely to bring on illness, pain, and disability. My definition, then, encompasses the positive and negative traits of "health." It also is far more limited than the famous 1947 World Health Organization definition of health, which encompassed "complete social well-being"—and thereby opened the way to turning all human problems into medical problems.[5] Following common usage also, illness may be defined as the individual's experience of pain, suffering, or disability, while sickness refers to society's perception of a person's capacity to function in the usual social roles.

Though much debated, the formal definition of health has remained static over the years. Yet one noteworthy feature of health as now understood has changed. Medical progress and shifting social standards have escalated the demand for good health while simultaneously raising the stakes for what counts as good health. Fatalism is no longer fashionable and no degree of pain or discomfort is thought beyond the medical reach or simply to be accepted as part of life. Greater progress brings forth greater demands. The phenomenon of "doing better but feeling worse," identified decades ago, is as strong as ever.[6]

The always unclear line between what ought to count as a pathology and what is simply life gets harder to find. If research can find a solution to what bothers us, it instantly incorporates the item—however untraditional its origin—in the medical armamentarium (to use an old war-redolent term). The history of mental illness shows this progression, as do many of the efforts to overcome the burdens of aging, substance abuse, and learning problems in children. Moreover, since nature throws up a steady array of ways to make our bodies hurt and to bring us down, the improvement of health is, like science itself, to use Vannevar Bush's 1947 phrase, an "endless frontier."

THE GOALS OF MEDICINE AND HEALTH CARE

At one level, the pursuit of health focuses on the individual and organizes the provision of those essential elements—medical, technical, economic, and social—that constitute health care. At the other, it focuses on a population; if anything, public health is even more important than individual health. Whether people have good health or bad depends on many variables: their education, income, living conditions, genetic inheritance, and access to health care. The increased recognition of the socioeconomic determinants of health has added a fresh dimension and emphasized the inadequacy of good medicine alone in enhancing good health.[7] Obviously, there are many useful forms of research to improve health that go far beyond biomedical research, on behavioral and environmental threats to health (I return to them later).

A core discipline in the pursuit of health is medicine, the care of the sick its central vocation, and the preservation of health its ultimate aim. It is also the arena for intense research, aiming to understand the origins of diseases and then to cure them. Though American health policy focuses heavily on getting sick people well, not keeping them well in the first place, this illogic is perfectly understandable. Most of us run faster and more desperately from what hurts us than toward what does us good.

I propose here four goals of medicine, combining ancient and contemporary ends and drawn from a project I organized on the goals of medicine:[8]

- the prevention of disease and injury and the promotion and maintenance of health
- the relief of pain and suffering caused by maladies
- the care and cure of those with a malady, and the care of those who cannot be cured
- the avoidance of premature death and the pursuit of a peaceful death

While these succinct goals may seem obvious, even trite, there is a little more here than meets the eye. The first point to make is that members of our project culled them from some forty posited goals espoused by one group or another over the centuries, as well as current discussion. The second is that, we concluded, there ought to be no fixed, permanently set priority among those goals. Disease prevention is sensible when an individual is well, and beside the point if death is on the way. The relief of pain and suffering seems obvious enough as an aim, but sometimes the price of getting well is to endure therapeutic pain and suffering. As a physician once remarked to me, "we take sick people, already hurting, and make them hurt even more to make them well."[9] Our research group concluded, therefore, that there should be no set priorities for the goals of medicine; everything will depend on the stage at which someone comes into the medical orbit: sick or well, with acute or chronic illness. The first task of the clinician is to determine where the patient is now, just as (for health policy purposes) it is to determine if the greatest need in a population is prevention or care for those already sick.

Setting aside the larger issues of health care policy and the delivery of health care as not directly pertinent to this book's topic, I focus instead on the research implications of these four medical goals.[10] They do not stray too far from those articulated by ancient Hippocratic authors: "to do away with the sufferings of the sick, to lessen the violence of their diseases, and to refuse to treat those who are overmastered by their diseases."[11] Missing in that quotation is only the goal of curing disease, hardly possible in the fourth century B.C.; other parts of the Hippocratic tradition aimed to prevent it.

The prevention of disease and injury and the promotion and maintenance of health.   Perhaps health promotion and disease prevention were once the province of public health, not medicine. But recent medical practice—advanced by the American Academy of Family Practice and the American College of Physicians, for example, the two largest medical specialty groups—has come to put health promotion and disease prevention high on the list of physicians' duties. HMOs have also given them a lofty place, though the reality is not as strong as the rhetoric. Since some 50 percent of deaths can be traced to behavioral causes, the case for prevention as both a public health and medical priority is strong.[12] As a research aim, health promotion and disease prevention have never had the prestige of medical research for acute illness, but their importance has stimulated greater research interest of late.

The relief of pain and suffering caused by maladies.   The somewhat antique word "maladies" indicates that disease does not cause all pain and suffering. Accidents account for their fair share as well. The relief of pain and suffering as a medical goal can be traced to the beginning of medicine itself. Pain and suffering trigger an interest in our health in a way hardly anything else can and remain a classic reason for people to seek the help of physicians. Some years ago the physician Eric Cassell called attention to the difference between pain and suffering.[13] Pain (an unpleasant physical sensation that comes in many forms) and suffering (the psychological and spiritual meaning we attach to the assaults of illness or other problems on our lives) often go together, but not always. Pain can exist without suffering (if it is temporary and unlikely to recur), and suffering without pain (the knowledge of a malignant tumor as yet unfelt, or clinical depression). Both are obvious research targets.

The care and cure of those with a malady, and the care of those who cannot be cured.   The wording of this goal suggests the possibility of tension. The cure of disease is a highly prized medical goal, what we most hope for when we fall ill. But cure is not always possible, as with many chronic illnesses, and patients then need good social help and nursing or other forms of nonmedical care. The term "care" is meant to capture that latter need. Caring, however, has often been seen as second best, what is to be done when the search for a cure fails. That way of thinking, however, has often given a much lower research priority to the ways and means of caring, of which many can require health service research more than medical research. Since many diseases cannot be cured, and everyone is likely at the end of life to need caring, there is every reason to think that care and cure deserve equal weight, even if cure is likely to have a glamour that care will not.

The avoidance of premature death and the pursuit of a peaceful death. In this goal too is tension. A premature death—a notion relative to history and culture—may be understood as one that occurs before a person has had a chance to live long enough to experience the main stages of a human life cycle (life, love, work, for instance) and achieve or come close to achieving her or his life projects, or as a death that could be averted with no great burden to the individual or society. As the many arguments about terminating treatment have made clear in recent years, knowing if and when to switch from aggressive life-preserving treatments to a palliative-care effort for the dying person is by no means easy or clear. I argued in the previous chapter that death itself is not an appropriate enemy of medicine, but only premature death. As I assert in a later chapter on priority setting in research, research on palliative care deserves even more support, not simply because more can be known and done for the dying, but also for those not yet dying. With the dying, however, palliative care serves as a symbol of the medical need to accept death and thus clinically to come to terms with it.

None of these four goals has a permanent priority (although the relief of pain and suffering might come as close to that status as any). Everything must depend on people's health status as they come in contact with medicine and health care. For health care systems as a whole, different parts of a population will also be in those varied conditions. Determining which needs are the most important at a given moment ought to be a major determinant in setting health policy and must remain important for the future as a determinant of research priorities.

With goals of this kind in hand—none particularly controversial, and all reflecting the traditions of medicine—surely a determination of research needs and goals would be relatively easy. Not so. There are at least three complicating problems. One of them is the long-standing struggle about whether the goal of health care systems should be to promote good health (so that it is a "health"-care system) or pursue the eradication of disease and other maladies (a "sick"-care system). It seems to me a false dichotomy. To be sure, a greater emphasis on promoting good health might assign a much higher priority to behavioral and socioeconomic research with that end in view (one I would surely support). But people would continue to get ill at some point in their lives and come to need cure and care. We cannot banish illness by promoting health or combating illness. We should keep those who are well in good health as long as possible and treat those who are sick as effectively as possible. I do not see how it would be possible or desirable to design a system that would not have both ends in views, even if sometimes in tension with each other for resources.

More crucial are two other problems. Both bear on the important question of the appropriate scope of medical and health care and thus of the appropriate corresponding research aims. One of them is the question of research on what might be termed the nonmedical uses of medical knowledge and skills for purposes other than that of health; and the other is the extent to which research should seek, not simply to keep people healthy, but to improve and enhance their ordinary traits and capacities.

THE USES AND ABUSES OF MEDICAL
SKILLS, KNOWLEDGE, AND RESEARCH

The goals of medicine respond to diverse human needs. Yet the capacities of biological knowledge and medical skills to respond to needs and desires that bear on health only indirectly or not at all are significant and growing. Most of their capacities are good, but some can be evil. Medical knowledge can save lives and torture prisoners; relieve infertility and terminate pregnancies; eliminate pain and improve capital punishment techniques. Which uses are compatible with the primary goals of medicine and which are not? Or should we even raise that question: if medicine can give us something we want and find morally justifiable, what difference if any does it make whether it fits within the goals of medicine at all? A quick response to that last question: medicine itself will be at risk of internal incoherence and loss of direction if its applications float free of its appropriate ends (which may, however, integrate nonmedical purposes within its self-definition in ways not inherently at odds with its ends).

The potential use and misuse of medical knowledge can be divided into four categories, each of which admits of corresponding research goals: those that are fully acceptable, posing no serious professional, scientific, or moral threats; those that are unacceptable under any circumstances; those that fall outside the conventional goals of medicine but make use of medical knowledge and yet serve morally acceptable social and individual purposes; and those that are unacceptable under all but the most unusual circumstances. I leave for a much fuller discussion below the issue of using medicine to "enhance" human nature or traits since it is a complicated case not clearly falling into any of the above categories as a class of medical possibilities.

Acceptable and valid uses of medical knowledge. If research is directed toward meeting any of the four goals of medicine sketched above, it does not pose any obvious moral and social problems. On the contrary, that kind of research represents the main line of research, well tested and socially validated over time. Objections against various means proposed to carry out the research need not undermine its goals. There can, however, be two problems. One of them is to determine how intensively to carry out the research and what kind of resources to put into it. That requires, first, a sense of priorities within medical research; second, the priority of medical research in relationship to other kinds of scientific research of human benefit; third, the priority of funding for medical research over against already existing means of health care; and, fourth, the allocating of resources between health care and other social needs.

The other problem might be called the "how much and how far problem." If the struggle against illness, suffering, and disease ought not to be likened to war aiming at unconditional surrender of the enemy, are there any reasonable limits to the struggle? I refer here not to moral limits but rather to prudential limits. However much medical research progresses, it will run up against the "ragged edge of progress." Should research just keep going, as if we judge the earlier success and the improved health it has brought are not sufficient? That is the way the research community, with the public's assent, now operates. I have no doubt such a spirit will continue, but once progress has greatly (though not fully) pacified disease, society might not find it amiss to give other social priorities a higher status, higher than medical research. If, however, a society decides that there is no higher good than better health, and better and better health, then I suppose that decision would not be morally objectionable—though it would strike me as a strange kind of society, a paradise for hypochondriacs afraid of getting sick no matter how well they are, acutely unwilling to bear any ache and pain, and in daily dread of dying, no matter how long their lives already are.

Wrong and unacceptable uses of medical knowledge. A wrong or unacceptable use of medical knowledge is one in which the use's aim itself or its context is morally wrong. The use of medical skills to refine methods of torture—and the research leading to such skills—is a long-understood perversion of medicine, using knowledge to bring pain rather than to heal illness. The use of pharmaceutical or neurological techniques for political purposes, such as to improve interrogation outcomes, or to keep prisoners passive, or to induce dread or anxiety as a means of terrorizing people, is also intolerable. Research on the use of recombinant DNA techniques for the development of biological warfare is another, increasing threat. In each case the end itself is wrong, made all the worse by a perverted use of research of clinical skills to achieve it.

Physicians' cooperation with capital punishment is now widely rejected as incompatible with the ethic of medicine, as would be research to improve capital punishment techniques (even though it might reduce the suffering of condemned prisoners). The use of human subjects for hazardous research without their informed consent would count as an instance of the use of wrong means for what might otherwise be acceptable purposes. Far more controversial and notable for their lack of social consensus are the use of medical skills for euthanasia or physician-assisted suicide and for the performance of abortion.

Acceptable nonmedical uses of medical knowledge.   Medical knowledge has long been applied to areas of human interest quite independent of health needs. Cosmetic surgery is well established, used for the repair of facial injuries and deformities as well as for purposes of vanity and self-improvement. Contraception and sterilization may be used for health reasons but are far more commonly used for reproductive control. Forensic medicine is used in the criminal and civil justice system, making use of DNA techniques in bodily fluid identification. Within the military, medical means are used to assess personnel's capacity to take part in combat. The test in each case, though usually implicit, is whether the use of medical knowledge violates the ethics of medicine or affronts public values. Physicians are often willing to serve these assorted nonmedical purposes. Research to advance those possibilities and their clinical application can be judged by the same criteria, and in most cases the nonmedical purposes are supported more by the private than the public sector.

Uses of medical knowledge unacceptable under all but the most rare circumstances.   Predictive medicine, the use of genetic markers to calculate the likely health threats to a person, is already possible for forms of breast cancer and early-onset Alzheimer's disease. The use of family histories, for the prediction of both genetic and nongenetic conditions, has been around for some time, but predictive medicine will extend the scope of that kind of investigation. As relevant as this information may be—and as chilling as it may be for some—there is wide agreement that it should not be used for insurance or job screening, which constitutes misuse of an otherwise neutral technique. The application of eugenics promoted in the late nineteenth and early twentieth centuries, and lethally used by the Nazis, is another possibility with this technology, now universally condemned but by no means unimaginable in the future.

Coerced abortions and sterilization, mandated genetic screening and prenatal diagnosis, or excessive pressure to change health-related behavior are only some of the abusive possibilities. The temptation to use medical knowledge and skills to manipulate entire classes of people in the name of improved health or cost control (or assistance to private industry in one way or another) is real and could become irresistible—particularly in a culture that steadily escalates the value of good health and sometimes stigmatizes those who fail to toe the mark.

ENHANCING HUMAN LIFE AND HUMAN TRAITS

In 1637 the philosopher René Descartes said, "for the mind depends so much on the temperament and dispositions of the bodily organs that, if it is possible to find a means of rendering men wiser and cleverer than they have hitherto been, I believe it is in medicine that it must be sought."[14] That hope was not seriously pursued for hundreds of years. Of late, though, speculations about enhancing human nature, and improving on characteristic human traits, have gained momentum, stimulated in great part by genetic possibilities. Why could we not have better memories, higher IQs, more sociable temperaments, improved looks, greater resistance to disease, longer lives, and of course children tailored to our notions of better, more desirable offspring?

These are the questions being asked, at least by some, and the kind of aims and ideals that inspire them can only, or mainly, be achieved by research. How far, and in what directions, ought research to go in trying to enhance human life and human traits? I touched on that issue earlier, in my discussion about possible efforts to increase the human life span, but it is appropriate now to take it on more fully.

As with the concept of health, "enhancement" presents an immediate puzzle. A colleague of mine at the Hastings Center, Erik Parens, directed a project in the late 1990s to determine how public policy should deal with the possibility of human enhancements.[15] Though the project brought together a thoughtful group of people from a variety of disciplines, it could not settle on a clear enough, usable enough, definition of enhancement to provide any policy guidance.

Enhancement, like health, is general in scope and informal in usage. Isn't ordinary medicine an enhancement, taking sick people and making them well; or immunizing them against a disease such as measles or smallpox; or bringing a child with a growth hormone deficit up to normal height; or prescribing Prozac to allow people more psychological peace in their lives; or using cosmetic surgery to help ordinary-looking people look better?

Yet these ordinary medical improvements aimed at normalcy leave out what are commonly seen as real and dramatic enhancements, such as improving intelligence or choosing the traits of one's children to make them superior. Accordingly, to suggest the range of enhancements I once again use the three categories of normalizing, maximizing, and optimizing, not too far from ordinary usage but not quite the same either:

> The *normalization* of human life and traits is the traditional medical goal of maintaining or restoring individual health to what Norman Daniels has called "species-typical functioning," and what is popularly understood as either "making people well" or assisting them to live as normal a life as possible with their incurable diseases or disabilities.[16] By this standard, prevention would be part of ordinary efforts to normalize health as would strenuous efforts to find effective chemotherapies for cancer; both aim to bring people up to, or keep them at, average standards of good health, not to go beyond them.

> The *maximizing* of human life and traits would be efforts to choose the most desirable, highest standards of *present* excellence in human health and to bring everyone up to those standards. This aim would encompass plastic surgery for cosmetic purposes, working to make ordinary people as attractive as those acclaimed as the most beautiful, or the choice to have a child whose IQ was in the top 1 percent, well above where the parents are but where other people can already be found. Maximizing, in other words, does not seek to improve human nature as such but to help everyone come up to the highest observed standards (or those thought to be such).

> The *optimizing* of human nature seeks to go beyond the best that now exists, well beyond it. The vision is that of people living to 150 or 200, not the high present maximum of 105–122; of people who could get by with little or no sleep, or go far beyond the far end of the IQ curve, or live a lifetime without significant disease, or be always peaceful with themselves and genial with everyone else (with no deleterious side effects)— and able to fashion the child of their choice by the means of their choice, satisfying every fantasy of the perfect baby.

The Human Genome Project and the emergence of more serious possibilities of genetic engineering have added a fresh, often breathless, impetus to speculation about all these possibilities. As the various examples I have offered suggest, enhancement can be understood in medical and non-medical ways; as helping us draw boundaries around the legitimate use of medical skills; and as bearing on the most fundamental questions of all: what does it mean to be a human being, and what ought to count as a responsible use of research to shape and reshape our nature or our traits?

COMPLEXITIES OF ENHANCEMENT

There are, for that matter, those who think the idea of "normalcy" itself is suspect, apt to stigmatize those who are disabled or otherwise impaired, and others who worry that harmful cultural pressures (to look young, or be pretty) will drive people to ersatz enhancements.[17] The philosopher Dan Brock has carefully looked at problems of equity that enhancement research and application raise—allowing the affluent to improve their lot even more; widening the gap between rich and poor; creating two classes of people, the enhanced and unenhanced; and creating a situation where the enhancement will be useful to some only if unevenly distributed (for instance, the paradox of human growth hormone: if everyone uses it, the present distribution between short and tall people will remain).[18] None of those developments or a research agenda that made them likely would be welcomed by those who give a high place to equality.[19]

Is there an inherent difference between medical and nonmedical means of enhancement? Training for athletic events can use ordinary exercise and traditional training methods or supplement these with, for instance, steroids. Is it worse to give young people some performance-enhancing drugs than to employ a severe "natural" discipline over many years that drives out other things young people need for their full development? Gymnastics is notorious for its pressures on young girls. Even if we decide that all means of natural enhancement, whether in athletics, or appearance, or for memory improvement, are tolerable in principle, would not the means of enhancement, or its magnitude, make a difference?[20]

Rather than attempt to deal with each and every one of those questions, I work with a few examples and suggest criteria for ethical and social judgment that apply to them. Here are relevant questions:

will the enhancement be medically safe?

will it unduly widen the gap between rich and poor, the well endowed and poorly endowed?

will the enhancement pose significant harms to important social institutions and values?

will it give one person (or group of persons) too much sway over the lives and future of others?

will society as a whole benefit from the enhancement, or only some individuals—and does that distinction matter?

should certain enhancements be supported with federal research grants?

should certain individual enhancements be discouraged, even stigmatized?

I suggest two criteria in response to the need to pass judgment on enhancement research. First, the federal government should support only those forms of research that promise to improve ordinary health, that is, either to bring the sick up to ordinary levels of functioning or to enable them to live better with their sickness. Research of that kind is suitably directed not only to population health but also to *individual* benefit. Enhancement research, by contrast, should only be supported when there is a clearly defined *social* benefit in view; that is, a benefit that promises to help the population as a whole and to make a contribution to overall social well-being. Those social benefits should be more than merely speculative. They should have behind them a solid body of data and public debate to indicate that the research is meeting a recognized common need and that it promises to satisfy that need, in whole or in part. Individual desires for enhancement should never be sufficient to command governmental research support. Government-supported research, even if it would have certain population benefits, should not be undertaken if the results would clearly, or most likely, support only part of the population, and all the more so if it were likely to increase the gap between the affluent and the poor.

Second, private market-oriented research holds out many possibilities for enhancement-oriented benefits (and no doubt eventually for profit as well) but must respect standards of moral judgment about their social acceptability. Even if it is not made illegal, we should condemn research that will, in playing to individual desires, have the result of giving some people undue power over the lives of other people. A perfect baby fashioned to meet parental specifications (irrevocable by the child) would be a case in point. Research that would give some people a competitive or social edge over other people, but not available to those others, should not be acceptable either. We may well debate just which individual enhancements ought to be considered wrong. What we should not do is to assume, because they will come from the free choice of individuals, and be accepted by the law, that they will have no harmful social consequences. As I have argued at various points in this book, the aggregate of private choices by individuals can change not just those individuals but also the societies of which they are a part.

Performance Enhancement

I begin with what might seem to be the most acceptable kinds of enhancement, those that would improve our performance of valuable activities. My examples bear on athletics; on intelligence; on mood and attention; and on procreation. In each case, we already pursue "natural" means of doing so; that is, we usually add nothing artificial from the outside to our bodies but work only to develop what is latent within the capacities of the body or mind. To improve our athletic skills, for example, we get good coaching and then follow rigorous training regimens. Or to improve our memory, we practice and make use of various mnemonic devices, and to improve our intelligence (if that is possible), we read and think and, so to speak, exercise our mind (I do not count practicing for IQ tests as a way of improving IQ). If we already do those things and often commend others who do them, why should we not be free to pursue by genetic or other biomedical means those same enhancements?[21] And why should not research be devoted to helping those who aspire to such enhancements do so? Here I respond with a forthright "it all depends," and my four examples will help make that clear. In each case, my focus will be on government-supported research, with side comments on private research.

Enhancing athletics. I begin with this form of enhancement not only because it has loomed large in the debate over medical enhancements, but because it has been important culturally and poses many of the most difficult enhancement puzzles.[22] As a onetime competitive swimmer, moreover, I have had a great interest in the remarkable improvement in times over the years. Most of that can be traced to better stroke techniques, improved coaching, body shaving, much increased daily training distances, and, most recently, special swimming suits that reduce water friction. With the exception of the new swimming suits, all the other improvements are of the "natural" kind, and even the swimming suits are understood as a borderline case. As in all other amateur sports, however, the use of performance-enhancing drugs is forbidden even if many of them would not be forbidden in ordinary life.

The reason for such regulations turns in part on safety considerations, as with the use of steroids, but hardly less important are the traditional ideals of amateur competition. It is the playing of the game or the running of the race for its own sake that is most important, not winning. Drugs would give those who used them an unfair advantage, which would also thwart the ideals. The purpose of athletic competition is, as it should be and always has been, that of determining who, through a combination of natural talent, intelligent training, and discipline, is the best—but, we all recognize, competing is in itself part of the pleasure, not just winning; and, since most people cannot win, being the best would be foolish as a sole motive anyway.

Those ideals lose their sheen if, as the great professional football coach Vince Lombardi remarked, "winning isn't just everything, it is the only thing." Football (or any other paid sport) is no longer a "game" in the traditional sense, having changed its ends (from competing to winning) and broadened its means (to include the use of performance-enhancing drugs to enhance the likelihood of winning). Since the line between amateur and professional sports is now all but invisible (with cash prizes and other inducements freely available in both contexts), it is hardly surprising that the control of performance drugs is sought, but the results mixed. My impression also is that what might be called the "winning imperative" is stronger now than earlier, though in world-class athletes it was always strong—necessarily so if they wanted to be world-class—and always prone to pathologies.

One of those pathologies raises another question about performance enhancement: what after all is the real difference between a winning-obsessed parent or coach pushing obsessively to make someone a winner and an athlete who uses drugs? If we permit the one, why not the other? I offer two reasons. One of them is that, while we can hardly "ban" overly zealous parents and coaches, we can and do condemn them, judging that they appear to be more interested in their success than in the welfare of their child-athlete; and they should be condemned (now and then coaches of that kind lose their jobs). The other reason is that the pushy parent or coach is, after all, only pushing to maximize the natural potential of the athlete. The fault lies not in trying to bring out that potential, but in the bullying and domineering ways likely to harm other potentials of the child even if they improve the athletic potential. As Erik Parens noted, the means for choosing the enhancement do matter, even if those means are traditional.[23]

I do not want to minimize here the fact that there are many borderline cases, even if none of them seems to me to show, as some might contend, that there is no difference between normalizing and enhancing. The swimmer who takes caffeine tablets to increase the pulse and excitement level, or the runner who uses a blood transfusion of his own blood, or the marathoner who trains at a high altitude, could all be said to be going beyond established, conventional methods of training or competing. But there is still a difference: there are no threats to health or safety of any consequence, and the various techniques are open to all without blame—even as most observers concede that the line between convention and enhancement is sometimes very fine.

I have so far said nothing about the use of research, focusing instead on various current practices and debates about the use of various techniques. What makes the athletic case interesting though is that, unlike many other imagined enhancements, this is one that has been around for a long time and has been examined. We know, in other words, a little more about what we are talking about. No one in the American sports community has proposed the use of federal funds to find better biomedical or pharmaceutical means to improve athletic performance, or even the use of private funds for that purpose. I can think of no reasons to make such a proposal myself. Yet precisely that kind of research was carried out, under governmental auspices, in East Germany and China.

The improvement of athletic performance offers no likely social or individual benefit, even if it might please many ambitious nations and athletes. Nor would it offer the institution of athletics any benefit. Competitive swimming is much more sophisticated and demanding in its training methods than in my heyday, and the times are much better. But I see no evidence that it is any more fun to be a competitive swimmer or that the races are any more enjoyable to watch. Nor is it evident that a shift from an hour's practice a day to three hours is a useful way for teenagers to spend their time. Is it good for family life or the swimmer for a mother to drive her teenage daughter (my niece) to swim training at 4:30 A.M. every day, which is the time set for those kids who want to be in the "competitive" as distinguished from the "normal" swimming program? Research, using drugs, to achieve the same end would not be beneficial either.

Enhancing intelligence and memory. A high intelligence is something most people think they want, and all the more so if they want to do well in their society. No one—at least no one I have ever heard of—thinks it is better to have an inferior rather than a superior intelligence (even if a memorable argument was once made for a Supreme Court candidate, not notably brilliant, to be confirmed on the grounds that the Court would benefit from someone with average intelligence). But what is intelligence anyway?

One thing seems certain: it is no longer the simple model most of us were raised on. If what is called the general cognitive ability ("G") model is still alive and well despite many years of argument, more recent contending models have been introduced as well. Some efforts have been made to bring the different proposed varieties of intelligence together, and it has long been accepted that G intelligence has a number of features; it is not monolothic.[24] Howard Gardner's important 1983 book, *Frames of Mind,* and Daniel Goleman's 1995 book, *Emotional Intelligence,* have been two of the most striking efforts of late to put to rest the idea that intelligence is a simple concept, readily understood and measured.[25]

Gardner wrote that his purpose was "to undermine the common notion of intelligence as a general capacity or potential which every human being possesses to a greater or lesser extent," questioning in a fundamental way long-held assumptions about the value of standardized verbal instruments. Intelligence, he contends, encompasses a much wider range of competencies than previously understood and is best conceptualized as the ability to solve problems or accomplish tasks that are valued in particular cultural settings. Gardner identifies seven forms of intelligence: linguistic, musical, logical/mathematical, spatial, bodily/kinesthetic, and intra- and interpersonal. Moreover, "an individual's facility with one content has little predictive power about his or her facility with other kinds of content . . . genius (and *a fortiori,* ordinary performances) is likely to be specific to particular contents."[26]

This latter point seems obvious when we think about it: the brilliant politician, with great personal skills, is not necessarily capable of being a brilliant mathematician, or those good with language to be equally good in dealing with spatial problems. Part of being successful is knowing what kind of intelligence we have and then finding the right context in which to exercise it.

Daniel Goleman's contribution was to develop the idea of "emotional intelligence," which means a capacity for self-awareness, impulse control, persistence and zeal, self-motivation, empathy, and social deftness.[27] Invoking these two perspectives, people who discover the appropriate context in which to exercise their intelligence will (usually) need emotional intelligence to realize its full potential. Architects with a splendid spatial intelligence are not likely to have great success if they cannot work well with colleagues and clients.

While psychologists still argue about the views of Gardner and Goleman, the multidimensional view of intelligence has been generally accepted. The long search for genes that can be associated with intelligence continues, mainly using the G form of intelligence as its point of departure. Its main attraction is still what it has always been, a reliable and valid predictor of educational and occupational levels. There seems confidence that such genes will be found, even if there is considerable uncertainty about how much genetic variance among individuals will be accounted for by individual genes.[28] What needs to be distinguished here is the difference between doing research to further our knowledge of intelligence, and the role of genetics in it, and the use of such knowledge to improve IQs in general or individual IQs.[29] The first task seems valuable, the second more doubtful.[30] If the genetic research can turn up important clues to learning disabilities, for instance, that could be most valuable. It is the latter task that is more problematic. It is hard to imagine how research might go about enhancing G intelligence, much less enhancing one or more specific kinds of intelligence but leaving the others undisturbed.

There is, for openers, no way to know in advance what results enhancement might have, particularly whether it would enhance the overall welfare of a person as well as the specific intelligence that is the enhancement target. If we think, moreover, about the general well-being of society there is no way to predict what the outcome of such an attempt would be. It would surely require an unparalleled social experiment, and one that would have to be carried out with a number of people and require many years to measure its full possibilities.

However self-evidently valid it seems to carry out research on intelligence for its own sake, or to cope with learning disorders, I find it difficult to imagine why the government would want to sponsor research on general intelligence enhancement, with unknown consequences and no promise whatever of an improved society. Such support could easily smack of class or racial bias since lower IQs have long been associated with various deprived groups. In any case, given the debates about the important role of environment in intelligence, how much would those targeted groups actually benefit—and just *which* intelligence should be enhanced anyway?

As for everyone else, what evidence is there that higher levels of intelligence would produce a better society? The Nazi leaders were reputed to have had standard IQ scores over 140, and apparently Stalin and Mao, to mention two great political murderers, were not lacking in intelligence either. Few, if any, of our major social problems can be traced to intelligence deficiencies. In short, while intelligence in all its varieties seems highly valued—and why not?—there is no reason to call for a focused publicly financed research campaign much less to argue, as one article did, that "this research is morally required" (though it actually offered no social benefit reasons).[31] Again, a private market would probably find takers (as do private markets in just about anything); and even if I am skeptical, I am uncertain whether harm would necessarily come from efforts, genetic or otherwise, to enhance intelligence.

Memory enhancement is a different matter. The memory of most people declines with age. Would it be an advantage to everyone to have a better memory, to maximize memory so that all of us could, like the great mathematician John von Neumann, recall whole pages verbatim from books he had read only once years ago but (unlike some of what used to be called idiot savants) be described as a warm, sociable, well-balanced person? While the ability to forget troubling memories has its value, I have not read that a strong memory necessarily floods the mind with unwanted memories. Nor has it been shown that better memories in individuals would lead to better societies. These reflections do not lead me to think that memory enhancement would be a good use of public resources, but no doubt would find willing seekers in the private sector.

Enhancing mood and attention.   All of us know people whose temperaments are a delight. They are relaxed, outgoing, not easily ruffled, full of feeling but rarely distraught much less depressed. Why should not everyone aspire to be like that, happy with themselves and a source of pleasure to others? Or we might use our imagination at the other end of the spectrum, not with the clinically depressed but with those whose swings of mood, whose low points, and whose irritable personality can be a burden to themselves and others. Surely it would be nice to find a way to bring such people up to a higher level of temperament, not to displays of gaiety but simply to ordinary, balanced feelings, if never very high then again never very low.

There are many ways of trying to achieve these two states. To get to the high end of the spectrum, aiming to bring ourselves—or everyone—up to the most emotionally blessed among us, maximizing the possibilities, a campaign of reading uplifting books might help, or sustained psychotherapy. Those same methods might work with those who simply seek to rise to the ordinary level. But those methods have drawbacks. They take time and are unreliable. No book yet written can anywhere near guarantee to bring happiness, not even the Bible, which has other ends in view. Therapy helps many people, but not all, and does best with those living below average possibilities, not those who want to rise to the highest levels of tranquillity.

A supposedly better, more direct—but still controversial—way has been pursued for at least a few decades: drugs. They are faster than books and psychotherapy, safer than alcohol, and not out of step with accepted medical models. The debate has never been better characterized than as one between psychotropic hedonism and pharmacological Calvinism.[32] Should we be open to drug-induced states we consider desirable, or should we be wary and repressive? There are drugs addressed to problems of depression, schizophrenia, bipolar disorder, anxiety, phobias of various kinds, attention-deficit disorders, and those that are helpful to people who suffer from the blues, minor depression, and stress.

Those aiming at the clinically serious conditions have been around for a long time and are well accepted. Their success is precisely what has stimulated a thought: if drugs can work well for those with both serious and mild emotional and mental problems, why could not drugs be developed to take those at ordinary levels or slightly below and bring them up a notch and take those already reasonably well off and put them in the maximal range? Prozac has some of those benefits with some people; and other drugs are under research that will do even better with more people with fewer side effects.[33] Aldous Huxley's Soma, from *Brave New World*, has long been a talisman of that possibility. Moreover, if Ritalin can help those with attention-deficit disorder, adults as well as children, why not imagine a drug that would go beyond just helping, to achieve a focusing of attention akin to that of the greatest, most concentrated thinkers?

There has always been an uneasiness about these developments. Even though drugs work well with the most serious clinical conditions, schizophrenia and depression, there has been a lingering debate about the use of biomedical means that classify them simply as biological conditions. Old-fashioned psychotherapy, aiming for patient insight, has not quite been pushed aside and has its strong advocates, aiming for balanced therapies and long-term change. In almost every case as well, and even with those drugs aimed at milder conditions, side effects of one kind or another are usually present and particularly if the regimens go on for many years. No perfect drug—utterly efficacious results with no side effects—has yet been invented. Imperfect drugs are often the only ones available and eagerly used.

The uneasiness with a drug such as Ritalin or Prozac is of a different kind.[34] There is little worry about those instances where there is an identifiable psychopathology, no objection to bringing someone from a deficit level to something approaching the common norm. The objection is more subtle, though of various kinds. Diagnosis is one stumbling block, that of distinguishing between the mildly troubled but still within or close to an ordinary range—the difference between a lively, somewhat jumpy child who, as the saying goes, "can't sit still" but is otherwise productive and is a candidate for Ritalin, and the person who now and then has sad thoughts, often well founded in his or her life situation, who is a Prozac candidate. Should they be put on those drugs? Another stumbling block is how long the drug treatment should go on, as a temporary, bridging measure, or as a permanent way of life (as with insulin for the diabetic)? Then there is the question of what to do about those who are nowhere near serious problems and perhaps not even in a borderline situation but who want to live their lives with the kind of permanent highs that few of us enjoy without outside help.

It is this last category that is most troublesome, at least from the perspective of suitable goals for pharmaceutical research. Would it be helpful for us to have available a drug that would take us to, and keep us at, the highest levels of peace and calm with no physical side effects? A drug that could suppress feelings of grief and sadness or emotional pain at seeing the misfortune of others, and that could allow us to transcend the stress of interactions with other people? Objections to a drug of that kind depend heavily on a particular view of life—that it is good to feel grief and sadness on occasion—a view that not everyone may share.

"Whose life is it anyway?" some might ask in the face of any effort to ban the development and sale of such drugs. Psychotropic drugs with no known side effects, achieving on a permanent basis what banned narcotics achieve on a temporary basis, would probably pass legal scrutiny. While I believe there is still much to be said for the ancient idea that one has duties to oneself, the obligation to fashion a self of a richly human kind has come on hard times. But in fact laws against marijuana, heroin, and other controlled substances still embody elements of that way of thinking—that there are limits to what people may do with their own bodies—and the laws will not soon, if ever, be overturned.

Since there are no fundamental, well-founded objections to drugs designed to restore normality, there can be no serious objection to research, public and private, aiming to improve such drugs. Once they are available, their proper prescription is another matter, worthy of much study and efforts at the professional control of abuses, as is now the case with Ritalin and Prozac. Yet since there is no medical or social necessity for people to be in psychological heaven all the time—even if a few seem to be born that way—and since there are many reasons to worry about a society peopled with those who want to go beyond even the happiest among us, we do not need government-supported research to bring that about. Arguments that such drugs might reduce violence or help maintain social peace have as yet little evidence to support them (and many biological and evolutionary reasons to cast doubt on them). As for research in the private sector, impossible to stop and doubtless of commercial promise, some systematic scorn and public stigma would not be out of place.

Enhancing procreation.   Responsible parenthood, the leading idea of the family planning movement of the 1950s and 1960s, came on hard times from the 1970s on, pushed aside by the language of reproductive rights. The difference was not simply one of words. Responsible parenthood was meant to strike a balance between the needs and desires of procreating couples and the welfare of their child-to-be. Parenthood itself was to be a free choice, but the decision acknowledged that a child, eventually to be independent of the parents, was coming into an existence. The reproductive rights movement shifted the emphasis almost entirely to the woman's right to control procreation, and increasingly little was heard of responsibility to any hypothetical offspring. For many commentators, the right to have a child, and to space childbearing, extends to any kind of child the mother might desire by any means desired.[35] Using the word "choice," they would pull a curtain over that sacrosanct realm described by the word "private."

While I am quite prepared to accept the choice of contraception, sterilization, and a woman's legal right to abortion, it is quite another step to limit public discussion of procreation simply to the right to make such choices. What constitutes a good choice, and what kinds of choices might be irresponsible? Such questions should be part of the public dialogue. To decide whether to have a child is to enter a realm of moral responsibility. Parenthood is a paradoxical condition. It comes about to satisfy a parent but results in a life that the child, not the parent, must live and find satisfying. If it would be very strange for a person to want a child solely for the child's sake, it would be morally strange to think that only the mother's satisfaction with her life in having the child was of any consequence.

I say all this by way of preface because I believe that, under all but the most unusual circumstances, any discussion of "enhancing" a child ought to be tantamount to a discussion of the welfare of the child, not the pleasure or reproductive rights of the parent. There is a paradox here as well: if we believe that it is the welfare of the child that is finally at stake, it is also true that, for the serious and responsible parent, that welfare will be satisfying for the parents. Hence, a parent who asks only that a child be healthy, that it be loved and appropriately cared for, asks also for something that will satisfy the parent and benefit the child. This kind of foundation is not meant to set the parents' trajectory for the child's life but only to lay a foundation sufficient to ensure that the child will have a life.

It is easy to understand why parents could be drawn to enhancements of various kinds.[36] The protection of a child's health beyond the ordinary means of food, clothing, and shelter is one reason. Another is the avoidance or cure for a genetic disease or a physical anomaly, or a greater possibility of good intelligence and attractive appearance—everything, that is, that will allow a child to have an ordinary life.[37] Parents down through the generations have sought those benefits for their children and, when those children marry, have hoped that they will choose spouses likely to give them such children. Family genetic counseling may be a comparatively new professional discipline, but it is an old family practice. And it is in line with what I have been calling normalization. While there are interesting debates about whether human growth hormone ought to be used not just with children suffering from a deficiency of such a hormone, but also for those who may just be shorter than average, that is still a debate within the confines of normalization.[38]

Another step can be taken. Parents could aim to have superior children, healthier and smarter and better looking than average, up to and including traits identical to those most admired and envied—maximized children, so to speak. Many techniques are employed by many parents toward just those ends: private schools, tutoring, special classes, tireless parental stimulation, orthodontia, a little plastic surgery perhaps—a life, that is, focused on success and social triumph, a child to be (really) proud of. Up to a point, none of those efforts incurs disapproval. Parental ambition for a child may benefit both parents and child. We begin to take notice, however, when parents push too hard, too obsessively, when the purpose seems more to please the parents than to do good for the child (though no pushy parent is likely to admit that is happening). Even in an era when the abortion of a genetically defective child is widely accepted—sometimes even by those otherwise antiabortion—parents who would abort an otherwise healthy fetus because of the danger of a minor handicap are unlikely to evoke praise.

I am suggesting that one way to think about the biomedical enhancement of a child is to consider what we now think about the old-fashioned methods of enhancement used by excessively ambitious parents. We are prone to think they go too far when the spirit of their effort seems utterly that of their own gratification, a child made in, if not their image, then an image of perfection or excellence that will give them pleasure and indifference about what it might mean for the child to have this done to it. Parents who ignore or rationalize the potential harm to the child in furthering their ambitions are not admired parents—and often not even if the child seems content enough.

The philosopher Joel Feinberg has made a persuasive case that each child has a right to an open future, and that is exactly what the domineering parent compromises.[39] The parent simply will not let the child be what the child is, which is unknown but open to many possibilities. An open future can be understood as one that ought not be dominated environmentally by a parent bent on self-satisfaction through shaping a child, however ordinary and natural the means, or as one where the parent tries to impose on the child a genetic pattern otherwise unavailable.

A way of testing proposed enhancements for their moral and parental acceptability might be twofold. The parents ought to carefully examine their own motives, asking just whose interest is being served, and no less asking themselves whether they are perhaps the victim of cultural folkways, especially of a fashionable kind, that have given them a distorted vision of what will be good for their child.[40] Affluent, educated parents who think that nothing less than an Ivy league education for their offspring is tolerable, and who ceaselessly push their child to get in the right classes and get the right grades, are typical examples of what I have in mind. Yet since parents shape their child in some way, they have some ideals in mind in order to be good parents; they cannot simply do nothing. A second test is whether, whatever the parents do, it is reversible by the child without great psychological travail. Parents may, appropriately enough, nudge a child in one direction than another, but the child ought still be left free to shape his or her own future.

Parents who choose the sex of a child out of a desire to have a child of each sex are acting not for the child's benefit. It is not wrong, say, to want a girl after they have had a boy, but it bespeaks a proclivity toward wanting a child to satisfy parental desires, not to be accepted for its own sake. Parents who would use genetic means to get a child with a certain eye color, or to be of a certain height, or have other special physical traits, ought to fall under the same considerations: just whose good is being served anyway?

As with other forms of enhancement already discussed, it is just about impossible to make any kind of sane case for government-supported research to make enhancements (other than to further the chances that a child will be born healthy). That can be left to the private sector. Yet it seems to me that future children would benefit most from a campaign of parental education and persuasion that would have one strong message: do all you can to have a healthy child, give it the best circumstances within your means, but above all, help the child become what it can become, not what pleases you. And support only research to help make that possible.

UTOPIAN FANTASIES, SOBER REALITIES

I have taken a look at a few of the most discussed possibilities, and fantasies, for improving human nature—or if not quite that, at least for enhancing important human traits. Speculations about human nature seem as old as our species itself, and utopian dreams of improving that nature have a history almost as long. These dreams might be put in two categories. One of them is sweeping and revolutionary. It is the possibility of creating better human beings, more lovable, less violent, smarter and wiser and more sensitive, of enhancing the best traits and eliminating the worst. The other category might be called the individual design model, to give us much greater personal control of our lives, to allow us to fashion a body and a self of our own choosing.

The first dream has always had an intrinsic problem. How could we possibly know whether the successful scientific transformation of human nature would in fact give us a better nature? That would be the mother of all human-subject research initiatives, but we could not know the outcome for years, even centuries; and then it might be a bad outcome and we would be stuck with it. A certain amount of aggressiveness appears valuable for humans, and greatly enhanced intelligence might not produce nicer or more cooperative people; a loss of various anxieties and gloomy moods might deprive us of something essential, even if unpleasant. In short, perhaps blind evolution, knowing no ultimate goal, paradoxically knew what it was doing. Strikingly, the literature on genetic enhancement is happy to speculate about ridding us of disease, pushing death back many years, and improving our spirits with elegantly engineered drugs. But it says less and less about fundamentally changing human nature: no one knows just what that would mean or how it might be accomplished.

Far more attractive and more difficult to deal with is a kind of piecemeal tinkering—the individual design model—working to allow change in one or more traits, aiming not to change all of us in some fundamental way but allowing us to pick and choose to make of ourselves and our children what we will. The individualism of the left (it's my body and my life to do with as I please) and the market practices of the right (people should be free to buy what they want and manufacturers to make what people will buy) will join hands to facilitate the enhancement boutique. At the outer limit of that vision is what the French novelist Michel Houellebecq characterized in an argument between Bruno and Michel, the main protagonists in his novel *The Elementary Particles*, about Aldous Huxley's novel *Brave New World*. The argument was whether Huxley's picture of the future was utopian or dystopian. Bruno sees it as utopian, an expression of our unconscious wishes:

> Everyone says that *Brave New* World is supposed to be a totalitarian nightmare, a vicious indictment of society, but that's hypocritical bull shit. *Brave New World* is our idea of heaven: genetic manipulation, sexual liberation, the war against aging, the leisure society. This is precisely the world we have tried—and so far failed—to create.[41]

There is something to that view. The note of liberation from the nature-imposed restraints of the body and the glorification of unlimited choice is a strong undercurrent in much writing about the enhancement possibilities. Not all of us will want to take advantage of them, and some of us will want different ones than others; but that's just the splendidly permissive point.[42] A skeptic can readily point out that, while there is the scientific promise of enhancement possibilities, there are no promises that choice and self-manipulation will make us happy. But that lack has never fazed enthusiasts for optimizing choice. They say: use research to give us more choices, let us choose those we like, and allow us to judge for ourselves whether we want to risk bad outcomes (and we think it better to have more choice with possibly bad outcomes than no choice at all).

With the four forms of enhancement I examined above, only in the case of mood and attention enhancement would government-sponsored research seem justifiable. Such research would address recognized (even if at times controversial) health problems, and the main problems would probably arise more at the level of prescription and distribution than with the research itself. As for the others—enhancements of athletics, intelligence, memory, and procreation—they may be desired by many people, wisely or not, but their desire falls short of making a case that there is a national need for such research at public expense or that we will all, as a society, be better off if it goes forward.

That leaves any such research in the private sector and, as I suggested, there is little doubt that a market could be found for the many enhancement possibilities. I do not think it would be possible to ban such research, even if desirable. Much will instead depend on the cultural climate that develops in the future to determine how intensively such research will be pursued. I have no doubt that the research will produce expensive products, aimed primarily at affluent customers. Inequity is inevitable, but whether those unable to buy goods from the enhancement boutique will be worse off (other than lacking choice) will depend on how the enhancements work out. The worst threat I foresee is not just that the private sector will pursue this kind of research, but that it will aggressively market it, aiming to reduce resistance, generate enthusiasm, and in general convey the message that enhancement is a way to a better, more liberated, carefree life. It will not be, but many will believe it.

I predict the general reaction with a great sense of resignation. Purely libertarian solutions on the one hand, glorifying choice and freedom, and market solutions on the other come to the same thing: a judgment that some research possibilities, however controverted, should be left free of governmental intervention and regulation. As a practical matter, this is probably right. We neither can nor should ban, much less regulate, research on the myriad possibilities of human enhancement. If nothing else, many of the possible enhancements would come not as the result of direct research aims but as the side effects of otherwise valid research. Memory enhancement for all could well come from perfectly laudable efforts to preserve memory in Alzheimer's disease, or a pleasure pill without side effects from efforts to develop psychotropic drugs for the mentally ill. In chapter 6 I note that social stigmatization, simply involving public opinion, remains an option with enhancement therapies. Whether that possibility is feasible may be doubted; and whether it would work to slow or stop enhancement research is even more doubtful. But it would be well worth a try—a statement of principle, even if ignored.

Back Door to Eugenics?

It has been common for years now to deride the idea that a new eugenics is on the horizon. The old eugenics, a child of the false biology and genetics of the late nineteenth and early twentieth centuries—and culminating in the Nazi ideology and atrocities—is said to be dead and buried. The times, moreover, are different: because of the Nazis' experience, and particularly their desire for a master race, for genetically superior types of human beings, we have learned the dangers of going down that road. Now our science and our social values are better. It can't happen again and it can't happen here.

This confidence is misplaced. The sociologist Troy Duster over a decade ago came closer to the truth with his book *Back Door to Eugenics*.[43] He noted, as did other observers even then and earlier, that the backdoor route would be through work to improve genetic health in individuals and to rid ourselves of genetically defective fetuses. The intentions of such a move are fine: genetic diseases (and other sources of abnormality) are harmful to human life, the source of premature death and much misery. Is it not perfectly consistent with the traditional goals of medicine to try to cure lethal and harmful conditions, including those with a genetic basis? Does it not make sense, from a societal point of view, to reduce the incidence of genetically damaged babies, who may well live miserable lives and who will, in the process, be a burden on their families and society? The logic of that argument, now well accepted (if not by everyone) seems morally faultless—and hence the popularity of prenatal screening. Research to improve the screening is no less popular. This phenomenon might be termed a subcategory of normalization, a kind of single-minded dedication to health, using not utopian views of human possibilities as the model but instead ordinary, garden-variety models, that of a person or child or fetus without disabling or burdensome flaws.

The hazard here, the backdoor route to eugenics, has been to insinuate over the past few decades a combined individual and economic argument. Parents ought not to want defective children or even to run the risk of such children. If it is wrong for parents to run such risks, particularly risks known to be avoidable, then of course it is unfair for them to impose the burden of the care for such children on society, which is the likely result. There need be no talk of a master race or perfect babies, but simply healthy babies, unproblematic for their parents, for society, or for themselves.

Perhaps we can continue to walk the fine line between an attitude toward genetic disease, especially in the unborn, which has the good of the mother and child only in mind, not infected by fantasies of perfection, and genetic disease reduced to a noxious social and economic burden. But as the historian of science Garland E. Allan has noted in a discussion of eugenics, "We seem to be increasingly unwilling to accept what we view as imperfection in ourselves and others . . . if eugenics means making reproductive decisions primarily on the basis of social cost, then we are well on that road."[44]

Here is a fine instance of the way the research imperative, which legitimately pushes us to know more about genetic disease, can turn in a damaging direction. The more we treat genetic disease as a great evil, and genetically defective fetuses and babies as exemplars of that evil, the harder it will be to avoid going down the eugenics road—or going farther down it. There was a slogan that became popular in the 1970s, that of a "right to a healthy life," and it was advanced as a powerful reason to rid ourselves of genetic defects. To go from that kind of right for individuals to the right of society to have healthy individuals in the name of its economic and social well-being requires no long jump. It need not happen, but to argue that never again, and not here, will eugenics stage a comeback seems naive.

5   Assessing Risks and Benefits

The research imperative is a demand of human nature and an enormous social benefit. The drive for knowledge and the understanding it brings deserve strong public support. Even so, in its present manifestation, that imperative shows growing signs here and there of overreaching for success, of becoming obsessed in its drive for ever-greater scientific gains, of inclining toward that old god, Mammon. There are other, even more disturbing, signs of this trend. They include a keener aversion to moral limits or the serious social implications of research possibilities, and a proclivity for attacking or belittling those who question the research imperative and its purported benefits. A small cadre of philosophers, in my own field, have made a specialty of minimizing or denying risks.

As good a place as any to look for the research imperative in its unbuttoned form is a brief 1999 article in *Time* magazine by James D. Watson.[1] No scientist has been more celebrated in this country in recent decades than Watson who, together with the English scientist Francis Crick, discovered the structure of DNA (for which they won a Nobel Prize). In that article, Watson referred to the earlier public ambivalence about the development of atomic knowledge and nuclear weapons. He then described the recombinant DNA debate of the 1970s, noting that many scientists and nonscientists worried about potential harm. That was, in his mind, a great mistake, as demonstrated by the (ex post facto) results: no harm ever came out of research using the technique. The "doomsday scenarios" served only to impede scientists "itching to explore previously unattainable secrets of life."

"The moral I draw from this painful episode is this," Dr. Watson adds, "[we should] never postpone experiments that have clearly defined future benefits for fear of dangers that can't be quantified. Though it may sound at first uncaring, we can react rationally only to real (as opposed to hypothetical) risks." As an instance of a present impediment to research, he uses the widespread opposition to germ-line therapy—potentially useful for therapeutic purposes—that (to use his language) "might help redirect the course of future human evolution." Watson does not buy that kind of nervousness: "you should never put off doing something useful for fear of evil that may never arrive."[2]

This is a strange and careless position. It is strange in that it shrugs off the scientific community's hard-won recognition of a duty to warn the public of possible, and not simply demonstrated, dangers. It is even stranger in that it turns the single recombinant DNA debate and moratorium into a clinching case against warning of dangers and the hazards of "spurious arguments" in slowing research. But the carelessness can be seen in the language itself. It is, after all, easy to develop experiments that have "clearly defined future benefits" (for instance, the conquest of cancer), but their likely success is something else to show (much less in quantifiable ways).

Yet Watson treats aimed-for benefits of research as far more solid than "hypothetical risks," as if those benefits were not themselves hypothetical before the research achieves them. If they were not hypothetical, no experiment would be necessary. Why does a "fear of evil that may never arrive" have less serious status for consideration than a hoped-for benefit that may also never arrive? The history of biomedicine is filled with research that does not produce a "clearly defined" benefit. But in Watson's eyes, any projection of possible harms is a fantasy, a lack of nerve, while germ-line gene manipulations are presented in the most Pollyannish way: "The first germ-line manipulations are unlikely to be attempted for frivolous reasons . . . [but will instead] probably be done to change a child's death sentence into a life verdict."[3] Watson says nothing more about the possibility, which he himself noted earlier, of thereby redirecting "the course of future human evolution." Not important enough to raise some questions about? To worry about? To warn about their risks, to paraphrase Bentley Glass?

Watson was by no means alone in calling for less ethical hand-wringing. The *Wall Street Journal*, sniffing the likelihood of great future profit in the aftermath of the completion of the Human Genome Project, wrote in a lead editorial that "political backing will be needed to damp down objections to this kind of progress."[4] The editorial clearly did not have in mind Robert Merton's notion of the scientific ethic of communalism when it wrote, "If the potential of genetic research is to be fully exploited, it will need to be pursued by private interests seeking to develop proprietary products." Echoing the same theme, the Council on Competitiveness argued, "The enormous positive potential of biotechnologies to improve diagnosis and treatment of disease could be lost if it is overshadowed by fear."[5]

While there was much public opposition to the idea of human reproductive cloning, once Dolly appeared a quick phalanx of cheerleaders showed up to deride the worries. Writing in the *New York Times,* Kirkpatrick Sale referred to President Clinton's hesitations as putting "the government squarely on the side of technological alarmism."[6] The legal scholar Laurence H. Tribe wrote that a ban on human cloning would cut society off "from vital experimentation, thus losing a significant part of its capacity to grow."[7] The Harvard biologist Richard C. Lewontin assaulted the cloning report of the National Bioethics Advisory Commission—which called for a five-year moratorium on research—as an "attempt to rationalize a deep cultural prejudice," while mocking any religious viewpoint as "capable of abolishing hard ethical problems if only we can decipher the meaning of what has been revealed to us."[8]

Lewontin's article, however, which itself abolished human cloning as a hard ethical problem, showed that religion is not necessary to perform that feat. A self-confident scientist, forgetting Glass's responsibility "to discuss quandaries," can do it just as effectively. Lewontin was not the only person to mock religion as a source of opposition to new technologies—a historically inaccurate claim in any event. Even when religion is not mentioned in discussions of technology, any skepticism is met by the charge that, often hidden just below the surface, "religion" or "God" exerts a baneful influence, just one more item in the "simplistic moralism" that lies behind opposition to technological innovation.[9] As the historian of science Daniel Kevles put it, "As with so many previous advances in biology, today's affront to the gods may be tomorrow's highly regarded—and highly demanded—agent of self-gratification or health."[10] That is true enough, but Kevles did not take pains to promote further discussion, suggesting in fact that, if we don't carry out the research, then others will, a shopworn refrain when doubt surfaces: stop talking, and get on with it. Of course it is also an argument central to the entrepreneurial spirit, which sees a threat to profit and prosperity if the country falls behind competitively.

ASSESSING RISKS AND BENEFITS

My response to those who deride worries about risk should make clear that I consider their reaction wrong and inappropriate. Even if they turn out to be right in the long run on this or that projected risk, the reaction is still inappropriate now, at a moment when everyone is ignorant of what the long run will bring. It lacks a rational and prudent foundation on which to base such judgments. The possibility of a loss of profit, or the fact that other gambles in the past paid off, or that other countries will do it first, or the charge that religion motivates a lack of nerve, does not constitute such a foundation. They are little more than ways of stifling discussion.

Yet I must concede that the biomedical realm has no well-developed approach to the assessment of risks and benefits, much less anything like a solid theory about how to go about building one. In this it is unlike other scientific areas, such as analysis of environmental and occupational health risks and benefits, where there is a rich risk-benefit literature. Rather than try to develop a full theory to fill the biomedical research gap, in this chapter I lay out an array of considerations that would be pertinent to making reasonable risk-benefit assessments.

Here the emphasis falls on the means chosen to fulfill medicine's goals: what are the risks and benefits of a particular means chosen to achieve an otherwise acceptable end? Research to find a cure for a specific cancer, leukemia for instance, is ordinarily sensible, consistent with the goals of medicine. Research to achieve that cure must then choose some particular research strategy, perhaps to test a plausible scientific hypothesis. Perhaps the strategy's projected benefits may be great, but (let us say) there is some suspicion that the desired cure may have some hazardous medical side effects or may be exceedingly costly. At that point a risk-benefit assessment is imperative.

But isn't that obvious, hardly worth saying? Not so obvious, it turns out—otherwise, how are we to explain the various statements I cited at the beginning of this chapter, objecting to the idea of a ban on reproductive cloning, mocking those who mentioned potential risks, and slighting the need for assessment? But in any new scientific development, or research possibility, just what will truly benefit us in the long run or truly do us harm is rarely evident. Take the discovery of electricity, or the atom, or the invention of the airplane, the automobile, the transistor, the contraceptive pill, or the telephone; no one could predict, much less assess in advance, the long-term consequences of these new scientific discoveries or technological innovations. One change leads to another, and that to still another, and soon enough the world is different. And we usually don't see it coming. Biomedical advances have the capacity to change the way we think about the nature of medicine, about the meaning of health, and about the possibilities of living a life.[11] Those changes are almost impossible to predict as well. As often as not, it is their interaction with other social changes, often well outside biomedicine, that makes the decisive difference.

If the long-term results of research are unpredictable, and even the short-term results often highly uncertain, serious risk-benefit analysis would seem almost impossible—or, even worse, meaningless to the exercise of moral judgment or policy planning. That is not quite the case. At the least, there is now a wealth of historical experience with new biomedical discoveries and their technological applications; that is a source to be mined even if it offers no guaranteed insights into the consequences of new discoveries. It is possible to make reasonable calculations about the impact of some classes of research: the gain to life expectancies by the cure or control of cancer, heart disease, and diabetes, for instance; or the benefit to old age of effective drugs to mitigate the effect of Alzheimer's disease; or the effect on cancer death rates from a successful campaign to radically reduce or eliminate the use of tobacco products. In each of those cases, reasonably good data exist to make reliable predictions of research outcomes possible.

Far less certain are predictions about the economic results of such developments, or the increased life satisfaction they will bring about. Will they save money, or will other alternative diseases simply take their place, leaving the health care bill the same? The least certain outcomes will be those bearing on the possible development of optimizing or maximizing technologies. Lacking historical experience of any relevant kind, it is an exercise in science fiction to predict, for instance, what our collective social life, or our individual lives, would be, if we all lived to an average age of 110, much less to 150. Nor can we forecast with any certainty the effect on parenthood if people had far more control over the physical and behavioral traits of their children—or estimate the impact on children, created to their parents' specification.

Though more informally, people try to deal with uncertain research outcomes in other ways. Some spring from a specifically religious perspective on the world, one that sees God, not science, in control of human destiny and trusts in spiritual intuitions or traditions to supply the answer to scientific uncertainties. An analogous secular perspective, associated with environmentalism, runs along parallel lines. It sees a wisdom and sacredness in nature itself, sufficiently strong to look at interventions into the natural order and evolution as inherently dangerous. Both of these perspectives are prone to rely heavily on emotional responses of fear, or repugnance, or intuitive fittingness, as good indicators of lines we should not cross—even though a more sophisticated analysis would recognize that repugnance serves more to alert people about a possible problem than to prove its reality.[12]

The other response worth noting runs in the opposite direction. It seizes

on the uncertainty of many research outcomes, particularly of the optimizing kind, to argue that no meaningful collective judgment or political consensus is possible; and, in any case, that consensus or judgment does not
matter. Since many of the disagreements will rest on incommensurable
worldviews and controverted data, should we not in a pluralistic society just
leave it to up to the choice of individuals to encourage those lines of research
that appeal to them? Then, if the research succeeds, should not the market,
good old-fashioned consumer demand, see whether it is socially desirable?

Both of these alternatives for assessing research possibilities seem to me
defective. The religious alternative, whether of the traditional or ecological
kind, is unacceptable but not because we live in a pluralistic society. That is
not a good reason to reject it, since any sensible society should be open to
possible good insights whatever their source, and religion has contributed
many over the centuries. It is unacceptable because, even within the context
of those traditions, there is no way to judge the validity or truth value of
feelings or intuitions about interventions into nature. The term "playing
God" as an objection to some research possibilities is heard much less these
days than three decades ago (or is used as a convenient straw man to be
knocked down on the way to an embrace of a new technology). It is an idea
that made little religious sense to theologians when they examined it
closely and was always useless for policy purposes in a medical context—
which has always balked at that brute nature as it sickens and kills children
and ruins adult lives.

As for the individualist, pro-choice, market solution, it would be a foolish
solution if its impact reached beyond the individuals who wanted it to affect
everyone else as well. A society where some large number of people chose
permanent numbness through psychotropic drugs would be a different kind
of society, not just a society with different kinds of people. If some people
used market freedom to choose traits for their children—particularly ones
thought to give them social advantages—it would no less be a different kind
of society, not just a society with different kinds of children.

DEVISING STANDARDS OF RISK-BENEFIT ASSESSMENT

For all its uncertainties, then, some form of risk-benefit analysis is in order.
Neither religion nor the market offers reliable guides to public policy on
risk-benefit analysis. Specifically, the field of medical research needs something like the "precautionary principle" that now has a strong place in environmental law, policy, and thinking. To clear the way for such a principle, I
sketch out some important categories, or levels of analysis, to complement

those already suggested by the normalizing, maximizing, optimizing continuum.

The most common plea for a specific line of research is that it will benefit an afflicted group of individuals. And the most common objection against a line of research is that it may harm a group of individuals. At this "clinical" level—following the Hippocratic tradition—the focus is on the sick individual. Though surely important in some contexts, it is wholly inadequate when we try to assess the full implications of research, short-term and long-term. As the history of many other scientific discoveries and technologies shows, their impact can sweep through many dimensions of human communities, changing social institutions, cultural traditions, and economic possibilities. Accordingly, I want to identify five levels at which medical research can make a difference:

The *clinical* level: what difference could a particular line of research make for the health of individuals? What are the possible health benefits, and what are the possible health risks?

The *population* level: what difference will the research, if successful, make for the health of whole populations? Again, what are the possible risks and benefits, but this time to populations? Might the research lead to the solution of a problem widely agreed to represent an affliction of populations?

The *sociocultural/political* level: what long-term side effects, or unintended social, cultural, and political consequences (good or bad) might the outcome of the research have?

The *moral* level: what effect might the changes wrought by the research have on moral values and principles? Would those changes be offensive to some groups in the population?

The *economic* level: what economic benefits might the research have, and what would be the impact on the cost of health care, and on the equitable distribution of health care resources?

Gene therapy research (of the somatic kind) offers an example of how risk-benefit analysis would work. Based on what is now known, we can answer some basic questions. Would the research, if successful, help individuals afflicted with various genetic diseases? Yes. Would it make a health difference at the population level? No, probably not enough people would benefit from somatic gene therapy but might from germ-line therapy. Are there any important sociocultural implications? None have so far been advanced. Would somatic gene therapy raise any special ethical problems?

Probably not (but germ-line therapy would). Would gene therapy add to the costs of health care in a way that might threaten equitable access to care? It might, if made available to a large number of people.

A full and solid risk-benefit analysis should encompass all five levels. If the history of the effects of scientific discoveries and technological developments teaches us anything, it is that almost every important breakthrough eventually affects each of those five levels. We might as a society decide to ignore the economic implications, or to set aside the moral objections of some groups, or to give priority to individual over population benefits. But first we must carefully put all the levels on the table for full consideration.

At least six other topics are essential to risk-benefit analysis as well: the relative urgency of the research, its likelihood of success, its short- and long-term consequences, alternative possibilities for research, the range of scientific responsibility, and responsibility for decision making. I touch on most of these dimensions in later chapters but introduce them here in order to fill out the risk-benefit picture.

Urgency of the research.   How important is a particular research possibility in relationship to other possible research expenditures, and other health needs? Any answer to this question is bound to be influenced by different perceptions of individual and social needs. But it is fair to say that those diseases of a readily infectious and lethal kind, posing the danger of epidemics and pandemics, will elicit a great sense of urgency (e.g., AIDS, flu pandemics). So will those diseases and medical conditions that have a particularly devastating effect on children and mothers, as would those that lead to a high level of premature death. Urgent research will almost always open the possibility of using a different balance of risks and benefits than, say, research aimed at maximizing present health indicators or at optimizing human health, neither of which requires immediate attention.

With the possible exception of impending plagues and pandemics, there is bound to be a considerable difference of opinion on what counts as "urgent." This is an issue that requires a combination of scientific assessment and a gauging of public opinion. Public opinion surveys, appointed national commissions, and recommendations to the National Institutes of Health and other relevant research groups would seem appropriate.

Likelihood of success.   Research is by its nature uncertain—uncertain of success at all, uncertain in its immediate outcome, and uncertain in its long-term social impact. We cannot know a priori where it will eventually lead. Even so, the prudent allocation of research resources requires an assessment, however rough, of the likely success of a research initiative, particularly one aimed at better understanding or curing a disease. Scientists are often (though hardly always) able to have some sense of likely success with a given research idea. It makes sense then to think of success in something like the following terms:

- high probability, near certainty of success
- moderate probability of success, but not certain
- low probability of success, but plausible line of exploration
- exceedingly low probability of success, but not entirely implausible

Only scientists with a specialized state-of-the-art knowledge of research possibilities can make judgments of that kind. Since there may well be disagreement about the prospects of success, scientific consensus conferences may be helpful.

Short- and long-term consequences.   The implications and results of research may last for a short or long time, and it is pertinent to attempt a calculation of the effects over time. Inevitably, as with many of the other categories I have been outlining, considerable speculation and uncertainty will often mark such efforts. In some cases, it will be necessary to discern whether certain forms of research that might produce irreversible results will pose dangers to, or limit the opportunities of, later generations. Here are some ways of categorizing those effects:

Short-term and long-term health consequences are expected, but all of them are beneficial (e.g., reduction in the mortality and morbidity of heart disease). The consequences of those heart disease reductions would almost certainly be reversible (however unlikely a decision to reverse them).

Short-term consequences are expected to be good and reasonably predictable in nature, but the long-term consequences are considerably less certain. A case in point here would be germ-line therapy, which would pass traits along to future generations in ways that might be harmful and not easily reversed.

Uncertain short- and long-term consequences are expected. This might particularly be the case with human cloning, which would most likely affect the life of cloned individuals (assuming they knew about it), but whose psychological or social condition as a result could not clearly be known at first and could be even hazier over their lifetime; long-term consequences for human procreation are highly uncertain.

It is by no means clear who is in the best position to make judgments about the likelihood of research consequences, imperative though it might be to make them. No professional group can claim insight into the consequences of scientific advancement. My own preference—never so far tried, as far as I know—would be to have a carefully appointed public commission of medical and technological historians, technological analysts, epidemiologists, and cultural historians/analysts consider the specific problem at stake and ensure that their conclusions reached the executive branch or Congress, whichever was in the best position to make use of the developed insight.

Alternative possibilities for research. Many recent debates on controverted research have included arguments that there are other, less controversial, means imaginable of achieving the same goals. Stem-cell research, some assert, might be carried out in ways that would not require the use and destruction of embryos—the use of adult stem cells, for instance, could be an alternative to embryonic stem cells. In cancer research, there are many different research strategies in play at present. One way of classifying the possibilities of different lines of research might be as follows:

One and only one plausible, likely successful, research strategy can at present be envisioned.

While there are other imaginable research strategies, they have a somewhat lower probability of success but are still worth pursuing.

Other strategies have a significantly lower probability of success, making them a long shot at best.

Some conceivable strategies have an entirely unlikely probability of success.

Scientists alone are in a good position to make the necessary judgments here. In the instance of research that poses or could pose a risk, it would seem obligatory for them to use all their skills to see if alternative pathways can be conceived. A look at most research now going on reveals that, in almost every case, scientists are exploring many pathways, frequently in an argumentative, competitive way. Scientists working on such long-standing health problems as cancer or heart disease, or new ones such as HIV disease, rarely put all their research eggs in one basket. Of late research advocates (though not scientists) have often given the impression that some kinds of research necessarily take a single avenue (e.g., embryonic stem-cell research) or otherwise abandon all hope of success. The history of medical research offers no support for that narrow view.

The range of scientific responsibility in the face of possible risk.   Like other sets of thoughts and actions—in marriage, childbearing, voting, and the tilling of gardens—scientific activity has consequences. In seeking to determine moral responsibility for these consequences, I propose general, but defensible, moral propositions:

> Individuals and groups are ordinarily held responsible only for the consequences of those actions that are voluntary and intentional on their part. They may also be held responsible for the unintended consequences of their actions if, through negligence, they foresaw them but failed to take them into account or, because of negligence, failed to see what they could have seen.

> Individuals and groups cannot be held responsible for those actions of which the consequences are totally unknown. If, however, they fail to make an imaginative effort to explore possible consequences, they cannot totally disclaim responsibility for what happens.

> Individual scientists and scientific groups are subject to the same norms of ethical responsibility as are all other individuals and groups in society, and particularly in reference to the most central moral rule: a person bears moral responsibility for any act that foreseeably affects the life and welfare of others.

At the end of his important book *The Making of the Atomic Bomb*, Richard Rhodes contends "that science is sometimes blamed for the nuclear dilemma."[13] "Such blame," he responds, "confuses the messenger with the message. Otto Hahn and Fritz Strassman did not invent nuclear fission: they discovered it. It was there all along waiting for us, the turn of the screw." That is a strange conclusion. In sober and overwhelming detail, his book shows how theoretical physicists sought to discover fission, how they conceived of the possibility of creating a great bomb with that knowledge, how they then persuaded the government to put up hundreds of millions of dollars to get the bomb built, how they worked with engineers, chemists, and mathematicians to create the actual hardware of the bomb, and how, once the first bomb was exploded in New Mexico, and two bombs were dropped on Japan, they were pleased to accept congratulations for all they had done.

To be sure, a number of scientists refused altogether to work on the bomb. Robert Oppenheimer, in charge of scientifically organizing and managing the research, never for a moment denied responsibility for the deaths from the bomb or the permanent threat to humanity the development of the bomb brought with it.

It is always possible to dispute who is responsible for what. In science, as in most of the rest of life, people are eager, even highly competitive, to claim responsibility for whatever turns out well and merits praise—but no less eager to disclaim, or diffuse, responsibility when the opposite happens. Scientists are probably the best placed to know what they are or are not responsible for, and thus it should probably fall to the scientific community itself to determine responsibility. On occasion, when there is disagreement about responsibility, it may be necessary to bring in outsiders to adjudicate the conflict. But on no account should anyone ever go so far as to relieve scientists of responsibility for what they in fact did (or deny them praise where deserved).

Making risk-benefit decisions. I have left until last the question that applies to everything I have said so far. Who should decide about the risks and benefits of research? Which decisions should be left to individual scientists, to the scientific community as a whole, to the general public, to appointed administrators, to courts and legislators? The immediate feature of a list of the kind of considerations I have developed here does not readily lend itself to any single general procedure. Some decisions are best left to scientists, others to legislators and judges, still others to informal mechanisms of choice. Here is a range of options:

Leave risk-benefit decisions to individual choice, whether laypeople or scientists.

Leave risk-benefit decisions of any social consequence up to appointed agencies or commissions.

Leave risk-benefit decisions of important social consequence up to Congress for national legislation (making use of, but not being bound by, national commissions).

Leave risk-benefit decisions up to the public and informal social preferences and pressures, by working with public opinion polls and focus groups to determine the public's preferences, and communicating those preferences to Congress, research bodies, and the research community, but not attempting to legislate those preferences—in effect, using the power of public opinion to assign praise or blame for them.

Generally speaking, any research initiative that may well produce results that could influence population health and social or familial values and practices and affect the lives of future generations should have a public examination, preferably by commissions and expert panels. One of their tasks should be to determine the need for regulations or laws.

Risks, Benefits, and a Precautionary Principle

Not all the analytical tools I have laid out here are equally pertinent to each research case. But there are no good reasons to ignore, or deliberately to set aside, *any* of them. In dealing with the full panorama of the research enterprise—from manageable issues of physical safety for research subjects to complicated multifaceted issues of population and cultural consequences—we need an equally robust set of tools.

One strong tendency with many research issues is to act as if physical safety is the only serious consideration, whereas there are usually many others that deserve systematic examination. We need "research impact statements," an idea that Senator Walter Mondale proposed in the 1970s. Unlike environmental impact statements, they need not necessarily be *legally* required but should stand as moral mandates strong enough to force care and attention.

The now-standard issues of risk-benefit analysis need only brief mention here since the literature on risk—unlike that for medical research—is now broad and rich, generated mainly by considerations of the dangers posed by various technologies for human health and, in the environmental context, for both human and ecological well-being. The hazards of lead poisoning for children, or the use of seat belts and air bags to reduce the risk of auto injuries or death, the tolerable level of particulates in the atmosphere, and, in the medical context, various chemical and other occupational hazards are now familiar fare in the literature.[14]

In narrowly statistical terms, risk encompasses the probability of a harmful event affecting our life or other serious interests under various circumstances. For practical purposes it takes in both objective probability and subjective individual and cultural responses. Risk is one of those concepts—like "peace" or "person" or "progress"—that combines scientific information and value judgments. Such concepts are not entirely social constructs, for scientific data or other objective evidence is considered relevant. But that evidence is never decisive since evaluation in ethical or other nonscientific terms is no less necessary.

The psychological literature has long emphasized that people do not simply judge risk in terms of harmful probabilities. Even more important may be the severity of the danger should it materialize (the explosion of a nuclear power plant, or the birth of a severely damaged child); the familiarity of the danger (thus auto accidents receive less attention than airplane crashes); and the relative extent to which people feel they have some control over the danger (and hence fear dangerous obesity less than cancer). The international debate on genetically modified agriculture has also shown that supposed "safety" issues can actually masquerade as cultural values that seem threatened, such as the importance of indigenous food and wine traditions in Italy and France. Safety is also sometimes a stand-in for a larger fear of domination by uncontrollable international corporations, a threatening "globalization" of trade.

BALANCING RISKS AND BENEFITS: A HAZARDOUS ENTERPRISE

We can and often must talk of risk in terms of its nature: the probability of harm, the extent of the harm, the duration of the harm, and the social distribution of the harm. Correlatively, we can use the same category to speak of benefits. Are they not commensurable categories, and can we balance them? The answer is no, at least not in many cases. At one extreme are those instances where the risks and benefits do seem commensurable: if no harms are otherwise foreseen (and few have been projected), a cure will benefit, not harm, people at risk of cancer. A comparison of having and not having cancer allows ready and unproblematic balancing.

In other cases no such commensurability exists or the categories generate heated debate. One class of cases is where certain kinds of risks will not morally be tolerated because they offend some important and widely held values. It is no longer possible to argue that, in the name of saving lives, hazardous research without informed consent is acceptable, even if some people think it should be. That kind of "balancing" has been taken off the scales altogether—even if it can be shown that the number of lives likely to be saved would well exceed those lost by the research. In other cases, such as stem-cell research using spare embryos, one group of people thinks it poses no serious moral issue and thus easily lends itself to deciding that, as President Clinton put it (conceding the existence of a controversy), "I think that if the public will look at first of all the potentially staggering benefits of this research, everything from birth defects to Parkinson's, certain kinds of cancer, diabetes, spinal cord injuries . . . it's a potential chance for the future."[15] Of course, for the moral opponents of embryo use, no balancing at all is acceptable. Their reasoning is much the same as those who oppose human-subject research without informed consent: it ought never to happen. If the embryo is thought to have no moral value, then no balancing is necessary; it is nothing other than disposable research material.

Less difficult are those situations where some degree of harm is to be balanced against some degree of benefit for the same person. Sometimes a balance can be achieved (the development of life-saving drug with some serious side effects; or the development of kidney dialysis, keeping patients alive but not fully well). But sometimes it cannot, as when the beneficiaries of a drug may be different from those put at risk in research on the drug (a standard objection to using people in poor countries as research subjects for drugs they will never be able to afford). Putting one group of people at risk to help another group is an unfair, unjustifiable balance.

In sum, fair and meaningful balancing can take place only where commensurability is possible, and too often it is not. One person's satisfactory, morally reassuring, balance at the expense of my health or my values (but not his) ought never to be acceptable. It is relevant at this point to note an argument advanced during World War I on the morality of research to develop poison gas. A distinguished German scientist, Fritz Haber, justified his research to another scientist, Otto Hahn, as follows: "When I objected that this was a mode of warfare violating the Hague Convention [Haber] said that the French had already started it . . . by using rifle ammunition filled with gas. It was a way of saving countless lives, if it meant that the war could be brought to end sooner."[16] That turned out to be a false and bad balance.

A Precautionary Principle

In an effort to deal with the complexities of risk-benefit analysis, the environmental movement, particularly in Europe, embraced a "precautionary principle." It applies to a suspected health or environmental hazard where decisive scientific evidence to prove the hazard is lacking. Even in the absence of that evidence, can measures legitimately be taken to avert the hazards? Emerging first in West Germany in the 1970s, the principle achieved its most formal status in the 1992 United Nations Rio Declaration on Environment and Development: "Where there are threats of serious or irreversible damage, lack of scientific certainty shall not be used as a reason for postponing cost-effective measures to prevent environmental degradation."[17] The principle has been used in Europe to justify the banning of American and Canadian beef because of the use of human growth hormone and to delay approving genetically engineered agricultural products for sale there.

Within the environmental context, just about every formulation of a precautionary principle has been criticized. It is always difficult to formulate a principle of a general kind that will work well, and perspicuously, in each and every concrete situation. For that reason, rather than reject any attempt to formulate such a principle altogether, it is probably best to treat any specific formulation as an approximation only, meant to help organize analysis rather than produce a definitive decision. A precautionary principle for use in a health and research context will have to take account of various objections against its use in the environmental arena. The most common objection is to the vagueness of the principle: it has many versions and a bewildering number of ways to interpret them. How severe, for instance, should the possible threat of hazards be before precautionary action occurs? "Beyond a "shadow of a doubt," or "beyond a reasonable doubt" or by virtue of a "preponderance of the evidence"?[18]

At one extreme would be a standard so severe as to forbid any new technology, an implication of the 1982 World Charter for Nature, which held that "where potential adverse effects are not fully understood, the activities should not proceed."[19] At the other extreme would be a standard that held that action on a hazard should occur only where decisive evidence of harm already exists; speculative harms don't count. That might be called the "gambler's principle." In the passages quoted at the beginning of this chapter, Watson seems to hold that position, common in both the medical and environmental worlds. Research, or technological innovation, should always go forward, the gambler's principle holds, if someone—anyone—desires that it go forward, if anyone will (following market reasoning) buy the products of the research, and if no one can produce *in advance* hard evidence of harm. Since hard evidence of harm can never, by definition, precede the research itself, there are then no grounds at all for stopping it (or even, according to Watson, for a temporary moratorium to allow further analysis). If speculative harms (though *not* speculative benefits) are inadmissible, nothing stands in the way of the research imperative.

It is not, then, surprising that some commentators have seen the precautionary principle as incoherent and an impediment to progress.[20] Many forms of the principle are open to that criticism, fair enough game. Unless anything and everything research might develop is automatically to be understood as a benefit, and if no caution or prudence is entertained, then, yes, the principle could be seen to hinder progress. But it is no moral or cultural disaster to hinder or slow progress, and no moral absolute always to pursue it. It is also possible to recognize the value of a well-crafted principle of caution and to use the precautionary principle as itself a spur to better research. As an editorial in an environmental journal put it, "Responsible precaution requires that we accompany proposals for precautionary actions with a research agenda to decide if the actions, once taken, are justified."[21]

With those assorted reflections in mind, here is my suggested precautionary principle for use in risk-benefit analysis of biomedical research:

> When there is reasonable uncertainty about the possible risks of biomedical research—in the research process itself, or its outcome—full exploration of those risks should take place, if necessary by temporarily suspending or slowing the research, but *only* if there is a scientific understanding of the possible and plausible causal pathways of the projected harms. The more severe the possible harms, the more cautiously the research should go forward. If careful examination cannot reasonably substantiate those imagined harms, the research should proceed. Relatively minor possible harms should be acceptable. Contentions about the benefits of the research, ordinarily speculative as well, must not trump a full exploration of the possible risks. Situations of great urgency, such as rapidly spreading epidemics, should allow a shifting of the burden of proof onto those who perceive possible risks. Risk must encompass medical, sociocultural, moral, and economic hazards. A primary obligation of the scientific community is to take the lead in projecting risks and benefits, and not to intimidate those colleagues who foresee and publicize possible risks that may thus slow the research.

The aim of the precautionary principle stated this way is to find a middle ground between too rigid and too lax a standard and to encourage the scientific community to invoke the principle. The protection of scientists from the scorn of their colleagues would be an important part of any use of the principle—which one might expect those who see harms to invoke rather than those who see only benefits. Good research should aim for long-term benefits, those that can stand the scrutiny of later generations. If real scientific progress means anything at all, it is its capacity to bear that kind of scrutiny.

The trouble with the gambler's principle, displaying Watsonian scorn for "doomsday scenarios," is that luck, and luck alone, will avert harm if its potential is there, as is usually the case when we do not look before leaping. That is not good enough. A slowing of research is a small price to pay for responsible and reasonably cautious science. Moreover, it might be kept in mind, much if not most research will not, and need not, trigger a use of the precautionary principle. While it can elicit great media attention and public disputes, controversial research is still only a small portion of all medical research.

Not much research will be as dramatic, or terrifying in its implications, as research on biological and chemical warfare. The news in early 2002 that the Bush administration was tightening scientific secrecy to keep information on weapons of mass destruction from hostile hands met scientific resistance. The argument was that "secrecy policies will endanger the way open research on hazardous substances can produce a wealth of cures, disease antidotes and surprise discoveries." "It comes down to risk-benefit ratio," said Robert E. Rich, president of the Federation of American Societies for Experimental Biology; "the risk of forgone advances is much greater than the information getting into the wrong hands."[22] The precautionary principle I urge finds here a clear application against the claim of a research imperative for open research (and I agree with Rich on this issue). It is difficult to dissent from the conclusion of Matthew Meselson, a prominent scientist and biological warfare expert, "As our ability to modify life processes continues its rapid advance, we will not only be able to devise additional ways to destroy life but will also become able to manipulate it. . . . In these possibilities could lie unprecedented opportunities for violence, coercion, repression, or subjugation."[23] These possibilities make the strongest possible case for a precautionary principle.

A final caution is in order. Most risk-benefit analysis is consequentialist in its reckoning, looking at the likely results, good or bad, of a particular line of action (or in our case, of research) and attempting to determine whether the benefits exceed the risks. But in some cases there will be values, moral principles, at stake that ought not to be subject to that form of analysis at all. The principle of informed consent for human-subject research would, for many, be an example of a principle that overrides any other good, such as improved health. Similarly, those who believe human personhood begins at conception will not balance the good of the embryo against the good of research progress; for them, that too is not a morally licit trade-off.

As will become clear in the next two chapters, not only is it often difficult to balance risks and benefits even with consequentialist reasoning, it may also be necessary to debate when that kind of reasoning is wrong at the very outset. The trouble with consequentialist reasoning is that—apart from social convention and different ideologies—risks and benefits are inherently hard to weigh. It is all too easy for even the most conscientious people to disagree about the seriousness of a purported risk and the value of a projected benefit; which is why every serious risk-benefit analysis is likely to be a contentious effort. So too, in a pluralistic country, there will be differences about which good ought not to be subject to risk-benefit analysis at all. The enthusiast for scientific research, believing it to be the royal road to human welfare, is likely to see benefits and risks differently from someone with a more modest view of science.

6   Using Humans for Research

When I was a philosophy graduate student I sought relief one day from the tedium of it all by wandering about the library where I worked, looking for something, anything, to wake me up. Close at hand were the proceedings of the Nuremberg trial in 1947, bringing to judgment the doctors turned killers in the service of the Nazi regime. I woke up. The accounts were electrifying. Medical researchers had turned the ethics of medicine on its head, their goal not to relieve death and suffering but to inflict them.

Though I did not know it at the time, the use of human beings for medical research would put the research imperative at the center of one of the most intractable dilemmas of our times. To what extent, if any, can researchers trying to help many people use a few people as research subjects to gain that end? Clinical progress cannot move forward without human-subject research; it is a necessity. At the same time, there have been—and there must be—limits on their use to advance knowledge and clinical progress. Where are we to draw a firm line? When does the deeply felt urgency to find cures and save lives confront even higher moral demands? When does the benign research imperative begin slipping toward the hazardous imperative?

Earlier in this book I noted many recent examples of the way the research imperative has led some scientists and others to see ethical scruples and precautionary principles simply as obstacles to overcome. The cure of disease and the relief of suffering are taken by some to be moral imperatives of a higher order than moral principles devoted to respecting persons, or human dignity, or running risks with the greatest of caution.

The situation has generally been otherwise with human-subject research. Even if inconsistently and erratically—and nastily thrown aside in the Nazi era—that kind of research has moved in the opposite direction, resisting such rationales. I speak here of its animating principles. In practice human-subject research has been afflicted by the same stresses and strains that more generally infect the research imperative. Time and again during the twentieth century there have been scandals about abused or harmed subjects. A familiar ritual is then reenacted: the public is shocked, familiar moral principles are reiterated and polished up a bit, and revised regulations are put in place. Then everything is quiet for a time—until the cycle repeats itself. But it is striking how we still seek a center, and at that center is a great resistance to pragmatic arguments about the needs and benefits of research as moral excuses to set aside moral principles.

We are once again in the midst of such a cycle, which has seen a presidential commission in 2001 make recommendations for reform, and an upgraded federal office for the protection of human subjects put in place. Each new cycle, moreover, has brought forth some new variable. The rapid growth of for-profit organizations devoted to managing clinical trials and recruiting human subjects, and the no less rapid expansion of research efforts, particularly on the pharmaceutical side, have made clear the importance of the drive for new drugs, and the money they will bring, as factors working synergistically with the research imperative. Together they strew seductions in the way of the clinical researcher, and they beckon all the more insistently when the great cause of the relief of suffering seems to justify almost any means at hand.

Those temptations in human-subject research have also, time and again, run into a hard principle that admits of no compromise—the obligation to obtain informed consent from competent adults before recruiting them as research subjects. The language of a "war" against disease, otherwise so popular, has not in recent years gained the upper hand in this arena, although it always hovers nearby, trying to get in. The trajectory of the debates has been toward a stricter definition of protective principles, working to leave less room for the language of the moral imperative of research.

It has been an important struggle, but there are some puzzles. Why has the ethic of human-subject research, even if fitfully, always turned back time and again toward firmer rules, greater precautions, and a willingness to set research's needs to one side? And in those proclivities can we find a cautious model for the research enterprise as a whole, one that does not invoke the research imperative as a reason to put aside that caution? I return to that question at the end of this chapter.

FIRST STIRRINGS OF ALARM

Two episodes in the twentieth century are usually taken as taken as benchmarks for human-subject research. The Nazi medical experiments constitute one and the publication by Henry Knowles Beecher in 1966 of revelations of the postwar abuse of subjects in the United States is the other. Until the American reform efforts of the 1960s and 1970s it was thought that the issue had simply not been discovered earlier. It had been. As the research surge after the Civil War gained force during the balance of the nineteenth century, complaints surfaced with increasing frequency about dangerous research carried out without their subjects' consent. George Bernard Shaw coined the term "human guinea pig," and the early antivivisection movement (encompassing animals and humans) had brought the problem to public attention. The replacement of the family physician by the "scientist at the bedside," particularly carrying out nontherapeutic research, was a most worrisome image.[1]

The anxiety in the 1890s that the research enterprise might flounder for lack of interest, or not support the three American research journals started during that decade, proved unfounded. The advances of medical science, particularly in pharmacology, bacteriology, and immunology, and such technological innovations as the X ray and stomach tubes, expanded the need for research subjects. The research ideal, by then in full flower, encouraged physicians to see their patients as useful subjects. But the growth of research not only required more human subjects, it also brought out the numerous ethical problems that went with their use. As the historian Susan Lederer documents, the reconciliation of the "demands of scientific medicine with the traditional responsibilities of the doctor-patient relationship" was to preoccupy late-nineteenth-century medicine just as, to this day, it preoccupies contemporary medicine.

"I did not appreciate," a young oncologist wrote over a century later, in 2000, "the moral difficulty in navigating the tensions between patient care and research."[2] How, indeed, does a researcher explain with full candor, without subterfuge, to desperate, dying patients, that Phase 1 clinical trials for a new cancer treatment—testing only for safety—offer no therapeutic benefit to those who volunteer to take part, that the research may one day benefit others, but not them? The patients don't want to believe that and, understandably, researchers may not want to rub it in.

The physicians and researchers of the late nineteenth and early twentieth centuries were aware of these moral tensions. Hardly an issue now contested was not contested then: informed consent, risk-benefit ratios, vulnerable populations, and the like. But the arguments were just beginning, and there was far more early resistance to regulation than in the mid twentieth century. Claiming that "the limits of justifiable experimentation upon our fellow creatures are well and clearly defined," the celebrated physician William Osler said in 1907 that research on a new drug or procedure ought first to be carried out on animals, to assure "absolute safety," and could then go forward only with the "full consent" of patients.[3]

Not everyone agreed. In addition to the now-familiar refrain that many if not most patients are unable to give informed consent, there was considerable resistance to regulation. The integrity of researchers, it was said, is the only reliable bulwark against abuse. For such reasons in 1916 the AMA resisted the pleas of Walter Bradford Canon that it pass a formal resolution on the conditions for morally acceptable research (which took until 1946). The medical paternalism of the day, which included the belief that patients were better off without knowing the truth, needing only hope, provided a backdrop for evading the consent issue—even when Osler and others had in principle admitted its validity.

There was also research heroism. The effort to find a cure for yellow fever, a great need with the acquisition of Cuba following the Spanish-American War, and the building of the Panama Canal, saw the researchers themselves serving as subjects. To be sure, some Cubans were bribed with burial money to serve as subjects, but the yellow fever research was also marked by written agreements between researchers and subjects. The phrase "with full consent" was a feature of Walter Reed's published research reports. Nonetheless, despite lively awareness of the moral issues among researchers, the public was not so sure doctors could be trusted. The idea that hospitals were as important for biomedical research as for patient care was not always reassuring to patients. A still lingering fear among African Americans about hospital research, and medical research more generally, began in this era.[4]

All of the debates, however, as well as efforts to allay public fears, had a good outcome. The drama and benefits of research overshadowed some of the harm done in its name. "By the 1930s, the public's confidence in medical research and admiration for the medical profession in general," Susan Lederer has written, "made the task of defending medical research much easier than it had been at the turn of the century."[5] By that time as well, most of the conceptual and practical problems of human-subject research that are with us to this day were well known. How ought such research to be regulated and monitored? What is to be done with those unable to give consent or otherwise vulnerable? What does "informed consent" really mean? What is the difference between "therapeutic" and "nontherapeutic" research—if such a distinction is meaningful—and what distinct rules might apply to them?[6] What is an acceptable "risk-benefit" ratio and just what does "minimal risk" mean? None of these questions (which I deal with directly later in the chapter) has ever received a fully settled answer, and that failure—perhaps inevitable—is part of the early- and late-twentieth-century story.

THE NAZI ERA

Before examining those regulatory and definitional problems, I want to look at the history of Nazi medicine—a medicine that had its own research imperative. The opening sentences of Telford Taylor's statement at the beginning of the Nazi doctors' trial says it all:

> The defendants in this case are charged with murders, tortures, and other atrocities committed in the name of medical science. The victims of these crimes are numbered in the hundreds of thousands. A handful only are still alive. . . . But most of these miserable victims were slaughtered outright or died in the course of the tortures to which they were subjected. . . . To their murderers, these wretched people were not individuals at all. They came in wholesale lots and were treated worse than animals. . . . [Their] fate is a hideous blot on the page of modern history.[7]

The victims were killed in experiments on high-altitude exposure, freezing, malaria, typhus, starvation, seawater ingestion, sterilization, poison, and incendiary bombs. The instructions for assembling a Jewish skeleton collection were to photograph the victims first, measure them anthropologically, record vital data. And then, "following the subsequently induced death of the Jew, whose head should not be damaged, the delegate will separate the head from the body and forward it to its proper point of destination in a hermetically sealed tin car, especially produced for this purpose and filled with conserving fluid."[8]

Most readers will be familiar enough with that terrible history to need no more examples (although a reminder is always useful). More directly pertinent to this book is the ethical, political, and cultural context of this deadly research. There was an imperative behind it, that of "solving the Jewish question," as well as contributing to the wartime needs. The regime's racism was dressed up with scientific terminology, and Nazi doctors were well paid. For skills and legitimation they drew on earlier traditions of German medicine and, as the historian Robert Proctor has shown, the Nazis did not single-handedly politicize research much less force physicians to co-operate. "There were," he has written, "as many volunteers as victims." At the same time, Proctor plausibly adds, the horrors of this period cannot be traced to anything intrinsic to science and medicine. "It took a powerful state to concentrate and unleash the destructive forces of German medicine."[9] The complaint of an American doctor in 1900 that, for German physicians, "the patient was something to work on, interesting experimental material, but little more," suggests a virus lodged deep within the culture of German medicine, as did the massive starvation of mental patients during World War I.[10]

Yet it was not an unrecognized virus prior to the Nazi era. During the 1920s and 1930s complaints against German researchers became common. A 1931 report by a member of the Reich Health Office noted about the state of medical research that it was "marked by naked cynicism . . . mental and physical torture . . . martyrization of children in hospitals . . . [and] disgustingly shameful abominations in the name of science run mad."[11]

The complaints had their effect. In March 1930 the Reich Health Office organized a meeting to discuss "the permissibility of medical experiments on healthy and sick subjects," which eventually led to the promulgation of guidelines in 1931 for experimentation with human beings. There was subsequent debate about the legal status of those guidelines, and part of the doctors' defense at the Nuremberg trial was that the guidelines did not have the force of law. Yet they were promulgated and they surely suggest that human experimentation received high-level attention just before the Nazis took power. Most strikingly, the 1931 German guidelines were as forceful and detailed as the later Nuremberg Code and specifically stated that "experimentation shall be prohibited in all cases where consent has not been given."

Those guidelines were promptly brushed aside by the Nazis. In their Nuremberg defense, the Nazi doctors denied their legal validity in Germany. It was also noted in the trial that the AMA guidelines came into being only nineteen days after the December 9, 1946, opening of the trial. The United States could not exactly use itself as an exemplar, a point the Nazi doctors seized on. Those doctors had other defenses as well. Among them were the contentions that research is required during times of war, that no German laws had been broken, that the prisoners were in any case already condemned to death, that the use of prisoners for research had universal sanction (and the Japanese used prisoners too), that prisoners themselves often picked out the research subjects, that it is sometimes necessary to kill some people to save many, that no universal standards of research ethics existed, and that, as a clincher, "without human experimentation, there would be no way to advance the progress of science and medicine."[12]

That line of defense was decisively rejected by the prosecution. In addition to asking for the death penalty on seven of the defendants, the prosecution presented, as part of its judgment, what has become known as the Nuremberg Code. That 1947 code, which had as its first principle the necessity of voluntary consent by human subjects, became the foundation of later codes and, perhaps more than any other twentieth-century development, raised the issue of human-subject research to a high legal and moral status. Informed consent, experiments on animals before humans, an avoidance of all unnecessary physical and mental pain and suffering, and the prospect of meaningful medical benefits otherwise unobtainable, became the lodestone moral principles of human-subject research that have endured to this day.

The court rejected as valid many of the most common reasons advanced in wartime or in peacetime for the moral acceptability of using human beings against their will for some higher good, whether biomedical progress, the relief of suffering, or the needs of the state. The defense of the Nazi doctors was, on the face of it, outrageous, but their argument still echoes today. When all else fails, there is always some higher transcendent, or compellingly utilitarian, good that can be invoked; and that is what the defendants tried, and failed, to get away with.

THE POSTWAR AND COLD WAR YEARS

The United States was not utterly immune to such arguments and was by no means fully ready to take up the problem—as the slowness of the AMA in coming to grips with human-subject research even past the end of the war showed. There was, after all, a war to be conducted here as well, one that required new medical knowledge: to deal with the diseases—from gonorrhea to malaria—that American troops would be at risk for, to learn about managing the stress that battle would bring, and to better patch up and care for the wounded. The 1941 creation by President Roosevelt of the Office of Scientific Research and Development was meant to carry out both weapons research and medical research. The latter research, under the auspices of the Committee on Medical Research, was eventually to recommend six hundred research proposals for support.

Some of that research was hazardous and not all of it was sensitive to the rights and welfare of the subjects. In 1943–44 many children were put at serious risk without parental consent to test dysentery vaccines; homes for the retarded were used as sites to carry it out. Psychotics in a state institution were infected with malaria and given experimental therapies. Hospital patients were chosen for influenza research. Informed consent was not gained, and many subjects were injured. That said, the pattern of subject abuse during the war appears more erratic than systematic, and in many cases conscientious objectors and others willing to be subjects were told of the risks and given a choice about taking part in research. Still, as the historian David Rothman concluded, "Neither the growing distance between researcher and subject nor the inattention to principles of consent sparked critiques or expressions of distrust. To the contrary, all these characteristics were viewed as a necessary and admirable element in the home-front effort . . . well into the 1960s, the American research community considered the Nuremberg findings, and the Nuremberg Code, irrelevant to its own work."[13]

National defense needs were brought out again as the Cold War emerged. Beginning in 1944, with the prospect of the atom bomb at hand, systematic research with human subjects was carried out on the use of, or exposure to, ionizing radiation. Unknown to the public, it continued into the 1970s. The work of the Advisory Committee on Human Radiation Experiments established by President Clinton in 1994 brought to light a variety of experiments that, shielded by the protection of secrecy regulations and the exigency of the Cold War, had been known about only in a shadowy way. There were experiments on the hazards of plutonium, uranium, and polonium, on total body irradiation, and on the effects of atomic explosions. Whole populations were put at risk by the intentional release of radioactive material in the air.

Yet as the findings of the committee brought out, the dangers to which many thousands of people were exposed without their consent—military personnel, prisoners, and the general public—was not a subject of indifference to all the researchers. In many of the governmental agencies, and among many of those charged with oversight of the research, the ethical issues were recognized and debated. A 1947 letter written to Carroll Wilson, the first chief of the Atomic Energy Commission, by Robert S. Stone, a radiologist in favor of declassification of secret documents, upheld the need for secrecy but also held that, with plutonium exposure studies, informed consent was a basic requirement. As Jonathan Moreno has noted in his illuminating book on the radiation experiments, *Undue Risk*, that was the first time the phrase "informed consent" had ever been used (in contrast to the more common term "voluntary consent," used in the Nuremberg Code).[14]

Many of the federal agencies that carried out the radiation research debated the ethical issues. All too often they chose in the end to ignore them.

Efforts to publish data on the situation usually met claims about the need for secrecy. The overall impression is that the ethical debate was tepid at best, and that—time and again in the end—national security considerations favorable to research trumped concern for the rights of subjects.

Many of the recommendations of Clinton's radiation committee were aimed at bringing those rights back into focus and putting in place mechanisms to ensure that they would be taken seriously by governmental agencies in the future. In a separate statement, one of the committee members, Jay Katz, raised the question "When, if ever, should conflicts between advancing medical knowledge for our benefit and protecting the inviolability of citizen-subjects of research be resolved in favor of the former?" His answer is that only when voluntary consent, enunciated as the first principle of the Nuremberg Code "is firmly put into practice . . . can one avoid the dangers that accompany a balancing of one principle against the other that assigns equal weight to both."[15] Only with that principle in place, he added, can we fairly consider exceptional circumstances to go forward with research and reasonable means of determining them.

IMPROVING THE GUIDELINES

As the radiation experiments quietly went forward from 1944 to 1974, out in more public view there was a growing dissatisfaction with the Nuremberg Code. It had carried out its initial purpose, that of setting forth important standards to shape the future of human-subject research, and most specifically to put a solid barrier in the way of any return to the kind of experiments carried out by the Nazis. Further reflection on that code revealed many problems. In its first principle, the absolute requirement of voluntary consent seemed to close the door to research on children and the mentally incompetent, and perhaps on others, such as prisoners or charity patients in hospitals, whose context might make such consent impossible.[16] To what extent could consent be informed, when even the researchers might not be able to calculate risks and benefits? And then how could a code that provided for no review of researchers' action, relying entirely on them to make all the moral judgments, be taken seriously? As later events were to show, it was a code easily ignored and, if taken seriously, without bite or clarity.

As early as 1953, the Committee on Medical Ethics of the World Medical Association (WMA) began considering human-subject research. A strong motivation was the felt need for a code designed by physicians for physicians (the Nuremberg Code, by contrast, had been designed by jurists after a legal trial). An early result of that deliberation was the use of a distinction that has troubled researchers and their critics ever since, between "experiments in new diagnostic and therapeutic methods" and "experiments undertaken to serve other purposes than simply to cure an individual."[17] Important as well were resolutions requiring consent of the subject (or for an ill patient, the next of kin), and a spelling out of possible risks. The matter continued to be debated, and various draft codes were considered by the WMA. Finally, at its eighteenth annual World Medical Assembly held in Helsinki in 1964, what was known thereafter as the Helsinki Code I was passed.[18]

Though Helsinki I differed in many respects from the Nuremberg Code, the latter's influence was discernible. But the differences were important. The Helsinki Code called for consent in writing and sharply distinguished between clinical research, aimed at patient care, and nontherapeutic clinical research, where the aim is knowledge but not direct patient application. In a later version of the code, passed in Tokyo in 1975, and known as Helsinki II, the most important change was the added requirement of an ethical review committee, and even greater emphasis was laid on informed consent.

In response to the criticism that the Nuremberg and Helsinki codes are nothing more than voluntary sets of ethical principles, without true international sanctions, the World Health Organization (WHO) and the Council for International Organizations of Medical Sciences devised a set of international guidelines—though also without legal sanctions—in 1982.[19] They were meant to take account of cultural differences, vulnerable groups, and community-based research, among other things. Most important, the guidelines held that research carried out by scientists from developed countries in poor countries should adhere to the same standards that held in the initiating country. A 1996 draft Guideline for Good Clinical Practice aims to establish uniform standards for drug research.[20]

HENRY KNOWLES BEECHER: UPPING THE ANTE

What the concatenation of these different codes in the post–World War II world makes clear—each adding new refinements and clarifications—is that human-subject research is a far more complex problem in its ethical details than was recognized at Nuremberg. It took a gradual accumulation of experience, and some serious troubles, to move that process along. The revelation in 1966 in the *New England Journal of Medicine* by Dr. Henry Knowles Beecher of American research abuses in the postwar years came as a shock to a medical community and public that had, too comfortably perhaps, come to think that the Nuremberg and other codes had taken care of the problem. Dr. Beecher shattered that complacency.[21] M. H. Pappworth was doing much the same thing in Britain, admirably so (though meeting even greater resistance), but my focus will be on Beecher and the subsequent American developments.[22]

Dr. Beecher, a distinguished professor of anesthesiology at the Harvard Medical School, and I were indirectly linked in 1960. As a former competitive swimmer, I was recruited to take part in the clinical trials of a new drug, which turned out to be amphetamines. When I was taking it, and not the placebo, I had terrific times—but my wife had to put up with the great downer that followed each evening. Like many others in that era, I never even thought of informed consent, and I do not recall anyone asking for it. Not until the early 1970s, when Dr. Beecher helped me get the Hastings Center started, did I discover in looking through his CV that he had directed the trials of which I was a part. By the time I met him formally, in 1970 or so, he was already as revered an expert in the new field of bioethics as he was an excoriated figure among many of his medical colleagues. Those colleagues did not deny the abuses, but they thought it inexpedient to make them public, not helpful to the progress of research or the good name of medicine. Even in 1966 he saw what others have seen more clearly since then, that pressures to publish and to gain academic ascendancy would push ambitious researchers in the wrong direction; and those same pressures were behind the objections to his revelations. But there was no denying the force of his arguments or the facts he brought out, some twenty-two examples of harmful research (out of a sample of fifty he had collected).

Jay Katz, a Yale law professor I quoted above, and one of the most important pioneers in pressing the ethical dilemmas of human-subject research, began working with Beecher in the mid-1960s. They first corresponded and then Beecher took part with him in a seminar Katz organized in 1966 at the law school. The seminar, "Experimentation on People," was surely ahead of its time. Beecher had already published a book, *Experimentation in Man*, in 1958 but it did not attract the attention of his 1966 article, a recitation of a number of dubious and harmful experiments. The important common law legal doctrine of informed consent, affirmed by the Supreme Court in 1957 in *Salgo v. Leland Stanford, Jr.*, was barely five years old and had helped frame the issues that Beecher and Katz discussed.[23]

Beecher was bravely ahead of his time in exposing problems his medical colleagues did not want to hear about, but he was conventional in another sense: he wanted to keep them within the profession. He knew that improvement in the ethical use of human subjects was critical, but he did not believe in governmental regulation to bring that about. Only a researcher's integrity and conscience would avoid the kinds of abuse he had uncovered.[24] He was right and yet wrong. He was right that only researchers' integrity and peer pressure would eliminate all problems—a clever researcher can usually circumvent any federal regulation and get past local institutional review committees. But he was wrong in the implication of his position—that regulation could not work at all. Regulation *does* change behavior; more subtly, it also changes researchers' mores. In any case, regulation is crucial for public trust. Revelations of researchers' abuses are not quickly forgotten, and only assurances of strong governmental oversight are likely to clear the bad odor out of the room where bodies might be buried—or, more likely, where research subjects were put at risk and sometimes hurt.

What drew me to the analysis of what Beecher and Katz were up to in the 1960s was Katz's confrontation with the issue of most concern to me. That is the relationship between the aims of researchers and the rights of those who, as subjects, are needed for the research. Many researchers were at the time particularly suspicious of the first principle of the Nuremberg Code, voluntary consent, because of the potential obstacle it put in the way of research. Katz forcefully pointed to this problem in his later book, *Experimentation on Human Beings,* when he wrote, "When human beings become the subject of experimentation . . . tensions arise between two values basic to Western society: freedom of scientific inquiry and protection of individual inviolability. . . . At the heart of this [value] conflict lies an age-old question: When may a society, actively or by acquiescence, expose some of its members to harm in order to seek benefits for them, for others, or for society as a whole?" That question, he contends, has never been well analyzed, noting that Congress has "insufficiently faced up to the fact that the practice of medicine and the conduct of research are different enterprises."[25] The possibilities of research breakthroughs, of future lives to be saved by bold research, simply fade out in the clear light of the moral need to gain informed consent.

FEDERAL REGULATIONS AND NATIONAL COMMISSIONS

The medical and research community could not ignore Beecher's article—nor could the federal government. Three cases of abuse (two of them cited by Beecher), moreover, achieved public notoriety. The New York Jewish Chronic Disease Hospital case saw the injection of live cancer cells in patients there. The Willowbrook case (in a New York state home for mentally retarded children), encompassing an effort to understand the natural history of hepatitis, saw the injection of hepatitis virus into the children. The Tuskegee syphilis study, the most notorious of them all, saw a group of four hundred black men observed from 1932 until the early 1970s to determine the natural history of their disease; and, when penicillin became available during the study, they did not receive it—that would have spoiled the study.[26] There was no consent obtained in any of the three cases, the purposes of which were known only to the researchers and the doctors close at hand.

There has been debate over the years about the relative role of research ambition and racism in shaping and continuing the Tuskegee study. Racism has been the most common explanation, but David Rothman wrote in the early 1980s that a broader perspective "gives the styles and mindsets of the research scientist much greater prominence."[27] A number of major medical journals reported on the study. Most strikingly, when effective treatment became available, the medical and public health project participants urged that it be made available to the research subjects. The researchers rationalized, bypassed treatment, and continued. Both the Tuskegee and Willowbrook cases were observational studies and both took advantage of the social deprivation and vulnerability of the subjects. The research imperative, of the hazardous kind, was the driving force. Racism made it easier for that imperative to triumph.

By the mid-1960s the federal government had become a crucial actor in the regulation of research. As noted earlier, the AMA had directly addressed the research issue only in 1946. Except for the Nuremberg Code (written by American judges), American law, moreover, had little to say about it until the 1960s, though it was agreed that researchers could be held liable if harm came to their subjects.[28] A 1958 national conference on the Legal Environment of Medical Science focused heavily on medical experimentation, and a 1960 grant from the National Institutes of Health to the Law-Medicine Institute at Boston University chose to study the actual practices of researchers and research organizations.

As so often happens with governmental regulation, it took a major medical tragedy to galvanize Congress and the Food and Drug Administration to develop a policy on human subjects. The Drug Amendments Act of 1962 (known as the Kefauver-Harris bill) came about as a result of the work of Senator Estes Kefauver and his Senate investigation of the pharmaceutical industry. Its work was greatly helped by the well-reported harm done by a drug for morning sickness, Thalidomide, which in fact caused infant deformities. The FDA conceded that it had little control over clinical drug trials or even knew their extent; before 1962 there was simply no regulation of clinical testing at all. The Kefauver-Harris bill mandated drug testing for efficacy and safety, greater control of drug advertising, and the imposition on the FDA of comprehensive regulation of drug testing.[29] Informed consent was a key ingredient and, through the tough-minded work of the FDA's Dr. Frances O. Kelsey, the agency resisted pressure to waive the consent rule at times on the grounds that it was necessary to preserve the research design, or to protect the doctor-patient relationship.

By 1963 the other important federal health agency, the NIH, began to study the advisability of developing guidelines for its extramural research program. As a result, acting on the recommendation of the National Advisory Health Council, in 1966 the director of NIH promulgated a policy statement that required institutions applying for grants to carry out prior review "of the judgment of the principal investigator or program director by a committee of his institutional associates."[30] A number or revisions and clarifications quickly followed, and the present institutional review board (IRB) system for the approval of federal grants was put into place. The guiding policy statement specified a self-regulatory system in the universities and research institutions receiving grant money from the Public Health Service and the NIH. The guidelines for the system aimed to protect the rights and welfare of subjects, to require the gaining of informed consent, and to demand an assessment of the risks and potential benefits of the research.

While there was considerable muttering about the NIH policy, and many worries about regulations that would stifle and even stop research, the IRB structure was quickly adopted. Though it works well enough in many respects, there are myriad ways to obfuscate or evade its requirements and deride its way of defining terms and requirements. If Henry Beecher was wrong to oppose regulations, he was not far off the mark in noting the inherent difficulty of applying general guidelines to individual research projects. That is the clinician's—and then the researcher's—old lament about making the move from the general rule to the particular case, as much a problem with ethics as with medical care.

In subsequent years, complaints about the IRB system found a receptive ear in Congress. In 1974 it established the National Commission for the Protection of Human Subjects of Biomedical and Behavioral Research—its very name reflecting a general fear that the IRB system was not doing as good a job as it should. Recommendations for improvement were made, and the NIH paid heed to them, but still all did not go well. In 1979, the President's Commission for the Study of Ethical Problems in Medicine and Biomedical and Behavioral Research was created. Its much broader mandate nonetheless required still another look at the IRB system, and some fresh recommendations were made. But in the mid-1990s the system's recurrent problems surfaced once more, and by executive order in 1995 President Clinton established the National Bioethics Advisory Commission, a central part of whose charge was to conduct a thorough review of research on human subjects.

During these nearly forty years of activity, going back to the action of the FDA and NIH, interest in human-subject research rarely flagged. In 1979 the Hastings Center established a journal, *IRB: A Review of Human Subject Research* (still the only such professional journal), a steady stream of articles on the topic appeared in medical journals, and the media were able to pick up one problem after another in the use of human subjects. In addition to all the other activity, in 1991 sixteen federal agencies adopted the NIH rule (45 CFR 46) for the protection of human subjects, known as the "common rule." And while private-sector research has not been bound by the federal regulations, many companies voluntarily have adopted its standards. The FDA, in contrast, has jurisdiction over private-sector pharmaceutical research that will be marketed to the public as a biologic, drug, or medical device.

Special note must taken of a document that emerged from the work of the 1974 commission, called the Belmont Report.[31] Reflecting the work of a major group of bioethicists, lawyers, and physicians with particular ethical interests, the report advanced three ethical principles for the use of human subjects in biomedical research, each said "to be generally accepted in our cultural tradition": *respect for persons*, encompassing the requirement to acknowledge autonomy and protect those with diminished autonomy (it underlies the requirement for informed consent); *beneficence*, insisting on the avoidance of harm and the maximization of possible benefits and the minimization of possible harms (which underlies the requirement for risk-benefit assessment); and *justice*, advocating a fair distribution of the benefits and burdens of research (which supports the requirement for fair procedures and outcomes in the selection of research subjects).

Moral theories rarely receive the blessing of the federal government. Hence it is noteworthy not simply that a particular set of ethical principles—now known as principlism—were drawn on for the report, but that the federal government formally accepted them as the "philosophical underpinnings for current federal laws governing research involving human subjects."[32] Over the years, moreover, those principles have received international sanction and support, though, as we will see later, not without puzzles and problems. Why were they popular? One obvious reason is that the principles are, as the report stated, consonant with our culture and, in themselves, not controversial in the American public forum. They are also relatively easy to work with, and if over the years they have received much criticism by those in bioethics, including me, they have nonetheless proved convincing and workable to clinicians and biomedical researchers (who grumble even so about the difficulty of making the move from a general principle to a specific case).

John Evans, a sociologist of medicine, has made a good case that their real attraction has been twofold: they push aside the moral clutter of confounding facts and values that exists in any serious ethical problem, and they lend themselves nicely to the need for crispness and objective transparency that appeals to policymakers faced with the need to limit subjective decision making.[33] In sum, what many of us find to be the main drawback of principlism—its excessive simplicity and seeming indifference to context and complexity—is just what makes it congenial to government-run regulatory systems. That much said, there is no doubt that the concept of respect for persons, and informed consent, has served well in limiting the force of a hazardous research imperative that looked on persons simply as research material.

THE PRESENT ALARM

Despite the Belmont Report, and despite two earlier national commissions, human-subject research has been subject to a new, and even stronger, round of criticism in recent years. Neither the principles themselves nor the organizational structure of institutional review boards seem able to deal with the force of a heightened research imperative or the adequate management of a large, even overwhelming, number of research protocols. The increasing importance of for-profit contract research organizations has heightened the alarm, raising questions about conflict of interest and indifference to patient welfare.[34] I characterized the earlier struggles over human-subject research as a constant tension between the desire to move research along and the need to protect subjects. Again and again, fortunately, the necessary reforms have always moved in the direction of greater, not less, protection for subjects as against "balance" between research and protection. Yet again and again over the years the pendulum has swung back either openly in favor of giving greater force to the research drive or, in practice, permitting a laxity of oversight and monitoring of the work of IRBs, which in effect achieves the same end.

Now a new, even if familiar, struggle is pitting many of the same ideas and interests against each other. In 1969 Dr. Francis Moore, chairman of the Department of Surgery at the Harvard Medical School, wrote, "we must always insist that [subject protection] guidelines protect society by enabling a continuous advance of biomedical sciences. . . . [By] protecting the individual patient, [the researcher] is subjecting society to the hazard of a static rather than dynamic medicine."[35] The 2000 Declaration of Helsinki, however, refuses to recognize such a priority: "concern for the interests of the subject must always prevail over the interests of science and society."[36] Dr. Marcia Angell, pointing out the implications of that standard, wrote that "whether research results are important is immaterial in judging the ethics of the research."[37]

Though separated by some thirty years, the tension between Dr. Moore's view, focusing an ethical lens on the interests of science and society, and the Helsinki Declaration, looking after the interests of the individual subject, remains the central issue. Despite the clear and unequivocal force of that declaration and other similar international statements, it has never fully pacified the research imperative. "It has become common," Dr. Beverly Woodward has written in a masterly 1999 analysis of the present situation, "to read or hear statements by medical researchers that assert the primacy of the interests of science and society and that place the burden of justification on those who would put any obstacles in the way of scientific and social goals."[38]

By the end of the 1990s it was clear that many things were amiss in human-subject research, and that something urgently had to be done about them. The inspector general of the Department of Health and Human Services (DHHS) reported in 1998 that "the long-established system for protecting human research subjects has vulnerabilities that threaten its effectiveness."[39] A relatively temperate attitude did not last long. If the 1999 death of Jesse Gelsinger in a gene therapy research trial in Philadelphia was the most notorious instance of a problem, there were plenty of others to catch the eye, particularly the federal eye.

The pace of reform quickened. Jane Heaney, commissioner of the Food and Drug Administration (and the principal agency with responsibility for oversight of the gene therapy trials), noted that "some researchers at prestigious institutions have failed to follow good clinical practices" and then went on from there to list ten different kinds of failure to meet established ethical standards, ranging from conflict of interest to a failure to report adverse research events.[40] Donna Shalala, secretary of the DHHS, wrote in late September 2000 that she felt compelled to take action because, among other things, there was evidence that subjects were not being fully informed about the risks and benefits of research, that clinical researchers were not adhering to good standards of clinical practice, and that potential conflicts of interest were increasingly arising.[41]

A number of cumulative events had led her to write that statement, including the Gelsinger case. In 1999 the NIH Office of Protection from Research Risks placed a number of restrictions on a variety of important research centers, including Duke University, as punishment for a number of oversight failures. And as a warning signal to the research community, that office acquired a new title in 2000 (Office of Human Research Protection), a new home (in the DHHS rather than the NIH), and a new director (Dr. Greg Koski). No sooner had Dr. Koski taken office than he fired a loud warning shot: "Institutions failing to meet the highest ethical standards would simply not be allowed to continue doing research."[42] A bipartisan congressional group introduced the Human Subjects Research Protection Act of 2000, extending informed consent requirements and prior review for all human-subject research to the private as well as the public sector.

All these developments have fed into what Jonathan Moreno has called the end of "moderate protectionism." That kind of subject protection is heavily reliant on researchers' integrity, which is where the original emphasis lay a century ago. A move to strong protectionism—increased regulation and greater governmental oversight—now hopes to end the long-standing tension between subjects' interests and scientific progress.[43]

What explains the new crisis and the new urgency to do something about it? Is it simply the flare-up of an old chronic ailment, or has the ailment itself changed? I believe it is the former. In upholding strong standards of human-subject protection, we may always encounter almost intractable problems and difficulties. I say "almost intractable problems" not because they seem in principle insoluble but because in practice high standards and the organizational mechanisms to enforce them are exceedingly hard to apply.

No doubt the research imperative to relieve suffering and fight disease is one of those chronic forces, but now it is at an especially high pitch, pulling the pendulum back in the direction of research interests. Other reinforcing motives support it. Henry Beecher picked up on some of them in noting the pressure on young researchers to be productive if they were to advance in their professions. From all reports, that pressure is greater than ever, intensified by floods of money for research, public and private, by competitive pressures in the private sector, and by the greater fame and fortune that research success can now bring.

The net result entails more research, more subjects, and more access to human biological materials and patients' medical records.[44] I have not seen a full account of the attempt at gene therapy that ended in Jesse Gelsinger's death, but the most plausible explanation is that the nascent field of gene therapy desperately needed a success story (after ten years of virtual failure); that the University of Pennsylvania, which had invested university funds in the Institute for Human Gene Therapy, needed to show some kind of payoff; that the part ownership by the director of the institute, James Wilson, in a company that stood to make a profit from gene therapy success may have played some role; and that the ordinary drive, and impatience, of ambitious researchers led them to cut some regulatory corners. In short, it was a combination of background pressures and circumstances that led to Gelsinger's death, no one failing alone.

PERENNIAL TENSIONS AND SERIOUS PUZZLES

A persistent issue over the decades has been that of specifying crucial definitions and meanings. The primacy of consent has, as noted earlier, been recognized for well over one hundred years. At first, the language was that of "voluntary consent," but it gradually evolved, in the aftermath of the Nuremberg Code, into "informed consent." But from the first as well, each fresh attempt to specify more clearly just what "consent" means, and what "informed" means, seemed to both add clarification and multiply confusion. How can that be? One reason is simply that people can interpret the same words in different ways, and all the more so if they have normative ingredients.

Each effort to clarify informed consent has entailed spelling out its implications, usually by means of an articulated principle, and in turn has opened that principle to some further degree of uncertainty and debate. The federal common rule, for instance, specifies "a description of any reasonably foreseeable risks or discomfort to the subject," as an element of informed consent.[45] There is plenty of room for disagreement about what the word "reasonably" means (or better, means to different people), and the old story of the princess and the pea shows the wide range of possibilities for "discomfort."

That is not the end of the complications. The Belmont Report tried to show that the rule of informed consent is rooted in the broader principle of respect for persons, of which their autonomy is a core value. But in some cases there is further room for conflict between autonomy and some other important value, such as beneficence.[46] Is it always wrong, for instance, to set aside some individual's autonomy for the medical benefit to others, which beneficence might seem to require? The research imperative, aiming to relieve suffering, might well be understood in many cases as nothing but an expression of beneficence. The tradition and common interpretation of the principle of informed consent, however, is that it must never, not ever, be overruled by beneficence, however much suffering might be relieved by doing so.

At the same time, however, I must note two difficulties. One of them is simply that there is room for considerable, and perhaps intractable, debate about the meaning of informed consent simply because of the above-noted interpretive problems, built into our use of language. According to the common rule, informed consent requires an explanation of the procedure, the possible benefits to the subject or others of the research, the absence of coercion or undue influence, a right to withdraw from the research—among other conditions.[47] There is plenty of room for quibbles there. The other difficulty is even broader: some forms of research on some subjects may not be open to obtaining full informed consent. This difficulty can reflect either the scope of the research (epidemiological studies of whole populations) or the research subjects it requires (a vulnerable group: prisoners in some circumstances; or one unable to give consent: children, the retarded, the demented).

The troubling question is whether, and to what extent, and under what circumstances, there can be exceptions to the principle of informed consent—exceptions that recognize the force of the research imperative in its benign sense and can operate without danger of allowing the imperative in its hazardous sense to take over. Even Jay Katz, as firm as anyone in asserting the priority of informed consent, has agreed that it may be put aside when "the urgency of the situation demands it and there has been a full prior review."[48]

In this context an odd and unsettling case of deception research in social psychology deserves mention. The famous, or infamous, study of Stanley Milgram in the 1960s, testing how people would react to commands to inflict pain on others, entailed the use of deception: for the research to work, the subjects could not be allowed to know they were part of an experiment.[49] Despite a great deal of criticism over the years, the American Psychological Association has defended the legitimacy of such research when the prospective scientific gains warrant it, when there is no other way to gain the information, and when there is unlikely to be any harm to the subject.[50] Using an argument that would be dismissed out of hand in the medical context, defenders of the research have used the term "presumptive consent." The supposed acceptability of such ex post facto consent has been based on interviews with people after the research was completed that elicited neither an objection on the part of the subjects to their participation nor the report of any evident harm.

It is of course ironic that Stanley Milgram's study was in part designed to understand how ordinary people, which most Nazis were, could be led to do such terrible things to other people—and in the process Milgram violated the first principle of the Nuremberg Code. If that is ironic, it is curious that the American Psychological Association has never understood that there can be higher values than scientific knowledge. Or is it, less grandly, a desire not to thwart a whole field of social psychology research? Or because, as an expression of an interest group's power, that is just what some researchers want to do?

The social psychologists' argument that there is little or no risk to their subjects has often been used in biomedical research. Two conditions pertinent to risk must be met in biomedical or behavioral research: that risks to subjects must be minimized, and that the risks be reasonable in relation to anticipated benefits.[51] Here again are problems inherent in the use of language, particularly general terms such as "risk," which is open to many interpretations and differing personal responses. So too is the word "benefits," which has usually been interpreted to encompass individual and social benefits.

Beverly Woodward, citing many studies, concluded, "Current trends in research and research regulation continue to erode the requirement of consent, while the notion of minimal risk has become, as a commentator put it recently, 'upwardly mobile.' "[52] A 1996 decision by the FDA to allow drug research on patients with a life-threatening condition when informed consent could not be obtained from the patient or his family met with a shout of protest as a basic assault on the principle of informed consent.[53] A series of calls to make it more possible to conduct research on children, shifting the interpretation of minimal risk, met with a similar response, but researchers, who see the changes as the removal of unnecessary impediments to research, welcomed it.

The use of vulnerable subjects. The first problem with the very first principle of the Nuremberg Code, calling for voluntary consent, was that it left out a large portion of humanity. Many of us may not be competent to give consent, not always competent or wholly competent, or competent but in a position where the conditions for assuredly free consent are missing. Young children, the mentally retarded, those with severe mental conditions, and the demented elderly, are typically not competent. Some older children may be partially competent (enough to say "no" to research), while some mentally ill people will have variable competence. Prisoners as a class are open to undue institutional influence even if otherwise competent. Vulnerability, in short, comes in many forms.[54]

Here, then, are situations where the benign research imperative—the need to carry out valid research designed to help the vulnerable—and the possibility of exploiting them for research purposes not necessarily in their interests are in tension. The aim need not be the malevolent one of using the vulnerable as subjects simply because they are vulnerable, and thus less trouble than the competent. An old-fashioned paternalism could simply be at work: the researcher is the best judge of what will and will not be harmful to, or in the interest of, the research subject. That is a tempting stance to adopt in determining what counts as a "minimal" risk, or a good balance between risk and benefit.

The regulatory details for managing research on the vulnerable need not be examined here. But there are three general requirements. In each of the general classes of cases noted above, IRB review and prior approval is necessary. Surrogate decision makers, ordinarily families, may be used in the case of the incompetent and their standards may be that of the "best interests" of the patient; and the IRB must decide if there is a good balance for the research subject of risk and benefit.[55]

This last point causes the most trouble. Competent subjects can decide (unless there is great danger) what is an acceptable risk-benefit value. With the incompetent, someone (or some group) must make that judgment. Not surprisingly, researchers often want—and sometimes must want—to press beyond what other persons might consider acceptable. Unlike the situation with competent subjects, whose power to say no is absolute whatever the quality or motive of their reasoning, with the incompetent there is no corresponding fixed boundary. It then becomes the judgment of one group, say an IRB, over against another group, the researchers.

Put another way, the research imperative has no moral status at all to coerce the unwilling competent person to take part in research. With the incompetent, there is no comparable and clear barrier. As the IRB negotiates the murky waters of risk-benefit judgments and decides the risk of a research protocol is too great, then incompetent subjects may lose out on research of possible benefit for their particular disease. Alexander Morgan Capron has argued that patients with mental disorders need *greater* protection than others, noting a trend toward what some researchers call a "minor increase" in risk occasioned by allowing guardians or other surrogates to permit them to take part in nonbeneficial research; sometimes the intent is to give the patients other medical benefits. For Capron and other critics of research with the incompetent, these incremental benefits are little more than "the camel's head and neck following the nose of 'minimal risk' into the tent."[56]

Capron may well be right, but it seems even more evident that once we move beyond the category of the competent subject into that of the incompetent or partially competent, there are no clear rules to balance research possibilities and subjects' protection. The ethical issue would surely be easier to handle, for instance, if no exception had ever been made to research on children, and if that exception had not employed the term "minimal risk" as the standard for allowing such research. But in that instance, each side was able to make a plausible case to bias the balance in its favor. The research put children at greater risk and yet could gain valuable knowledge at a small cost. I am ambivalent on this issue, at least to the point of refusing to attribute wrong motives to researchers who wanted some exceptions to the consent rule.

In the end, I believe, we must develop general lay community standards of risk-benefit ratios, and of minimal risk. IRB oversight is a necessity, but it can do its work only within the broader context of some consensus on the right moral balance. Whatever that consensus, there can never be an automatic deferral to the claim of research benefit, or an automatic dismissal of a research possibility because of some degree of risk. Instead there must be community discussion, an assessment of experience in carrying out research on the incompetent, and a willingness to change the standards when necessary. Nothing less seems sufficient. This is not a wholly satisfactory solution, but that is what happens when there are no standards other than the considered judgment of people with different legitimate interests in complex situations. If these matters are hard when the research will have no benefits for the subject, they are no less hard when there is a mixture of (alleged) therapeutic gain for the subject and scientific gain for the field.

Therapeutic and nontherapeutic research. Inspired by the German model in the late nineteenth and early twentieth centuries, we recall, scientific medicine made a concerted and successful effort to turn ordinary physicians into researchers. It aimed to take research from the laboratory bench to the hospital bedside. That mixing of roles has brought many more clinicians than might otherwise be the case into the research enterprise. It has also occasioned a running battle about the mixing of those roles. The Advisory Committee on Human Radiation Experiments, commenting on a total body irradiation experiment—defended as therapy—judged that "there is evidence of the subordination of the ends of medicine to the ends of research." It then went on to ask whether "the ends of research (understood as discovering new knowledge) and the ends of medicine (understood as serving the interests of the patient) necessarily conflict and how the conflict should be resolved when it occurs are still today open and vexing issues."[57]

A physician trying out an experimental therapy with a patient, aiming only to benefit the patient, is not required to gain IRB approval to do so. But a physician carrying out "therapeutic research" on the patient—loosely defined as a systematic effort to gain organized knowledge that will be beneficial to other patients—must gain approval.[58] The problematic part of the distinction is twofold. Is it a valid distinction?[59] Many would say no and would like to see even the innovative effort by a physician with a patient, but with no larger research aim in mind, brought under IRB procedures. Is it conceivable that a clinician researcher could manage the clinical and the research role without tension, even severe conflict, especially from a patient's point of view?

The term "therapeutic misconception" applies to the most disturbing and subtle part of the dual role. It arises when a clinician researcher is carrying out research of no expected or intended benefit to a patient (as in Phase 1 drug trials to test safety only), but which the patient (often with the physician's tacit support) believes will offer a chance of benefit. Two contrasting views tend to dominate the debate. One insists there is a conflict, never perfectly resolvable, and the clinician researcher must live with it. The answer is a much stronger effort to develop standards of integrity for the researcher to help manage the conflict.[60] Whether that is possible—requiring the cultivation of diverse, often conflicting skills—is by no means clear, but there is no doubt that there is a strong push in that direction (and perhaps all the more so at a time when clinical research itself is experiencing a decline, the victim of economic pressures).

The other view, advanced most bitingly by the legal scholar George Annas, agrees that some clinician researchers make conscientious efforts to juggle both roles responsibly but sees corruption within the practice: "Even a cursory history of modern experimentation demonstrates the pervasiveness of three doublespeak concepts: experimentation is treatment, researchers are physicians, and subjects are patients." Since patients want to believe the doublespeak as well—which is why they persist in hoping for, or expecting, benefit even when explicitly told not to expect it—it is useful for both researcher (doctor) and patients (subjects). But Annas goes farther, contending that the doublespeak is too often deliberate and the therapeutic misconception systematically insinuated. Annas would do away altogether with the concept of "therapeutic research," which only obscures what is really going on, the systematic confusing of the ideology of medicine and the ideology of science.[61]

The successful effort by AIDS activists to gain access to drug trials only served to strengthen the confusion by conflating research and treatment, misleading the activists and offering an irresistible pool of subjects for researchers. Noting that it will probably always be impossible to eliminate self-deception among desperately ill patients hoping against hope for benefit from nonbeneficial research, Annas proposes that only minimal-risk research be permitted and that physician researchers recruit the patients of other physicians for their research. That makes sense, with the qualification that Miller and his colleagues underlined, that it will be difficult for sick people to distinguish between the obligations of their own physicians toward their well-being and the obligation of the researcher, also a physician.

Research in developing countries. The very first issue of the *Hastings Center Report*, in June 1971, contained an article by Robert M. Veatch exposing a situation little known at that time, the use of developing countries as handy venues for research.[62] Veatch's article looked at contraception research in Puerto Rico, part of the United States of course but otherwise at that time much like a developing country. The advantages of those countries, or Puerto Rico, were principally two: the possibility of much less expensive research, and the even more attractive possibility of doing an end run on human-subject regulatory systems. The practice of turning to developing countries as research sites persists to this day, steadily growing all the while, and the motives remain much the same. Its most active promoters are for-profit contract research organizations that organize research trials in developing countries. The great difference now is that the practice attracts more notice and takes the research protocols and subject protection rules more seriously. Many groups have made a systematic effort to set the entire issue within the context of global standards of health care justice and access to care. In that respect, the problem is now understood at two levels. One of them is that of devising appropriate ethical standards for clinical trials in developing countries, and the other is the pursuit of greater equity in the relationship of rich and poor countries.

Both levels figured prominently in a debate that captured attention at the end of the 1990s and the start of the new millennium. Probably the most significant triggering event was a sometimes nasty argument about the conduct of clinical trials in Africa to test a short-course AZT (azidothymidine) treatment with pregnant women to reduce the birth of children with HIV (human immunodeficiency virus). That battle centered on two issues, one being the use of placebos when the value of AZT in a standard long-course procedure was already known to be efficacious. The other was the underlying "standard of practice" with research in developing countries—should it embody the same standards used in developed countries or standards more context-dependent and resource-realistic?

Meanwhile, as that dual struggle was taking place, the World Medical Association was working its way toward a revised Helsinki Declaration, one that would turn out to be the third such declaration to reflect important changes. Between them, the AZT and Helsinki battles set the stage for a fresh look at research in developing countries, at a time when the disparities in health care between developed and developing countries became all the more known, and embarrassingly, shamefully, so.

The loudest and most noticed salvo in the complex battle that followed was the attack in the *New England Journal of Medicine* by two physicians long associated with Ralph Nader's public advocacy group Public Citizen, Peter Lurie and Sidney Wolfe, on short-course AZT trials being carried out principally in Africa. The trials were said to display a double standard, displaying practices that would not be tolerated in the United States, particularly the use of placebos.[63] An accompanying editorial by Marcia Angell, then executive editor of the journal, supported the attack and took the argument a step further. "The justifications for the research," she wrote, "are reminiscent of . . . Tuskegee," particularly in the defense that the women in the placebo group, receiving no treatment, were no worse off than they had been before the research, and thus had not been harmed.[64] There is something to the comparison, but what was most objectionable with Tuskegee was the fact that the four hundred men in the study received no penicillin when it became available and was inexpensive to use. There was no parallel in the short-course AZT trials, whose aim was to test efficacy, not to see what would happen without treatment.

Harold Varmus, the director of the NIH, and David Satcher, the surgeon general, issued a brisk defense of the study.[65] For one thing, they said, it had been supported by the Ugandans, who approved and carried out the trial—though with support from the NIH and the Centers for Disease Control and Prevention (CDC)—and, for another, only a placebo-controlled trial would turn up results usable and feasible in poor countries. A comparison with the full-course AZT treatment would be irrelevant since that was not a financially viable option for those countries. Barry Bloom, chair of the UNAIDS Vaccine Committee, echoed that thought, asking how there could ever be efficacy trials on AIDS vaccines or other interventions of use to a country if the "best proven standard" of the developed countries was applied.[66]

In a fine survey of the debate two years later, David Rothman came down on the Angell side, noting a variety of dubious trials then under way, as well as the financial and other incentives to use poor countries for research. "Abject poverty," he noted, "is harsh enough without people having to bear the additional burdens of serving as research subjects"—adding, as many were by then, that it is not enough that investigators should not leave their subjects worse off; they should be left better off. [67]

By October 2000 the World Medical Association had finished its revisions of the Declaration of Helsinki. Those revisions were strong and far-reaching, representing a clear victory for those who wanted firmer protection of subjects and a more equitable outcome for those who become subjects. It recognizes that medical progress requires experimentation on human subjects (article 4) but reiterated the principle that "the well-being of the human subject should take precedence over the interests of science and society" (article 5). It stressed the need for informed consent and a careful assessment of risks and benefits and addressed with nuance the use of those who cannot give consent as subjects.

The most radical and far-reaching part of the revisions, however, centered on the question of benefits of research participation for the subjects and for the host country of research projects. No group, it stated, should be included in research unless the research is necessary to promote the health of that group, and be likely to benefit from it (article 19). Any new therapeutic method should be tested against the best available method, and that placebos should be used only when "no proven . . . therapeutic measure exists"(article 29). At the end of the study, it insisted that every subject should have access to the best treatment identified by the study (article 30).[68]

It is an old axiom in ethics that "ought implies can." It is thus reasonable to ask whether the new Declaration of Helsinki and the philosophy it represents are likely to effect the changes sought in the whole structure of research in poor countries. Those changes can easily be summarized: research should treat subjects just the same as, and perhaps even better than, subjects in affluent countries; it should aim to benefit the group of which its subjects are a part; and its results ought specifically to benefit those in the group after it is over. By adopting as the "standard of care" that of affluent countries, the declaration states that cheaper, somewhat less effective treatments cannot be pursued and that, in any case, placebo trials cannot be used when there are effective treatments already available. No one who might benefit from an available treatment ought to be denied it by being enrolled in a placebo control group.

On its face, then, the revisions appear to be a clear defeat for the research imperative, as sometimes practiced in developing countries. Or perhaps a bit more precisely, that imperative will in the future have more obstacles in its path and be more expensive to pursue.[69] There are three serious problems here. The first is that placebo trials still represent the best scientific method for measuring the likely impact of a new treatment on a particular population (not to mention the fact that FDA policies permit placebos). The benefit to some subjects of a denial of placebo trials in a research protocol may well lead to harm in others, denied the possible knowledge that a treatment might not be good for them. There was a response to this objection: that the science would have been better if the new regimen had been used, which could then have been compared with the accepted 076 regimen (the standard regimen in developed countries). A placebo arm for the trial was, moreover, simply not needed. I remain uncertain on this point. The issue in the AZT trials was not just, as the critics alleged, whether the new, cheaper regimen compared well with the 076 regimen, but what other effects it might have. A placebo arm is one traditional way of making such a determination.

The second problem is whether the revisions—which are in any case voluntary guidelines only—will make it financially difficult, if not impossible, for research to be carried out at all in many cases. The political aim of the revisions is to put pressure on those supporting the research, or financially benefiting from it, to improve the lot of those they have used as subjects. In some cases that pressure can work, as is now the case in Thailand where an AIDS vaccine is being tested and an agreement reached that any successful vaccine will be made available to the subjects. It is surely imperative, at a minimum, that the subjects themselves be able to benefit and thus receive free drugs. Should all those in a country who come down with a disease in the future for which the research has proved successful receive a like benefit? That is less likely to be feasible without considerable external support from affluent governments, and not just from, say, pharmaceutical companies.

In sum, the Helsinki revisions represent a bold political move, the success of which will for a time remain uncertain. The international resources exist on paper to support the provision of even expensive drugs to poor countries. One of the great dramas of coming decades will be to see whether in fact those resources can be transferred to poor countries. The revised Declaration of Helsinki represents an important opening wedge, as do recent efforts (as with AIDS treatments in Africa) to induce the for-profit sector to allow free or inexpensive licensing arrangements, or to guarantee free or inexpensive distribution of beneficial products.

The third problem is one that has, so far, not drawn comment. Do the Helsinki guidelines effectively bar altruistically motivated subjects from volunteering to take part in research that will not benefit them (now allowed in affluent countries)? Or allow them, as is also possible in affluent countries, to receive a small fee for their participation in nonbeneficial research? Would they preclude, as is now common, the gaining of consent for research from community or group leaders, or would the standards of informed consent have to match those in affluent countries, not always easy to achieve even with well-educated groups in some cases (for instance, chemotherapy trials for cancer treatment)?

The answers to those questions are not clear, but they touch on the issue of paternalism. The assumption that all poor people are potential victims of exploitation, to be protected from their own bad choices and not allowed the range of free decision making allowed in affluent countries, is paternalistic, perhaps even patronizing. Whether there will be a reaction along those lines from the developing countries remains to be seen. If that kind of reaction comes from politicians and local researchers possibly influenced by financial inducements to approve research, the unpleasant complexity will rise to high levels. There was, it might be observed, a note of indignation in a letter written to the NIH in 1997 by the chairman of the AIDS research committee of the Uganda Cancer Institute when he said that "these are Uganda studies conducted by Ugandan investigators on Ugandans. . . . It is not NIH conducting the studies in Uganda but Ugandans conducting their study on their people for the good of their people." Two commentators noted, however, that the important role of the NIH and CDC in helping organize the studies belied that claim; and they dismissed as an outdated and dangerous cultural relativism the notion that, even if Ugandan-run, the studies were exempt from criticism.[70]

While the charge of Western imperialism, or Western paternalism, was not directly raised by the Uganda chairman, its possibility has been noted by at least a few seasoned observers. Two widely respected physicians, one from South Africa and the other from Canada—writing just before the publication of the revised Helsinki Declaration—made two points of importance. One of them asserted, "it has been incorrectly assumed that the standard [of care] set by developed countries can be considered the norm," adding that "little attention was paid to the fact [in the AZT short-course trials] that there were many differences between pregnant women in developed countries and those in countries where the 'best proven treatments had been established.' "[71]

As for placebo controlled trials, "these should be considered on their merits rather than be precluded by a bluntly designed exclusive clause in a declaration." While "the highest achievable standard of care should be the goal . . . the objective should be to ratchet the standard upward rather than to set utopian goals that cannot be met." It is important to "distinguish moral relativism from the morally relevant considerations of context."[72] The two physicians then go on to propose a set of norms for "redefining" a standard of care they think more suitable for international health research—but which is, in fact, not all that different (if less peremptory) than the Helsinki guidelines that were to appear a month after their article was published. If neither directly addresses the issue of imperialism and paternalism, lurking in all such guidelines, I find it noteworthy and reassuring not simply that international guidelines are being worked on and promulgated, but that they have on the whole met a warm reception. They will hinder some research, but they should in the long run advance the cause of research. The developing countries desperately need the benefits of medical research, and the only cautionary note would be to add that they need good research.[73]

Human-Subject Research as a Model for All Research

I began this chapter by raising the possibility that human-subject research might serve as a model for all research as an antidote to an overweening research imperative. I noted the contrast between trends in human-subject research toward firmer norms and a decisive priority given to subject protection over scientific or social needs, and the contrasting movement in other areas of medical research toward research imperatives impatient with regulatory road blocks and ethical hand-wringing. The trend in human-subject research has been toward a firm, uncompromising position on the need for informed consent from subjects; rejection of utilitarian arguments in favor of research even it might save lives; greater care and protection of incompetent subjects; a great suspicion of the practices and motives of for-profit companies pursuing or organizing research in developing countries; and in the international arena generally, the carrying out of research that is helpful to various research populations but also makes a contribution to greater international health care equity.

The trend has been different with other forms of research: too little resistance to for-profit research; a focus on potential individual benefits and expansion of personal choice rather than community, much less international, benefits; too little concern for the progress-driven rise in health care costs and a consequent threat to equitable access; a seemingly systematic campaign by technological enthusiasts to find a way of legitimating just about any new development that comes along; and a bias toward what I identified in chapter 5 as the "gambler's principle," far more attractive than a nervous-Nelly precautionary principle. Human-subject research has seen a precautionary principle pushed about as far as it can go; while in other forms of research, many efforts have been made to deride and dismantle it.

Two explanations for the difference seem plausible. The first is that human-subject research has the Nazi experience as part of its history—as striking a cautionary tale as can be imagined—followed by Willowbrook, Tuskegee, and other domestic atrocities. A lesson taken to heart from those experiences is that nothing less than a hard, tough principle of informed consent can prevent abuses and atrocities in the name of research, for good or bad motives. "Without autonomy," Robert Veatch has written, "there is the abyss."[74] When autonomy is not possible, nothing less than eternal vigilance and the most demanding kind of precautionary principles will suffice to justify the use of incompetent subjects.

Human-subject research has developed, in short, an uncommonly solid moral anchor, firmly resistant to moral relativism, to the attraction of relieving the suffering of the many at the cost of risk to the few, and prone—when standards and practices become lax—to move back toward the highest, most demanding ethical standards (of which the revised Helsinki Declaration is as good an example as any of this impetus). It should be obvious also that the protection of autonomy—the negative liberty afforded by informed consent, the right to be left alone from the uses to which others might put one—is a principle highly congenial to both the liberal left and the market-oriented right. It is probably the only imaginable principle that can stand up against a research imperative that might visibly do harm.

The second explanation is that the rest of research has no equivalent moral anchor, no single, strong, and clear principle that can say no to the research imperative. While there is certainly some worry about dangers from research possibilities, individual and communal, and various moral principles that can be brought to bear in thinking about them, none has the stark clarity, the unyielding solidity of the informed consent principle in its most common articulations. The lessons of history show us the opposite. During the eugenics movement of the late nineteenth and early twentieth centuries, the worship of scientific knowledge and the faith in its applicability to various social ills led to many evils. But many people resolutely *rejected* its lessons: the times were different, the science was bad, the new eugenics is clean (or so they say). The fact that it began in good enough faith (for the most part) and then went downhill does not mean it could not happen again. Perhaps it may well never happen again, but at least one minor sign of the force of the present research imperative is that even imagining a similar trajectory for the present genetics movement becomes, for many research enthusiasts, a sign of outright, irrational hostility to recent scientific developments.

If the present research imperative in general lacks a moral anchor that is the equivalent of the informed consent principle for human-subject research, it ironically has in the principle of autonomy one of its main allies. The research imperative often uses that principle to celebrate the possibility of, and right to, personal choice, which is a variant of the right to be let alone. As the next chapter tries to show, many of the most controversial lines of research find their final justification in the value of open and free research and in the right of individuals, not society, to decide what use to make of the fruits of that research. They usually minimize (or simply accept) claims of possible societal harm. Their net result is to force the research imperative back into the space of "balancing" risks and benefits—where disagreement is likely always to exist as to what counts as risk and benefit.

The backdrop of that effort is the ethos of pluralistic societies that aim not to discover what the good of humans is (thought to be an inherently dangerous venture) but how those with different visions of the good can live together in some kind of harmony. That means it is difficult to have any meaningful probe of the social implications, or the human meaning, of the scientific ambitions and possibilities. Even worse, as I will develop in the next chapter, the now-standard strategy for dealing with moral disagreement has been to fashion an understanding of pluralism and public reasoning that all but guarantees that most serious struggles will favor the research imperative. What in theory is meant to be a level playing field is in fact sharply tilted.

7   Pluralism, Balance, and Controversy

Hardly anyone denies that medical research may along with bringing great benefits also on occasion open the way to harm, medical or social. What is to be done when debates about that possibility break out? The history of research, medical and otherwise, has notoriously been marked by controversies. Some turned on the scientific validity of research projects, while others turned on political, social, and ethical disagreements. The Galileo case, Pasteur's work, Darwin's theories, early experiments with anesthesia, or the struggle within physics over the use of nuclear weapons, are obvious examples. Even if controversies are not more numerous now, they certainly seem more public, sometimes focusing on dangers in carrying out the research and sometimes on ominous ethical and social implications. With some frequency of late, governmental commissions have been appointed to deal with them. Characteristically, partisans of the research imperative are pitted against those who have anxieties about or objections to some research. One side sees the research as benign, the other as hazardous. Freedom of scientific inquiry, often with the aid of disease advocacy groups, says go. The critics say stop or slow down.

How ought disagreements be dealt with in democratic, pluralistic societies? What does it mean to "balance" moral concerns and scientific possibilities? What is the proper role of religious, ideological, and medical interests? First I summarize a number of debates that have taken place over the past thirty years or so (but emphasizing the most recent), grouping them in different categories. Then I try to tease out the various threads that run through them.

SOME IMPORTANT CASES

Recombinant DNA. While it might be something of an exaggeration to say, as did a reporter for *Science* in 2000, that the 1975 Asilomar conference on recombinant DNA research "was the Woodstock of molecular biology: a defining moment for a generation, a milestone in the history of science and society," it was surely a significant opening round in the debates that continue to this day.[1] A group of leading molecular biologists organized the conference to discuss the exciting new technique of "gene splicing." That technique, the cutting of DNA strands in a precise way in order to splice them into the DNA of other organisms, promised to open the way to a whole new order of genetic understanding. It also carried with it, at least in speculative theory, the possibility of turning otherwise benign microbes into pathogens such as cancer-causing agents or harmful toxins. A voluntary moratorium called in 1974 in response to that worry was to be discussed in California in 1975 at the Asilomar conference center.

With that conference, the moratorium was lifted, but strict controls were proposed for future work.[2] At the first meeting of the National Institutes of Health's newly established Recombinant DNA Advisory Committee, held right after the Asilomar conference, a number of precautionary guidelines were put into place and a monitoring system established. The ethical focus of the moratorium and of the events that followed was the safety of the research, not its broader social implications. As it turned out, while the worst scenarios did not materialize, there has been persistent, though unpublicized, evidence that gene splicing can easily produce unanticipated pathogens.[3] A number of scientists, led by James D. Watson, were sorry that the issue had ever been made public and—since none of the projected harms materialized—could and did repeatedly say in effect afterward "we told you so."[4]

As the years went by, and no obvious hazards appeared, the recombinant advisory committee was gradually marginalized and almost eliminated entirely in 1998 by Harold Varmus, then NIH director.[5] Narrow in scope, the recombinant DNA debate was the first serious public debate about the new genetics. It would hardly be the last.

The violence wars. The 1960s and 1970s were times of social unrest and, noticeably, rising rates of violence, not only protest events but also general criminal violence. Some scientists proposed research on violence. The prominent black psychologist Kenneth Clark speculated in the 1970s on the value of developing a pill to reduce it. That proposal drew more jibes than serious interest, but two other projects of a more systematic kind appeared. Public protest eventually shut them both down.

In 1972 Drs. Louis Jolyon West, director of the Neuropsychiatric Institute at UCLA, and James M. Stubblebine, director of health for the state of California, wanted to establish a center for the study and reduction of violence. That initiative was mentioned by Governor Ronald Reagan in his 1973 State of the State address as part of his mental health program. At first there was great enthusiasm for the idea, but opposition soon developed, some of it centered around rumors of planned psychosurgery on prisoners and other "undesirable" people. In the summer of 1973, a meeting was held in the apartment of Huey Newton, leader of the Black Panthers, to see if a compromise could be reached. It could not and efforts to stop the center moved from the state to the federal level. Senator Sam Ervin, chairman of the Senate Judiciary Committee, declared that the federal Law Enforcement Assistance Administration should not support the center (though an earlier grant application had been approved). By early 1974 the project was dying.

The protests had succeeded, but not because of direct attacks on the scientific validity of such research. Instead, in Dr. West's view, plausibly enough, the protests reflected the paranoia of the times, the fear that a covert plot was under way to do harm to minority groups. He did not seem to consider the possibility that minority fears were not altogether a fantasy. A most successful tactic employed by opponents of the center, one supporter conceded, "centered on the abuses of the knowledge that might follow from our work."[6]

The other project to meet a similar fate was research on the XYY phenomenon, the supposed link between males with an extra Y chromosome and a predisposition to violence.[7] The discovery of the extra chromosome went back to 1961, but it was not until 1970 that research began in earnest to see if there was a behavioral link to it. Stanley Walzer, a Harvard psychiatrist, developed a simple and inexpensive karyotyping test and began randomly screening newborns in the Boston Hospital for Women that year. He lectured and published on the subject without much problem for a time but in 1974 became the target of a concerted attack by various activist groups, most notably Science for the People and two of its important scientific organizers, Jonathan King of MIT and Jonathan Beckwith of Harvard. "Although the correlation between genetic constitutions such as XYY is not a scientific fact," a Science for the People publication said, "it gives pseudoscientific backing for the current ideology of 'blaming the victim.' "[8] The objections ranged from worries about stigmatizing the carriers of the XYY genotype through belittling the scientific claims about an alleged syndrome

to criticizing the informed consent procedures used to gain research subjects.

A formal complaint lodged at Harvard against Walzer and the project led
to several committee reviews. Though the Harvard faculty eventually voted
to support the research, a media campaign and personal vilification of Dr.
Walzer, together with an attack by the Children's Defense Fund and threats
of a lawsuit, led him to stop screening in May 1975.[9] A well-known scientist, Bernard Davis, appalled at the demise of the research, was to write in the
aftermath that "the XYY story . . . raises the old problem of how a democracy can protect itself from those who would use freedom of speech to deprive others of significant freedoms—in this case, freedom of inquiry, and
the patient's freedom to know."[10] Around the same time an NIH-supported
project on the XYY condition was shut down because of a lawsuit even
though it had won peer approval and passed IRB inspection.[11]

That was effectively the end of XYY research, which in any event did not
gain scientific support for the idea of a causal connection between violence
and the extra chromosome.[12] But it was not the end of violence research,
which continued, unremarkably, in a low key. An official of the National
Institute of Mental Health would warn, some twenty-five years later,
"Efforts to try and identify people who are likely to be violent . . . could result in labeling people."[13] By then, that was an old story.

Behavioral genetics.   Looked at generically, what I call the "violence wars"
were actually local skirmishes within a long-standing battle, summed up in
the term "behavioral genetics." That battle, for and against such research,
began in the 1960s and continues to this day. As that term implies, the research aim is to see what relationship exists between human behavior and
genetics or, put more technically, between genetic variation and behavioral
phenotypes. I liken the controversy to a cold war: the stakes are high; the
contest has endured for many years; and each side is strong in its supporters and arguments, yet neither side for many decades was able to achieve a
clear victory. Of late, though, it appears that behavioral genetics is gradually
outlasting its critics, finally gaining some respectability[14]—even if solid scientific gains remain scant.

Behavioral genetics has had difficulty achieving acceptance for one general reason and many particular ones. The general reason is this: almost
everyone is prepared to grant the truth of a bland truism, that human behavior has a mix of genetic and environmental causes—but that leaves
plenty of room to make claims about the relative weight of the causes in
particular instances. Often enough, neither side can achieve a decisive scien-

tific victory. Almost always it is a matter of finding the right mix, and almost always that target is elusive, shifting from year to year as research advances (as with the relationship between genetics and IQ). Among the more particular sources of controversy are the volatility of issues that behavioral genetics has looked into: violence (as we have seen), race and IQ, and homosexuality, for instance, along with more personal traits like impulsivity and shyness. There is no obvious socially tolerable way to examine the behaviors and traits that upset people without risk of offending or stigmatizing any groups.[15] The domain of inquiry and the social mud it can stir up are hard to tell apart.

As the research on violence demonstrated, the worries about behavioral genetics bear more on the possible misuse of the knowledge generated than on the safety of the research. The possible misuses (many of them cited again and again) are stigmatization of, and discrimination against, those found to have a particular gene or combination of genes; reducing life to genetics; putting money into genetic research that would be better invested in social programs; and explaining away social problems by blaming them on our genes (as well as "blaming the victim"). Not only the media, but some scientists are now and then enthusiastically capable of saying that a gene for some trait has been discovered, implying that the related behavior has been thereby explained, with a direct causal relationship between gene and behavior. At the other end of the spectrum, the most extreme claim made by the leaders of Science for the People in the 1970s was that the smuggling of social assumptions into science without acknowledging that it had been done (as with race and IQ, for instance) nullified any claims to freedom of scientific inquiry.[16]

In an eloquent response to such worries, and to threats to behavioral genetics as a whole, E. O. Wilson wrote in 1978 that "to agree to a policy of ignorance is merely the equivalent of surrendering discussion to uninformed ideologues."[17] I would amend his judgment by adding overly enthusiastic genetic researchers and their lay acolytes to that group. Writing many years later, Erik Parens noted that two errors have long held sway in the field. One of them is to posit a Cartesian-like split between mind and body, holding that genetic tampering with human life poses no serious problems for human dignity and rationality, since whatever happens to the body cannot harm the mind. The other error is to assume that the use of genetic facts inevitably harms good values and promotes bad ones.[18] Neither need prevail.

The embryo and reproduction wars. Another, even larger and more complex, conflict with few signs of thawing overshadows the waning battles of behavioral genetics. I call these the embryo and reproduction wars because, one way or another, they draw on two deep issues in our society, abortion and reproductive rights. When these issues are combined with the research imperative, they cut across many ideological party lines; various efforts are then made to find compromises or accommodations that will allow research to go forward. Unlike the violence struggles, they have attracted a great deal of congressional attention and occasioned federal commissions.

The first, a short-lived debate, came in 1973 over a proposal to allow medical research with newly delivered live fetuses. That debate did not so much get resolved as swallowed up by the proposal to establish a national commission for the protection of human subjects, finally approved by Congress in 1994.[19] The first really serious debate in recent years was occasioned by a 1987 request from researchers at the NIH to use tissue from aborted fetuses. The director of the NIH then sought approval of this fetal tissue research from the secretary of the Department of Health and Human Services, Louis Sullivan. In response, the secretary established a federal moratorium on grants for such research in 1988 until an advisory committee was formed to make recommendations on future research. That summer, a twenty-one-person panel was assembled, which reported its findings to the NIH director's advisory committee. The report said that the use of fetal tissue could continue as long as some guidelines were put in place. The committee concluded that "the consensus of the Panel reflected the consensus of the country itself."[20]

If there was such a consensus, the Reagan administration ignored it and, in 1989, indefinitely continued the moratorium established a year earlier. It set various regulations, among them a prohibition on the sale or purchase of fetal organs and of any payments for tissue that might serve as an inducement to have an abortion for that purpose. (One of President Clinton's first acts in office in 1993 was to lift the moratorium on research grants. In the aftermath of Clinton's move a fairly vigorous commerce in fetal tissues already in place accelerated, supposedly to be tempered by a requirement of "reasonable payments" only for the purveyors of tissue.)

In what might be termed the first salvo in a now-familiar ritual, to block the use of fetal cell tissue from aborted fetuses the Reagan administration went right to the heart of a recurrent theme, that of the abortion debate. Among the objections to the use of the tissue was the charge that it could encourage abortion for the purpose of tissue retrieval, that it would be an act of complicity with the evil of abortion, and that it amounted to a commodification of human life. Supporters of the research argued that, if a woman was legally free to have an abortion for any reason whatever, it should be her decision whether to make tissue from her fetus available; that the tissue (which would otherwise be discarded) could be put to altruistic use for research and therapeutic purposes; and that research would have scientific benefits.

Fetal tissue use was hardly new, even in 1988. Fetal tissues from aborted fetuses had been used for research and therapeutic purposes since at least the 1920s, and in 1988 the NIH itself spent $8.3 million for such tissue.[21] Fetal cells offer a number of advantages for transplantation: those cells do not elicit an immune response in recipients; the tissue cells continue to grow and divide; and they are able to differentiate after transplantation. Tissue transplants to the pancreas, thymus, liver, and brain have been used for therapeutic ends. With the exception of successful transplants for DiGeorge's syndrome, a congenital birth defect, the various other efforts have had mixed results.

The use of fetal brain tissue to relieve Parkinson's disease has received the most attention and considerable research. Many researchers have welcomed—and strenuously lobbied for—its potential as a source of knowledge. As its backers said—transforming promising research possibility to virtual certainty—it was just a matter of time and research money. Well over a decade later, the heralded research imperative to treat or cure Parkinson's disease with fetal tissue transplants has shown relatively poor results, with some scientists now arguing that it may never prove to be a viable treatment and that embryonic stem cells and other alternatives are more promising.[22] The virtual failure of the research made the earlier zeal and confidence temptingly easy to forget.

The step from fetal tissue research to embryo research, technically known as ex utero preimplantation research, was a short one. The British led the way here, making embryo research legal up to fourteen days of gestation based on recommendations of the 1984 Warnock committee.[23] Embryo research encompasses a number of possibilities: research on embryos left over from successful in vitro fertilization (IVF) attempts, creation of embryos specifically for research purposes, and the division of embryos into more than one part. Embryo research, its advocates speculated, might lead to knowledge valuable for the relief of infertility, to a better understanding of the development of early-stage embryos, to techniques for preimplantation diagnosis of genetic and chromosomal abnormalities, to the prevention of miscarriages, and to increased knowledge of cancer and its metastasis.

In 1979 the Department of Health, Education, and Welfare's Ethics Advisory Board (EAB) issued a report on embryo research, granting permission for such research but requiring approval by the board, which would regulate the research. Its reasoning in support of embryo research was that the moral claims made on behalf of the embryo must be balanced against the potential therapeutic and research benefits of the research, and that "health needs of women, children, and men must be given priority."[24]

The Reagan and Bush administrations, however, withheld funds from the board (which lasted only two years, from 1978 to 1980), resulting in a de facto moratorium on the use of any federal money for embryo research. Over a decade passed before research prospects revived. In June 1993 Congress passed a law nullifying the requirement for EAB approval, and NIH then undertook to establish its Human Embryo Research Panel to make recommendations on NIH policy. The panel issued a report in December 1994 recommending NIH support of such research, including the creation of embryos specifically for research purposes. President Clinton, however, overruled the creation of embryos for research purposes, and Congress followed suit in 1995, barring funds for any research that threatened the survival of embryos. That prohibition affected only federal support for the research, leaving the private sector free to pursue it, without federal oversight, and it has done so. Opponents of the research had won the day, heavily but not exclusively led by conservative religious and political groups.

By the mid-1990s the controversies were heating up. The most sensational of all—the possibility of human cloning research—though by no means the most important, was occasioned by Ian Wilmut's announcement in 1997 that in 1996 a cloned sheep, Dolly, had been born, created by the technique of somatic cell nuclear transfer (SCNT). That technique encompassed the transfer of an adult sheep's udder cell nucleus into a sheep's egg from which the nucleus had been removed. This feat, soon used with other animals, showed that an adult (nonreproductive) somatic cell contained all the genetic and biological information necessary to reprogram an unfertilized egg into developing into a completely new living being. The possibility, long debated, of using the same technique to clone a human being, became at once realistic. That possibility set off a huge clamor in scientific journals, among the public, in the Oval Office, and in Congress.

President Clinton's quick response was to announce that there could be no federal funding for research on human cloning, and a number of bills were introduced in Congress and many state legislatures to ban any such research. The National Bioethics Advisory Commission concluded in June 1997 that there should be a moratorium on human cloning research for a period of five years, after which the matter should be reexamined.[25] On the surface, then, it appeared that the research hardly stood a chance of being carried out in the public or private sector. That appearance was somewhat misleading. Efforts to pass a bill in the U.S. Senate to bar research met a well-organized, and successful, effort by leading scientists to kill the bill, and Congress did not pass a general ban in the years immediately following Dolly's birth. A number of scientists, some citing the deleterious opposition of "religion," held that the research could have valuable benefits, and a variety of ethicists devised arguments about how some needy or desirous couples might benefit from the ability to clone a child.

In the summer of 2001, however, the House of Representatives passed a bill to ban cloning, for either reproduction or research. In December 2001 a less restrictive bill was introduced into the Senate (S1758) to ban reproductive cloning but to permit what has been called "therapeutic cloning," cloning for research purposes only. In addition to a strong consensus among scientists that reproductive cloning was almost certain to produce abnormalities, there was as well the motive of preserving, and legitimating therapeutic cloning (perhaps more accurately called "research cloning"). A report by the National Academy of Sciences also urged a ban on reproductive cloning, a most unusual stand for a committee of scientists.[26] In addition to the Senate bill to ban reproductive cloning only, there is another that would ban all forms of cloning (S1899, sponsored by Sam Brownback, a Republican). As this book goes to press, no bill on cloning has yet passed both houses of Congress.

Tellingly, the National Bioethics Advisory Commission proposed a moratorium but could reach no consensus on most of the ethical issues of reproductive cloning, falling back only on moral worries about the safety of the research for children so procreated. Opponents of the research declared that to allow couples to clone a child was an unwarranted extension of reproductive rights, a threat to human dignity, and a violation of a child's right to its own genetic future, not one selected by its parents. When in the spring of 2001 a new round of debate on cloning broke out in Congress, the precipitating event was an announcement by the Raelian religious group and some Italian scientists that they would attempt to clone a baby. Around the same time, scientific reports began to appear indicating abnormalities in all cloned animals, including Dolly.[27] A strong consensus seemed to emerge: because of the potential physical harm to a cloned child, the research to create such a child should not be undertaken at all; there was no such consensus on therapeutic cloning.

If the possibility of human cloning caught the public imagination, the prospect of stem cell research had generated comparable scientific interest in 1998. The term "stem cells" ordinarily refers to cells in the human body that renew tissues, but of greatest interest are those found in an early-stage embryo. Embryonic stem (ES) cells have the capacity to develop into almost any cell type, while embryonic germ (EG) cells, with properties similar to ES cells, come from the primordial reproductive cells of the developing fetus. Though ES cells are *pluripotent,* able to develop into all the cells and tissues of the human body, they are not *totipotent,* because they could not develop into full individuals. When two researchers in 1998 reported the successful isolation and culturing of ES and EG cells, the excitement was intense. Suddenly a theoretical way lay open to the use of those cells not only for embryogenesis research and gene research but for important therapeutic purposes as well, most notably, the generation of new cells to treat injuries and disease, with Alzheimer's, Parkinson's, heart disease, and kidney failure frequently mentioned.

Once again a battle broke out between more or less the same combatants who had appeared in the earlier struggles over fetal tissue and embryo research (and, in fact, the possibility of stem cell research had been an ingredient in the second case). Stem cells have a number of potential sources: human fetal tissue following elective abortion; human embryos created by IVF but no longer required by couples undergoing fertility treatment; embryos created through IVF with gametes donated for the purpose of providing research material; and possibly various cloning techniques.

The reported cultivation of stem cells quickly provoked alarm and excitement among its allies and opponents. Coalitions formed for and against the research and some on each side lobbied Congress.[28] In January 1999 the NIH determined that the restriction of federal funds for embryo research did not apply to research using stem cells; they are not embryos. But the ban did seem to prevent NIH from deriving stem cells from embryos. That opened the way for federally supported research with embryonic stem cells provided by private sources. Current law already allows for the derivation of ES cells from an aborted fetus because it is already dead but does not address derivation from a live embryo; ES cells' removal kills the embryo (though some advocates would prefer to say "disaggregates" rather than "kills").

Yet for the research to go forward in practice with federal funds, the NIH had to draft guidelines and did so with an eye on the recommendations of the National Bioethics Advisory Commission (NBAC). The NBAC recommended that research involving both the derivation and use of human ES cells from embryos remaining after IVF treatment should be eligible for federal funds. The NIH guidelines followed the NBAC recommendations but differed in one significant respect, disallowing federally funded researchers to derive stem cells from human embryos. NBAC recommended that the private sector should follow its different rules, which would allow researchers to derive and use stem cells. The Geron Corporation and Advanced Cell Technology most notably have made an investment in private research, and their supporters have argued that applying the same rules to the public and private sector would speed research and obviate possible abuses. Others, also in support of the research, take a contrary approach, arguing that the absence of federal regulation in the private sector is a blessing in disguise, freeing the research from regulatory oversight.[29]

Germ-line research. The last case I cite is that of germ-line research. Though discussed as a speculative possibility earlier, germ-line research—called "inheritable genetic modifications" by some—refers to the manipulation of the germinal cells, the sexual cells, the egg and the sperm: in effect, the fertilized egg.[30] A genetic alteration in the fertilized egg would be copied into every cell of the adult, including the sexual cells, and thus ordinarily passed along to future generations. This kind of research is different from somatic cell research, where the aim is to replace a harmful gene with a healthy one, in a limited set of tissues or organs, by what has been called gene therapy. The changed gene does not affect the next generation's genetic material. The latter therapy has occasioned little ethical concern (other than the possibility of accidental harm to germ cells), but difficulty in making it work (reports of the first successful cases date from 2000) and the death of Jesse Gelsinger have slowed its progress.

The attraction of germ-line research is the possibility of its use someday to cure disease and do so perhaps more easily than somatic cell therapy. If it could cure a disease in a person, that same capacity could exempt the next generation as well, whereas somatic cell therapy could not. A more futuristic use is that of enhancement of various human traits or capacities, such as intelligence and memory, though so far the greatest emphasis has been placed on the likely health benefits, a powerful form of preventive medicine for genetic diseases that get passed along from generation to generation.

At present the federal government does not accept proposals for germ-line therapy research. The reasons for its policy go back some years, to the early 1980s. Citing potential hazards from the research itself to the persons who would have such therapy, the unknown consequences of passing genetic changes along to future generations, and the whiff of eugenics that would come from the elimination of "bad traits," the president's commission in 1983 said that there are "strong contraindications against therapy of fertilized eggs or embryos becoming a useful clinical option in the future."[31] Of late an affirmation of the need for careful animal studies before any effort with human beings and of the research value in the effort with humans have countered the objections, along with minimization of the technique's social implications as simply another form of medical progress, with altered genes not necessarily posing greater problems than unaltered genes.[32] Even more broadly, emphasis on the fact of ignorance about the consequences— for some, a reason not to go ahead—is turned into an argument that, knowing so little, researchers have all the more reason to proceed. It is the "gambler's principle" at work.[33] Others have noted that no such technology can be transferred with impunity from one species to another, and that to use untested methods to generate new human beings is inherently hazardous and therefore unethical.[34]

Unlike the other cases I have cited, germ-line research has not led to a specific federal commission to study it, or to any persistent public or legislative hostility. The debate has been quiet and academic in flavor, perhaps because there is little or no such research under way.[35] Nonetheless, it is an important issue because of a shift from outright resistance to the research among scientists in the 1980s toward favor for it in the 1990s. In the absence of notable scientific breakthroughs pointing one way or the other, the change seems to me best attributable to the growing power of the research imperative in the 1990s, which I speculate has shifted the imagination away from research dangers toward beneficial possibilities. And unlike the struggles over fetal tissue, embryo, and stem cell research, it has not inspired the opposition of any particular group even if there remain many doubters.[36]

SOME ETHICAL ARGUMENTS

As I analyze these debates I have summarized, I want to distinguish between the substantive ethical issues at stake and the policy assumptions and strategies that have been brought to bear in managing them. In general (though not always), heavy-handed research advocacy or bias has given short shrift to the ethical issues, and various policy strategies have not encouraged a fair and open debate.

Three important ethical issues provide a good place to start searching for the threads that run through the examples I will offer: arguments on the research imperative, on safety and the social implications of research, and on abortion and the embryo's moral status.

The research imperative.   In the context of the debates I have described, the research imperative generally takes two forms, the one benign and the other hazardous. The logic of the research imperative's benign form is this:

scientific researchers propose to pursue a particular line of research and often have a preferred direction in which they want to go (without implying it is necessarily the best or only way to go); they (and their lay supporters) hold that the research may be valuable in its results but do not say that it is morally obligatory; if there are objections to the research on ethical or social grounds, the researchers try to modify their work to respond to the criticism; and if the results prove not to be promising, the researchers move in another direction.

The morally hazardous form of the research imperative responds differently. The proposed research is called morally obligatory, and it is either said or implied that the chosen research direction is the only or the incontestably superior way to go; its proponents dismiss critics of the research as ignorant, fearful, or biased and make only superficial changes to mollify them; and when the research fails to pan out or is slow in coming, they take that fact to show that more research money is needed or that ethical hand-wringing and groundless anxieties have stood in its way.

Strikingly, for all the hostility it generated, research on violence in particular and on behavioral genetics more generally has not relied on the moral imperative language even though its supporters believe it can be of great value. At the same time, the researchers have been sensitive to the main line of criticism, that the research results can be misused, and they have been quick to object to media distortions or the excess enthusiasm of some of their colleagues.

The flavor changes with fetal cell, embryo, and stem cell research. The scientific claims grow more extravagant, the moral language rises to the highest register, and objections to the research are mainly explained away rather than being taken seriously. "Therapeutic cloning (or cell replacement by means of nuclear transfer) is a new medical technology that has the potential to transform medicine . . . this research is not only ethically permissible but imperative."[37] The National Bioethics Advisory Commission held that "research that involves the destruction of embryos . . . is *necessary* to develop cures for life-threatening or severely debilitating diseases and when appropriate protections and oversight are in place to prevent abuse" (emphasis added).[38] The implications of that sentence are that no other line of research can be fruitful, and that there is no abuse in destroying embryos. But the former claim is excessive, and the latter at the very least contestable. That same report did say that, in a broad way, the potential benefits of research are not necessarily sufficient to morally justify it, and that limits on science are sometimes necessary. But it did not set many limits to this kind of "necessary" research, at least none that will hold up in a serious way.

In chapter 3, I laid out some reasons why, with the exception of combating a society-destructive disease (such as a plague or AIDS), there is no moral obligation to carry out medical research. Such research is worthy research, valuable for the welfare of individuals and society to pursue, and worth a large research budget. But it is not the only worthy way to spend money, to pursue scientific research, or to work to benefit human life. "Imperative" is inappropriate language to use in seeking public money to carry out embryonic stem cell research; it is even less appropriate to use as a moral trump card to beat down ethical objections. A British physician and medical editor, Richard H. Nicholson, noted how, in Great Britain, the director of the Wellcome Trust claimed that 10 percent of the population would benefit from stem cell research. He added that, "however outrageous the claims, government ministers and members of Parliament alike believed them . . . the wider risks to societal beliefs about the value of human life, if one devalues the embryo, were hardly considered."[39] The same has been true in the United States, with excessive hype for the research (few informed scientists and enthusiastic ethicists or legislators urged caution in evaluating the claims), and a campaign to discredit opponents—and nothing could do that better than calling them the "religious right."

Social implications and safety. As the hostilities that developed in response to the XYY controversy and the development of the field of behavioral genetics demonstrated, a fear of the misuse of scientific knowledge has marked many of the debates. An objection to human cloning is not simply that it could deprive a cloned person of his own genetic identity, but also that it will move even further in the direction of "boutique babies" and the dehumanization of procreation. While I noted earlier that the social implications of research are surely worthy of consideration, and relevant in judging its value, two qualifications are in order. One of them is that it is difficult to know whether imagined social implications will in fact turn out to be true; and the other is that the way we deal with the implications—even if they come true—may make a great difference in their eventual social impact. The massive use of prenatal diagnosis in India to eliminate unwanted female children could not easily have been foreseen, for example, even if some use for that purpose could be. Looming over these two qualifications is a still more important question: how are we to measure potential risks and benefits of the research, particularly when the benefits are social and not more narrowly medical?

Save for historical precedent, if there is any, nothing is more difficult (but not impossible) than trying to predict the social implications of gaining new knowledge or developing new technologies, whether the discovery of electricity, splitting the atom, the invention of the airplane, or the impact of saving lives that once would have ended much earlier. While I do not think human reproductive cloning, for instance, offers any prospect of benefit to anyone except perhaps under rare circumstances for a tiny minority of infertile couples, I have no idea just what it might mean for the procreation of children. (I have an imagined scenario, not favorable, but it is an act of imagination, lacking any good precedents to work with other than parents who try excessively to dictate their children's lives.) But then neither has anyone specified the benefit that cloning will bring to the lives of children. The discussion of alleged benefits is parent-centered, not child-centered.

Those critical of behavioral genetics have, by contrast, the historical experience of the ill-fated eugenics movement to cite, and plenty of evidence about the way people can get stigmatized and marginalized by alleged genetic traits or predispositions. Those worries should not be decisive in stifling any and all behavioral research, but they do offer an empirical base for concern about the harmful potential use of the knowledge, and a strong incentive for the researchers to take great care in describing the meaning and value of their research. Of course most researchers try to handle their findings cautiously and articulate them sensitively to guard against their misuse. But there is no way, finally, for them to control what others do with the knowledge or techniques they develop. That is a good reason to be both cautious and realistic—cautious about potential harms yet realistic that not much may be done to avoid some of them even with the best will in the world. But the potential for misuse of otherwise valid research, conducted for serious reasons, does not in itself provide adequate grounds to stifle it.

The safety of a proposed line of research raises related problems. To this day many recall the worries about safety that marked the early work on in vitro fertilization. The theologian Paul Ramsey was one of the most eloquent writers on the danger that such research posed for any child so procreated. But when baby Louise Brown was born in 1978 and developed in a normal and healthy way, those worries were blown away in an instant, even though the researchers never did reveal how many missteps it took to get to Louise Brown. The failure of recombinant DNA research to produce any flagrant safety problems for the researchers or the general public in the 1970s was, as indicated above, taken as a cautionary tale by many scientists about the damage done by taking private worries to the public.

It was hard not to recall those incidents when NBAC called for a five-year moratorium on human cloning research solely on the grounds of a threat to the health of children so cloned. Possible harms are easy to project but their chances of materializing are not (though later work with both sheep and other animals shows how realistic the fears were). Moreover—to recall another feature of the early IVF research—in the early 1970s when the researchers clearly realized that there was a great deal of opposition to their work they went underground; or, more precisely, they continued the research but released no preliminary findings or did anything else to call attention to their work. If they were betting that success would silence the critics, it was a bet that paid off handsomely. Will anyone be astounded to hear, a few years from now, that researchers working in the private sector, free of bans, have managed to clone a healthy child—and that the failures along the way (or likely to occur later) will not be revealed?

Since there is no known social benefit in reproductive cloning, even if successful, there is no warrant for running any of those risks. Yet my crystal ball is no better—but no worse—than anyone else's. Nor should the proffering of inventive scenarios about benefits sweep away worries. Humanity in the past has produced many evils and still does into the present. The absence of human reproductive cloning does not appear to be the cause of any of them. Hence, the social risk of research that might change basic human institutions for the worse in order to gain small, very small, social benefits—in this case procreation—is worthy of the most careful attention. It is also the most difficult kind of assessment to carry out, if only because—as history has amply shown—nothing is much harder than judging the long-term consequences of new knowledge. Yet it is important to attempt such assessments, and a fine research project would be to see if some sophisticated methods could be found for doing so. It is not necessarily a less plausible project than stem cell research.

That much said, in 2001 I testified in Congress in favor of the House bill to ban research on human cloning for either research or reproductive purposes. I accepted the premise of the bill that research on human cloning opened the door to further genetic manipulation. It would be to take a fateful step toward the manufacture of human beings and of no notable good for them. A ban on therapeutic cloning is necessary since it would generate the knowledge and scientific techniques to make the further step of cloning a human being possible.[40] I reluctantly modified that position to favor a moratorium on cloning research, a politically more promising outcome. As it turned out, a compromise could be reached on cloning, and Congress has passed no bill on a ban.

Abortion and the embryo's moral status.　　I come to the place of abortion in the arguments over fetal tissue, embryo, and stem cell research with a personal history and a deep ambivalence. The first full book I wrote about health policy was on abortion in 1970, just prior to *Roe v. Wade,* but subsequently cited by the Supreme Court in a supportive way in that decision.[41] In the book I argued that, with early pregnancies, women should be left to make the choice for or against abortion. That much seemed clear to me then and still does. I also argued, no less strongly, that abortion remains a profound ethical issue and that the fact that it may be understood as a "private" decision does not make it any the less a moral decision. There are good and bad reasons for having abortions, just as there can be good and bad reasons for many other personal decisions in life. For me, an abortion is morally justifiable only if there is a serious health or family reason to have one; simply an unwanted or unplanned pregnancy is not a sufficiently grave reason (even if abortion is legally available).

I did not for a moment imagine that a pro-choice legal commitment to abortion would come, for some, to morally legitimate a use of embryos for research; and it is a move I resist, even if not in terms strong enough to satisfy any pro-life group. I believe that the use of embryos for research purposes is profoundly distressing and wrong. The more I listened to the debate, the more I felt that way. For reasons I develop below, the claim that embryonic stem cell research is a moral imperative came to appear less and less credible: the prospects of the research are less likely than advocates make them appear, alternative forms of research to achieve the same ends are possible, and even the mildest respect for embryos is sufficiently strong to reject using them for research purposes.

My main purpose here, however, is to try to correct a bias, to encourage at least a more nuanced, less self-interested, argument in favor of the embryos, and to make their use more of an uphill struggle. Opposition to the research is commonly characterized as coming from "the religious right," true enough, or the organized pro-life groups, true enough, but they are a part of our society, worthy of respect, and there are many people opposed to abortion who are not religious. "Abortion," some prominent ethicists once wrote in this context, "should not be permitted to hold every related issue of medical ethics hostage."[42] That is probably right, but another statement should complement it: "the research imperative should not be permitted to hold every related issue of medical ethics hostage" either. Public opinion, I concede, seems strongly favorable to federal funding of research with stem cells derived from donated embryos and thus supports the research imperative in this case.[43] I hope that climate changes.

I focus on three features of the debate in the abortion context: that of the "respect" to be accorded the embryo; that of the bearing of some contradictory currents in the pro-choice movement and their pertinence for the issue; and that of the research imperative as a justification for favoring embryo research.

Two federal commissions and one federal advisory group have taken what they considered an intermediate position on the moral status of the embryo. They rejected one extreme, that the embryo has no moral worth at all, and then the other extreme as well, that it has the same moral standing as children and adults. Instead, they chose what has been called the developmental view, according to which the embryo, and then the fetus, gradually acquires the properties of personhood and eventually, but not at first, the full moral status of persons (a position I took in my book). Accordingly, the NBAC report on stem cell research said that "the embryo merits respect as a form of human life," but not enough to prohibit its research use.[44] The 1994 NIH Human Embryo Research Panel spoke of "respect . . . for their special character," while the earlier 1979 Ethics Advisory Board said the embryo merits "profound respect."[45]

Since research on embryos, requiring their destruction however derived, is a decisive, nonreversible action ending the existence of the embryo, the language of "respect" in that context is hard to understand. My *Webster's Dictionary* defines the transitive verb "to respect" as "to consider worthy of high regard," and "to refrain from interfering with." I presume that those who justify the research use of embryos as compatible with respect did not have in mind the second definition. Even with the first one, however, can we have a high regard for that which is to be destroyed for research purposes— that is, solely for our benefit with none for the embryo? That's what some would like to show.

The most nuanced article by two philosophers defending the "respect" usage sees no incompatibility.[46] In some other cultures, the authors note, those who are to be killed are the subjects of elaborate rituals of respect (in Japan with abortion, and in Native American tribes with animals to be hunted, for instance), and we ourselves have long held that special respect is due newly dead bodies and cadavers.[47] But the citation of anthropological examples makes a strong moral argument only if there exists an impartial moral standard to judge such practices. Various cultures have done just about everything possible, both saintly and evil: the Incas were given to human sacrifice, and they showed proper respect for those to be killed; and widowed women consumed by suttee in India are "respected" as well.

Nor does the treatment of the newly dead or the research cadaver quite work as a parallel: their life is already gone and those respecting them—unlike researchers with research embryos—do not cause their deaths. The authors make some interesting points about how to manifest respect: serious scientific purpose, no other option, and the use of as few embryos as possible. But that kind of respect focuses on embryos as a class, not as individuals, which is the point of serious respect. The authors do not say whether those lacking such respect deserve banishment from research or ethics lectures. In the end, in any case, the *possible* benefit at some unknown future time for some unknown group of patients becomes more important than the certain death of the embryo. If "respect" for the embryo means respect for each and every embryo, that would imply some kind of *benefit* for the embryo at least as strong as that for a statistical and hypothetical population of the sick who will, someday, maybe, be saved. None of the commissions says what that benefit might be.

What of the contention that the embryos to be used for research purposes would otherwise be destroyed or (amounting to the same thing) kept frozen indefinitely? This argument is probably the most effective with otherwise pro-life legislators who nonetheless favor stem cell research. While I remain ambivalent about this argument, I cannot work up much enthusiasm for it. First, the spare embryos have come from highly flawed infertility relief procedures within an unregulated industry. Ideally, they need not exist at all for IVF to succeed. Moreover, they are spares, not because of some defect, but because their mothers do not want them implanted. While in many cases implanting them may not have been possible or prudent, freezing them when they will almost certainly be discarded cannot be called an act of respect. Second, since gestation only is needed for the embryos to become like the rest of us, they merit respect. Potentiality is not nothing: an important trait of human life at whatever stage is not just what it is now, but also what it can become. We mourn the death of a child not simply because it was a human being but because it lost its potential to develop and have a full life.

If we do not mourn the loss of an embryo (ordinarily we do not know there has been a loss), we can, with little imagination, envision the developed person it could become. However nascent that form of life, we ought to respect it, but in this case the respect should have a far reach: do not destroy it for research with a highly uncertain outcome. The "promise" of research is not enough to justify using an embryo as research material. There are other, less problematic, ways of seeking to cure disease. In the case of permitting the killing of an embryo, or fetus, in abortion, there is a difference. We are respecting a woman's right to decide whether her well-being is threatened, and we leave that judgment to her; but the threat is much more concrete and immediate than speculative research benefits.

That understanding of respect can still rest on the developmental view that the value of life increases with the length of gestation, but that the embryo even has value at the outset. Yet two little-noticed strands of the pro-choice abortion position are in potential conflict in the embryo debate. One view says, in effect, that the killing of an embryo for research purposes can be justified if there is a good moral reason to do so, such as promising research; some regulatory restrictions put in place; and if there is no other way of gaining the necessary knowledge. The other view holds that the decision to have or not have an abortion rests with the woman alone, as does the disposition of any embryo she produces: there are not, nor should there be, any moral standards whatever whereby to judge, coerce, or even influence a woman's decision. Whatever value an embryo has, if any, is solely determined by the woman's evaluation, including its worthiness of respect. This view logically entails that there can be no publicly acceptable grounds for prohibiting a woman from getting pregnant and having an abortion to contribute embryos for research, to sell them if she likes, and to specify more generally what may or may not be done with them.

The first view, presupposing the validity of the developmental position and the validity of some respect for embryos, has a catch. Directly or not, it takes a stand on the morality of abortion and the moral status of the embryo by in effect saying that not any reason whatever is a good reason to destroy an embryo. The legalization of abortion with *Roe v. Wade* emerged as a way of helping *women* with troubled pregnancies, not that of legitimating the killing of embryos in other contexts. The use of a sliding scale of personhood for abortion, directly and immediately affecting a real woman's welfare, is by no means equally justifiable as a rationale for the destruction of embryos for speculative research possibilities. To give any public moral status at all to the embryo, even one that calls for the mildest respect, is to fly in the face of the view that no one but the woman has any right whatever to make such decisions. The commissions have implicitly put that view to one side, just as they have put aside the strictest pro-life positions. But by trying to chart a middle course, they run into other difficulties. By being biased toward the research imperative, they have been driven toward finding rationales to make the use of embryos acceptable, and that turns out to be a variant of the standard pro-choice position. And by speaking of a necessary respect for the embryo, they undercut a key part of that position, which does not legally require women to have *any* respect for embryos.

To say that the embryo deserves respect, that there can be no commerce in embryos, that the informed consent of the woman whose embryo it is is necessary, seems like applying cosmetic ethics—that is, the researchers get the embryo and can do with it what they please in the name of research while a paper-thin wall designed to avoid "abuses" gives the appearance of a sensitivity that the embryo's lethal denouement belies. It is a tactic that surely will not satisfy those opposed to the use of embryos for research, any more than respectfully improving the last meal of someone about to be executed would mollify opponents of capital punishment.

The language of balance and consideration of all viewpoints appears frequently in the efforts to advance fetal tissue, embryo, and stem cell research. In its stem cell report, NBAC said that it sought "to develop policies that demonstrate respect for all reasonable alternative points of view and that focus, when possible, on the shared fundamental values that these divergent opinions, in their own ways, seek to affirm."[48] But to achieve those policies it eliminated from consideration the position of those who hold embryonic life to have full moral worth, excluded the other extreme that holds the embryo to have no moral standing at all, and posited a supposedly overwhelming research imperative.

Pitted against the cure of disease, the value of the embryo is found wanting. A more extreme version of the same logic exists in an article defending the language of balance, though arguing for a far less nuanced approach than that adopted by NBAC. The authors contend that "if ethicists or the public would restrict the use of embryonic stem cells, then they must bear responsibility for those patients they have chosen not to try to save by this means."[49] There is no such responsibility. Scientifically or otherwise, no one has proven that the destruction of embryos is necessary to develop cures. The authors imply (falsely) that cures can be achieved by no other means; or that those who try to find cures by other means are culpable because they do not go the stem cell route; or that there is a moral obligation to do stem cell research at all, when there are other valuable ways to allocate public and private resource for worthy causes.

NBAC did not help its case by speaking of the "tensions between two important ethical commitments, to cure disease and to protect human life."[50] That statement suggests that they are equal ethical values, while the Western liberal tradition has always given a priority to the protection of life. As I noted in chapter 6, the ethic of human subject research has repeatedly rejected that kind of balancing. I contended that the principle of informed consent in human subject research serves as a strong moral anchor, one that (with competent patients) admits of no compromise and no balancing of that moral principle and research needs or possibilities. The disputes I discuss in this chapter also have been saturated with the language of balancing. For my part, I conclude that there should be a flat moral prohibition against embryo research resulting in the death of the embryo for any reason whatever. That prohibition would serve as the moral anchor in the realm of reproductive and genetic research and therapy, playing the same role as informed consent in the human subject realm.

I say this not because I believe an early embryo is fully and clearly a person, which I do not, or that the killing of embryos should count as murder, a position that seems to me inconsistent with most religious and philosophical traditions. Instead, I take seriously the idea of respect for embryos and for their potential, as argued earlier, but take no less seriously a major problem with any form of embryo research: once the principle of research on embryos has been accepted, I see no way—other than arbitrarily—to draw a line against the creation of embryos for research purposes. The various commissions' notion of respect seems much too thin and inconsequential to long hold off that move—and, with only one dissent, the 1994 NIH Embryo Research Panel supported embryo creation for research. It saw that a middle-ground "respect" notion (toward which it nodded) did not have the power to resist embryo creation.

To put my position in a slightly different way, the "promise" of research, even if great, is still a speculative claim and thus has a weak moral claim on us. It is all the weaker when there are alternative research routes to the same goals. In the case of the possible benefits of embryonic human subject research, the NIH has invested and continues to invest millions of research dollars in those alternatives, whether for heart disease, cancer, Alzheimer's or Parkinson's disease. If the moral claims of the embryo are, as sometimes put, weak claims, then the moral claims of promising research is even weaker. There is no moral imperative to carry out human subject research, only (seemingly) a research imperative; and they are not the same. I am not, I should add, making a case for the banning of embryo or embryonic stem cell research (though a denial of federal research money would be appropriate). I doubt that a ban could make it through Congress but, in any case, would probably be unenforceable. A moral condemnation by at least some significant portion of the population would be enough. Reportedly, in 2002 some candidates for director of the NIH were rejected because of their support of embryonic stem cell research. That strikes me as excessive zealotry in a debate that puts reasonable and conscientious proponents on both sides; no one should be denied office for coming out on one side or the other.

NBAC dodged its balancing dilemma by raising the ante for the research to the "necessary" level and reducing the status of the embryo to the accommodating, flexible "respect" level. That's one way of getting out of a tight corner. It is rare for any of the commissions to spell out a theory of balancing, other than to say in a vague way that they are seeking some kind of pluralistic middle ground acceptable to a majority of citizens. Its definition of a middle ground often seems like a paraphrase of a famous line of George Orwell, "all middle grounds are equal, but some are more equal than others." The balancing seems nothing other than a statement of the commission members' values since obviously commissions with a different mix of people would either have more dissents or come out differently.

COMMISSIONS AND POLITICS

I have talked about NBAC and its work, but it is useful to step back a bit and look at the role of commissions more broadly. Francis Fukuyama has proposed the creation of a federal regulatory agency with "statutory authority over all research," and modeled on the British Human Fertilization and Embryology Authority.[51] But the history of federal commissions in the United States does not reflect the diversity of opinion a serious regulatory agency would need in order to be politically plausible and acceptable. To make matters worse, if it could represent a real diversity of viewpoints, it would be hard put to achieve the consensus necessary for firm regulations.

With one exception only, every one of the commissions has achieved a balance that (though with qualifications) chose the research imperative over moral objections. Dissents have been rare, and any brakes put on research mild. NBAC's report on human cloning was the exception: there was no serious dissent, but it did come out in favor of a moratorium on human cloning research, on the narrow ethical ground of safety for the clone; and it left open the possibility of a reconsideration in five years. That mixed outcome could not have hurt the lobbying efforts of a powerful group of scientists to stop any congressional ban on cloning. The earlier NIH embryo panel supported embryo research, including the creation of embryos for research purposes; and there was only one dissent from that latter position. So did the NBAC stem cell report support embryo research, though it did not approve the creation of embryos for that purpose.

Two points might be made about the politics of the commissions. With the exception of President Bush's Council on Bioethics (see below), they have represented the mainstream of educated, generally progress-minded liberal scientists and laypeople; but it is not the American population mainstream. If it were, the gap between congressional attitudes and the commissions would be smaller. No doubt some of that difference reflects the power of the religious right and the lobbying power of the Roman Catholic bishops, but that is too convenient a target and not the whole story.

The second point is that the mainline ethic about research in the United States comes down to this: unless there are some overwhelming reasons not to carry out research, it should not be stopped. That is not a bad principle, but if many positions are unrepresented among commission members, then in practice opposing viewpoints are bound to lose. My critique here is not directed at individual commission members. They themselves did not decide on a commission's makeup and were acting on their own conscientious convictions.

My critique is aimed at the selection process, one that—the prevailing pattern suggests—puts together groups unlikely to give much trouble to the research imperative. Until the Bush council came along, only one federal group—the NIH fetal tissue panel—had openly vocal pro-life members. How can that be justified in a society where at least 20 percent of the population falls into that group, as do many members of Congress?[52] Critics from the left, who also have a strong national following, have not been represented either. Jeremy Rifkin and his allies, persistent critics of many genetic research forays, were not to be found. As the detectives usually say in mystery stories, "I don't believe in coincidences." But I am *not* proposing a conspiracy theory. The committees were put together by research-inclined administrators, comfortable that good sense was on their side; and they chose people they believed would not stray too far from centrist positions.

As the sociologist John Evans has argued, federal bioethics commissions have eschewed serious wrestling with substantive ethics, settling instead for procedural approaches that tend to sequester questions of ends, with their place taken by a "thin" ethics of means. This approach, Evans contends, is most congenial to governmental panels and no less congenial to many scientists, who are unlikely to relish a direct confrontation with politics and the public. It no less tends to push aside the more serious, and deeper, problems of the human good.[53] Whether the Bush-appointed President's Council on Bioethics, created as part of the president's response to the stem cell debate, and chaired by Leon Kass of the University of Chicago, will move in a different direction is not clear as of the early months of 2002, but the press reports indicate that Kass's interest is not in reaching consensus but opening up a substantive public discussion. The composition of the council, though generally conservative, points to considerable diversity on the issues it is to examine.

It should go without saying that the only strong political blocs are not just those opposed to research. The scientific community is a powerful actor, as various ad hoc pressure groups put together to lobby for particular causes make evident. Richard Horton, editor of the important British medical journal *Lancet*—hardly an anti-medicine journal—has written, "just as scientists do not have ultimate control, despite their intense efforts to the contrary, over the interpretations others place on their work, so it seems ludicrous to impose a moral imperative on their motivations. Medical science is just as self-serving as any other branch of human inquiry. To claim a special moral purpose for medicine or even a beneficent altruism is simply delusional."[54]

Though research advocates often dismiss criticism as an intrusion of politics when their own interests are threatened, scientists and research universities can mobilize every bit as effectively as the religious right can. They did so in 1978, effectively helping scuttle some sixteen separate bills introduced into the Senate to make the NIH guidelines on recombinant DNA research mandatory for both public and private research; in 1997–98, helping kill proposed legislation banning research on human cloning; and in 1998–2000, working to get NIH to loosen its guidelines on embryo and stem cell research and to forestall any congressional ban.[55] Research advocates persuaded President Clinton to lift the NIH ban on fetal tissue as one of his first acts of office in 1993.

The Recombinant DNA Advisory Committee (RAC), one longtime science observer, the MIT historian Charles Wiener, has noted, "has been friendly to research and dominated by their interests."[56] A particularly effective lobbying group, CURe (Patients' Coalition for Urgent Research)—representing thirty-four patient and disease advocacy groups—was particularly effective in Congress in favor of stem cell research. The actors Michael J. Fox and Christopher Reeve were recruited to help the cause. "Stem cell research," CURe said in its press releases, "could help as many as 128 million Americans," a number that included all those suffering from cancer, cardiovascular disease, diabetes, Alzheimer's, and a few other common diseases.[57] Understatement has not been a trait of skillful Washington lobbyists. The recruitment of one hundred university presidents to sign a statement in favor of stem cell research was a brilliant political move (even if it was hard to believe that they personally had done the research to minimize the value of adult stem cell use, part of their statement).[58] The National Research Council and the Institute of Medicine contributed an enthusiastic endorsement of stem cell research, citing its unprecedented opportunities for developing new medical therapies.[59] The otherwise distinguished panel that wrote the report was not notable for encompassing dissenters; in fact there were none.

The legal scholar Lori Andrews, in her book *The Clone Age*, recounts how a group she chaired as part of the Human Genome Project, the ELSI

Working Group, assembled to advise the NIH and other governmental agencies on the prevention of harms from genetic technologies, was gradually whittled away when it began "asking some tough questions of our federal sponsors." She quotes James Watson, the originator of the Human Genome Project, as saying "I wanted a group that would talk and talk and never get anything done . . . and if they did something I wanted them to get it wrong."[60] Watson could serve as a poster boy for Richard Horton's judgment about researchers (though many scientists are as uncomfortable about his statements as I am).

BLESSING, REGULATING, AND BANNING RESEARCH

Beginning with the recombinant DNA struggle of the 1970s, every subsequent case I outlined earlier in this chapter has been marked by demands to either ban some research or regulate it. How might these demands best be understood? One way to begin is by looking at the positive incentives to do research and then look at the variety of disincentives available. Too much of the debate over the years has focused on the problem of bans, often suggesting a neat dichotomy between banning some research and leaving it utterly free to go on. In fact, just as there are many incentives for research, there are a variety of disincentives and braking mechanisms, most of which will allow the research to go forward, though more slowly.

There are four powerful incentives to support a proposed line of research: enthusiasm among scientists and well-articulated claims about its importance; media notice of the claims and their amplification to the public; generous governmental grant support for the research, with strong congressional backing; and correlative private-sector enthusiasm, with money to spend on it. The best example in recent years would be the support provided by Congress to the NIH for the Human Genome Project, which had all four of those incentives working in its favor. A fifth incentive can come into play as well on occasion, that of some very direct and dramatic health problem, begging for a research response. The work on HIV disease and breast cancer would be examples of that kind of incentive working together with the others.

This reading of research incentives, however, should not be taken to imply that all four or five of the ingredients are necessary: that is the best-case scenario and the one most liked by researchers. But much important clinical research that goes on is of interest to only a small number of researchers, or it is on some esoteric line of basic research with no promised clinical benefits but esteemed as scientifically important, or it is pursued in the private sector because of a potentially profitable product. If some research idea does not excite many scientists or engage Congress or the NIH or the private sector, then funding for the research faces an uphill, but not necessarily impossible, struggle. Stories of scientists with novel theories or half-plausible, half-kooky notions abound in the literature, sometimes making it difficult to separate the cranks from the visionaries; and sometimes they are the same.

There is no less variety in the obstacles and disincentives to research. They range from outright bans and refusal of federal research support through tight governmental regulations and close monitoring all the way to self-regulation and professional stigmatization. Proposals for outright bans on research, in both the public and private sector, have been common enough over the decades but have almost always, after early enthusiasm, fared poorly (save for some exceptions at the state level), abandoned by early supporters as well as persistent critics. A mid-1970s issue of *Daedalus* in the context of the recombinant DNA debate, "Limits of Scientific Inquiry" (and still as good a discussion as there is), did not turn up one outright proponent of a ban on the research, even though some of the authors (Robert Sinsheimer for one) saw serious dangers in the research.[61] And the furious battle within the Cambridge city council at that time, where banning the research was first supported, finally led to a regulatory compromise solution, almost always thereafter the solution of choice when a middle way had to be found between research enthusiasts and doomsayers.

Resistance to bans has commonly taken two forms. One of them, typically heard in the fetal tissue, embryo, and stem cell research context, has been simply to deny that the research is morally threatening enough to merit such treatment but not to take up the question of whether research should ever be banned.[62] The other form of resistance has been to hold that any ban on research, even if threatening, would be a major and unacceptable challenge to the freedom of scientific inquiry. That value has been legally defended as part of the protection of speech clause of the United States Bill of Rights, and morally backed by reminders of the harm done by the throttling of research, from Galileo to the present.[63] More practical arguments have been advanced as well, including the economic benefits of research that would obviously be harmed by bans.

The Nobel laureate David Baltimore wrote in the *Daedalus* volume that it makes no sense to ban a particular kind of research since there is "no way that major breakthroughs, even of a threatening kind, can be programmed."[64] Robert Sinsheimer commented, "science rests on faith that our probing won't displace some key element in the universe" and a challenge to that faith is not readily accepted.[65] The distinguished historian of science Gerald Holton noted apprehension among scientists about public fears of science and the possibility of limits on research; not a good development, he concluded.

Even though I supported a ban on human cloning research—and then modified that in favor of a moratorium—I can think of no other case in which a ban would be prudent. Bans have never fared well and probably never will, posing almost insurmountable constitutional and practical problems. If nothing else, someone can always say—and, history shows, individuals have said over and over again—that "if we don't do it someone else will," and that, with a modicum of ingenuity, any scientist can find a way around any ban; and some will be single-minded enough to try. Of course, once the metaphor of a "war" against disease is invoked in defense of research, then it is most unlikely any ban can succeed. I do not consider any of those reasons solid moral arguments but here bow to a reality principle: research may be slowed and encumbered, but if there is something in it of human interest (serious or pecuniary), it cannot for long, much less forever, be stopped. On occasion, however, a moral stand can usefully be taken in favor of a ban, even if doomed to fail: it is a necessary statement of moral conviction in the face of realpolitik.

More pertinent are the variety of other means that can be used to deal with the threats, real or simply feared, of research. Two principles need to be brought into some kind of equipoise; the supposed benefits of a kind of research and the social and political necessity of dealing with worries about, and sometimes objections, to it. The latter have usually fallen into two categories: safety concerns (recombinant DNA, human cloning, gene therapy research) and other moral objections (embryo and related research) and, in the case of the violence research, anxiety about the misuse of the research.

The research on violence—and on behavioral genetics more broadly—has never had to cope with federal or NIH committees, but if it had, it would probably have elicited what is by now the classical response. That response is to put together a committee or commission to look into the issue, devoid of extremists on the right or left (the most likely large-bore opponents of the research) and confidently expect it to propose a middle way. That way is governmental research support but with some restrictive, regulatory rules and (more or less) close monitoring. In the instance of a worry about safety, the standard response is a combination of tight rules, strict reporting requirements, and the threat of a loss of grant support for failure to meet the set conditions (gene therapy research).

Less considered, but conceivably no less influential, are a number of more informal approaches to controversial research. These include self-regulation (e.g., private researchers voluntarily accepting governmental guidelines), peer pressure (treating some kinds of research as despicable), and public condemnation (marshaling petitions, protests, boycotts). Self-regulation does not have a robust history (which is why most professions and much research get governmental regulation in the end), but peer pressure combined with public condemnation may work on occasion. Companies prominent in embryonic stem cell research might be less enthralled with their research if their scientists were condemned by other scientists, and if (to rub it in) there were picketers outside their doors every day. Protest advertisements in *Science* (if it would take such ads), the *Wall Street Journal*, and the *New York Times* would have an impact among venture capitalists, even if they disliked them.

My guess is that the opponents of research could not raise enough money to pay for such campaigns, and surely not nearly as much as those who stand—in any (predictable) countercampaign—to profit from the research, either monetarily or because of scientific prestige or as patients promised a cure. But to cast the debates in terms only of thwarting bans misses the point: there are many other ways of influencing the direction of research, for it or against it. President Bush's decision, in the summer of 2001, to allow federal support of stem cell research with presently available stem cell lines only was criticized by the right and the left, which is to be expected with compromise solutions. Whether the research that allows will be productive remains to be seen.

I end this section with an example of how future debates may go. Robert Pollack, an eminent professor of biology at Columbia University and Watson's longtime colleague, has said of germ-line therapy research that it has "the elegance of a complete solution. Unfortunately, it is a solution that sacrifices the current generation for the next, and as such does not serve the purpose of medicine, that is, to alleviate or cure the suffering of a person already here among us . . . at worst, the child might be born with another, unrelated form of inherited disease."[66]

If he is right, what is the prudent response? Banning will not ordinarily do (despite an unusual agreement at the moment on a reproductive cloning ban). It is unacceptable in principle to the scientific community and probably most Americans, but can regulation and oversight deal with the threats Pollack notes? Not likely. A commission created to deal with the dangers he mentioned would, if recent history is any example, be reluctant to ban the research but would feel compelled to acknowledge the worries. Such acknowledgment usually comes in regulatory oversight, but is it possible to have such oversight over the lifetime of a child who might be at risk from other genetic threats because of the research or oversight over her children and their children who will carry the gene that may have saved the mother? That is not likely. That child would be on her own. In some cases, then, regulatory oversight will be a kind of Potemkin Village, looking good on the surface but concealing the lack of serious effect—even if there are conscientious efforts to make it work.

TECHNICAL OBSTACLES AND ALTERNATIVES

If there are many drawbacks in the composition of governmental commissions, and in the reigning vagaries of the term "balance," two other problems need addressing as well. One is the way technical obstacles to highly desired but controversial research are often slighted, and how alternative research possibilities to achieve the same ends are frequently belittled or ignored. The other problem is that of the political use of a theory of pluralism—requiring the legitimation of "public reasons"—as a way of disenfranchising those who have religious reasons for opposing research. The synergy of these two strategies turns out to be a most effective way to delegitimate criticism of the research imperative.

With almost every controversial case discussed in this chapter, it is possible to discover a significant minority of scientists who believe that, despite the enthusiasm, the research will be difficult and the fruits many years in the future. With some of the older cases, that judgment has proved correct. Research on violence, though seriously slowed by the 1970s criticism, has not after some thirty years made much progress, and any genetic determinants of violence have remained elusive. Nor, as mentioned earlier, has much progress been made in the use of fetal tissue transplants for Parkinson's disease.[67] It took ten years and one death to see any good results from somatic gene therapy, and even those have been scant, no more than two successful instances so far and with emerging evidence of possibly serious side effects. The difficulties facing successful stem cell research and subsequent clinical application remain formidable. A question familiar in much medical research surfaces here as well. "Can the dramatic findings," a report in *Science* asked, "that have so far grown out of work with stem cells taken from mice be repeated in humans?" The answer to that question was: who knows, and certainly not now or any time soon; and nothing else has appeared in the literature to challenge that judgment.[68] In each of these cases, there were great technical difficulties. In none of them were those difficulties much communicated to the public. Only the excitement about the research was.

One particular kind of puzzle needs to be separated out. I have in mind those circumstances where the alternative possibilities for disputed research are not medical research at all, but instead a wholesale change of socioeconomic conditions. Those opposed to research on genetics and violence said that society should look instead to a fairer distribution of resources, the elimination of poverty, and better social structures to reduce violence. There is reason to take that criticism seriously. It may well be right. Yet are proposed social alternatives realistic? To change long-standing social inequalities, which is to change a society, may take decades, assuming the will for such a change and the capacity to make it succeed. In the meantime, people will have needs—to eat, to live without violence. How to meet them and redress long-standing inequalities is a dilemma. If we work too exclusively toward a scientific solution rather than social change, the latter may never come. Science ought not to supplant or discourage social reform, but it is not clear how we are to resist the lure of technological innovation as a shortcut.

Embryo research for infertility assistance is a particularly apt case in point. The presently available methods of infertility relief have many drawbacks. They have a poor success rate, produce excessive spare embryos, are expensive and arduous, and pose some medical dangers for mother and child. Embryo research, the argument goes, could not only bring a better understanding of the sources of infertility but greatly improve the safety of the relief procedures; and so, it asserts, not to seek that kind of knowledge would be morally wrong.[69] But even if the argument is true in part, it could simply mean throwing good money after bad. A public health counterargument is that infertility is a public health problem, heavily (though not exclusively) brought about by sexually transmitted disease, late procreation, and environmental hazards. As Elizabeth Heitman writes, after making a comprehensive survey of the infertility literature, "If, as the data suggest, assisted reproductive technologies have had little effect on rates of infertility or on their differentials among subgroups, it is difficult to justify their apparent primacy among interventions against infertility. It is even harder to rationalize any future widespread application at public expense."[70]

Heitman's conclusion is surely plausible. Those taking the rhetorical high road about the need for embryo research might consider its implications, though few have done so. A public health approach could work as well or better than a medical approach, and it would have the added value of reducing the number of spare embryos, already an awkward matter for many. To be sure, the public health route has no corporate sponsors, no companies pursuing it. But there is no reason why the NIH and CDC could not sponsor research along those lines. It is a potential way around the infertility problem that could be cheaper, less offensive to many, and potentially more successful. That would hardly solve all infertility problems, but it would make gains in dealing with them. In practical terms, it brings up the question of a scientific versus a social solution noted above, and the latter would not be easy (but then neither is the embryo research route). Why isn't a public health strategy on the table for serious discussion?

Research on adult stem cells, as an alternative to the use of embryonic stem cells, is an even more salient case, but systematically belittled. NBAC, for instance, wrote, "although much promising research currently is being conducted with stem cells obtained from adult organisms, studies in animals suggest that this approach will be scientifically and technically limited, and in some cases the anatomic course of the cells might preclude easy or safe access." That hardly constitutes a definitive reason to minimize the value of such research, and NBAC supported a search for alternatives. It also said that embryonic stem cell research is *justifiable only if no less morally problematic alternatives are available for advancing the research*" (original emphasis). Nonetheless, it concluded, "we believe that on balance the ethical and scientific arguments support pursuing research . . . with ES cells from embryos remaining after infertility treatment."[71]

Yet there are alternatives and any balancing in favor of ES research is at least premature. NBAC took what seems a standard strategy in belittling adult stem cell research—yes, there is some promise there, but going in that direction also has hypothetical difficulties—and then "balanced" it off to the sidelines. A number of scientists, however, believe that adult stem cell research could be fruitful and adult stem cells have already been used to treat cartilage problems in children, to relieve systemic lupus, multiple sclerosis, and rheumatoid arthritis. They also had a part in the first successful use of human gene therapy, with eleven children in France. "Thus," as one commentator noted, "adult stem cells are *already* fulfilling the promises only dreamed of for ES cells."[72] Quite apart from adult stem cells, there have been reports of stem cells being extracted from the placenta and from fat tissue.[73] Those reports may not turn out to lead to promising results. The point, however, is that there are scientific alternatives worth exploring. To imply that there are no alternatives worth exploring before turning to ES research is unwarranted.

If a line of research morally offends many, and if it is admitted even by those in favor of ES research that some "respect" is due embryos, why is not the alternative of adult cell research given priority? No one has shown that the ES route will be easier or that its technical problems will be simpler to overcome. Nor has anyone shown that the adult stem cell approach is bound to fail. Meanwhile, by 2002, reports were emerging of the possibility of developing embryonic stem cells in ways that do not require the use of embryos. If those possibilities turn out to be fruitful, the debate might well come to an end.[74] To be sure, many scientists want to explore both embryonic and adult stem cell approaches at once. But in the name of deference to those offended by ES, could they not wait a bit to see what the possibilities of adult stem cell research are? Such deference to the sensibilities of our neighbors is rare, and thus it was commendably striking when a committee organized by the American Association for the Advancement of Science and the Institute for Civil Society made a strong case for embryonic stem cell research but was still able to say, "Although the derivation of human stem cells can be done in an ethical manner, there is enough objection to the process of deriving stem cells to consider recommending against its public funding."[75]

WHOSE PLURALISM?

For the most part, the federal commissions and most commentators award the major victories to those who want controverted research to go forward—and then add a few restrictive provisos of no great consequence in the name of respect for the sensibilities of those opposed. Though there is much talk of the need to take pluralism seriously, the least plausible element of that talk is the stigmatizing of research opponents as the "religious" at best and the "religious right" at worst, implying not only irrational opposition to progress, but a wrongful use of political power. To its great credit NBAC invited religious testimony in its hearings on cloning and stem cell research but received criticism for doing so.[76] One prominent commentator, Ronald Green, harshly opposed to the influence of religion, held that the only moral concerns with research should be those of health and safety, and that majority views and public preferences should be put aside if they sniffed of religious influence. These controversial matters, he argued, should be dealt with by scientific elites in a "more protected environment for expert panels in the policy process."[77] Political pressure, he added, should be kept out of the picture—though that apparently does not mean the political pressure of scientists who want to do the research, or those companies that will finance it, or one hundred university presidents. The "protected environment" would, in any case, filter out the unwanted public pressures.

I do not cite this rather bizarre proposal for elite, protected panels as typical. A watchword in recent public policy discourse is the need for transparency, particularly when controversial ethical decisions must be made, and Congress would probably not accept so flagrant a rejection of that principle. But it reflects a more wide-ranging tendency to find ways around the influence of religion, likely to cause trouble. For all the recent talk of finding a richer role for religion in American society, there is a hard core of opposition among many scientific leaders and their supporters in bioethics and political science. It surfaces with great force in the medical research debates, where some religious leaders and churches can be counted on to raise unwanted questions.

There are two reasons to be suspicious of the rejection of religion and the effort to marginalize its influence. The first is that it is often the only source of serious opposition to some research proposals. Thus when research proponents want to muzzle it, clearing opponents out of the way in one fell swoop, they appear to exercise a self-interested "our crowd" pluralism. The second reason is that religion's right to speak and be influential should not be inferior to that of any other group in society. Only bigotry and a mistaken view of pluralism could justify that position. When a particular moral or social position is taken by a church group that is looked on favorably by opponents of religious power, no complaints are uttered. The use of religious pressure against cloning and stem cell research is considered outrageous, just an illicit use of muscle, but opposition to, say, capital punishment is not only acceptable but welcomed.

This is not the place to discuss at length the difference between the separation of church and state and the separation of religion and society. The Constitution enjoins the first separation, appropriately enough, but does not demand the second. A majority of people in this country are religious (though I am not). They find in their religious beliefs a way of making sense of the world and charting the course of their life. I consider such beliefs mistaken but not irrational or deserving of the back-of-the-hand slaps common enough in some of the research debates. But it does not matter what my judgment is: believers are my fellow citizens and have a right to frame the large questions of life and human destiny as they conscientiously see fit. As the philosopher Martha Nussbaum has articulated it, "[religion] has typically been a central vehicle of cultural continuity, hence an invaluable support for other forms of human affiliation and interaction. To strike at religion is thus to risk eviscerating people's moral, cultural, and artistic, as well as spiritual lives."[78]

The principal theoretical objection to the religious voice in moral and political matters is that it represents a way of thinking about the world and ethics that is sectarian in nature, positing a comprehensive view of the human good. Such positions are not based on, or justifiable by, rational standards accepted by the rest of society. The late philosopher John Rawls called for a pluralism in public policy based on "the idea of public reason." It encompasses "a family of reasonable conceptions of political justice reasonably thought to satisfy the criterion of reciprocity."[79] In practice, the idea of public reason has come to mean that if religious groups frame their reasons in public and not in sectarian terms, they have every right to be heard in political and social matters. They are then in a situation of reciprocity with their neighbors.[80]

This is a coherent and sensible principle, a reasonable demand to place on religious groups who would be heard in a pluralistic society. There is, however, a common confusion here, as if a stand taken by a religious group is necessarily sectarian. That is not true. In testifying at public hearings, religious groups say, typically, that such and such is their position on some policy matter. But they also usually offer public reasons as well for their stand, not speaking the language of sectarian doctrine. Religious groups who believe human personhood begins at conception generally argue from genetic or similar grounds. They reject a developmental view on the ground that potentiality counts and that there are no reasonable places to draw a line on the beginning of personhood other than conception. They claim the authority of reason for their stand, saying that is why their church holds the position, not the other way around. Obviously many people do not share their reasons, but not sharing someone's reasons should not be tantamount to saying their reasons are not public reasons.

In most cases, then, the reasons given by religious groups are a mixture of narrowly religious and broadly public reasons; and so it was with the American civil rights movement of the 1950s and 1960s. No one thought that the religious voice, such as that of Dr. Martin Luther King, should have been disqualified because it blended secular and biblical themes. As Louis Menand noted many years later, the language used by Dr. King in calling for the 1955 Montgomery bus boycott "appealed as well to many white Americans who held the federal government and its courts in conspicuous disregard but who were susceptible to a moral appeal on Scripture."[81] Should we regret that such an appeal occurred or think that it undercut the public reasons also advanced for the boycott?[82] Religious groups who oppose some research almost always mix religious and secular reasons. They should be heard even when they do not do so, but if they want to be taken with full seriousness, then they should find accompanying public reasons to support the positions they take. Since most of the research controversies find reasonable arguments on both sides, and scientists on both sides, this demand should not place a heavy burden on religious groups. As often as not, the American public will benefit from the different visions they bring to bear on research.

Jonathan Moreno has written eloquently on the need for social consensus with diverse problems but acknowledges its difficulty in many circumstances. "An important element of a democratic society," he has written, "is the persistence of dissent, of a loyal opposition. As the questions become more fundamental and difficult . . . the importance of the opposition increases."[83] Unlike the extended debate on human subject research, which has the moral anchor of informed consent as a point of departure, the recent quarrels I have touched on in this chapter admit of no obvious parallel anchor for them. My complaint is not of voices heard and ignored, though they surely exist. It is of efforts to disenfranchise them. Commissions that achieve a smooth consensus, lacking serious dissent, commentators who see the moral imperative of research as trumping dissent, and a notion of balance that requires slicing away the groups most likely to dissent, do science no real service. Nor the rest of us as well.

8   Doing Good and Doing Well

There is nothing in business quite like the pharmaceutical industry. Enormously profitable, it is as widely praised as it is widely despised. It holds within its hands great health benefits and the power to corrupt in their pursuit. It brilliantly defends its turf and ruthlessly exploits its opportunities. It is the only industry that was able some years ago to capture the word "ethical" to bless its products, and the only one that has, without apology, defended its high, and always higher, prices as necessary to save lives and reduce suffering. Turning the research imperative into a high-powered generator of profits, it has brought the art of doing well while doing good to spectacular heights. And along the way it has made impressive, even stunning, contributions to our health.

That bewildering combination of traits makes the industry both an easy target for critics and a model of capitalist genius. When I take time out from my wonderment, I regularly use inhalers to control my asthma, antibiotics to cope with periodic attacks of bronchitis, Claritin to deal with some allergies, and ACE inhibitors to control my borderline high blood pressure. As I write this chapter, two of my colleagues are having their lives prolonged by chemotherapy.

Yet the simple, awful, problem with the pharmaceutical industry is that there is an inherent tension in it, between its ability to heal and cure (putting it in the company of medicine), and its need to make a profit (putting it in the business of business). Any industry with a similar tension might behave the same. Nonetheless, by virtue of its importance for health—and its own grandiose self-description—it almost begs us to judge the industry by a higher standard than others. "At Pfizer," as one large advertisement put it, "we're determined to find the cures of the future. A cure for your father's Alzheimer's, your sister's heart disease, your best friend's diabetes."[1] In case that statement was not broad enough, the phrase "Life is our life's work" appeared under the company logo. Of course every company has important social obligations: to its workers, its shareholders, and the community in which it operates. But next to the practice of medicine itself, nothing in health care so massively affects the well-being of the public as the development and merchandising of drugs. There is no alternative source in most cases, as the industry knows and won't let us forget.

The public can thus reasonably demand that it ought to behave differently from other industries, in its research agenda and in the way it mixes the need for profit (fair enough) with the need to pursue its self-proclaimed healing mission. Its defense is that it operates the way it does in order to pursue its noble work; they go hand in hand. Not necessarily, as I will try to show. It is vulnerable in four general areas—the pricing of drugs; drugs for poor countries; its ties to the universities; and research and health care costs—that bear on the main issue of concern to me in this chapter, that of using the research imperative as a rationale for industry practices and a defense against industry criticism. First I offer a snapshot portrait of the pharmaceutical industry.

THE PHARMACEUTICAL PAST

The history of drug development and the industries that have brought it about is too complex to relate here, but its trajectory is worth recalling. The earliest drugs, still pursued by both alternative medicine and mainline pharmaceutical research, were leaves, roots, bark, and berries.[2] The early American colonists brought medicinal plants from England or learned of them from the Indians. In the early nineteenth century "proprietary drugs," as they are still called today, were widely advertised, aiming to relieve coughs, constipation, aches and pains, and fatigue. Many of those drugs contained alcohol, morphine, opium, or cocaine, but that fact was not known to their consumers and no law required that it be revealed. Excessive advertising claims for these drugs—using outright fraud or deceit—got the fledgling industry off on the wrong foot, initiating a long (and continuing) history of consumer complaints and governmental investigation. The Pure Food and Drug Act of 1906 was a response to criticisms of the proprietary industry, setting a pattern of governmental regulation that led eventually to the formation of the Food and Drug Administration in 1930.

Three great pharmaceutical developments marked the nineteenth century: the use of alkaloid chemistry to extract useful compounds from plants; the development of synthetic dyes from coal tar; and the formal use of research to develop new drugs (as happened in the case of aspirin, an offshoot of other research). The Germans were responsible for most of these advances and for the emergence of the pharmaceutical industry as a combined research and marketing enterprise. Their mix of a scientifically oriented system of higher education and partnerships between the pharmaceutical industry, government, and higher education was highly effective; its strong echoes can still be heard in the United States and other countries. The American industry lagged for many decades and began to catch up only during World War I, when the export of German drugs and drug ingredients was stopped.

By the late nineteenth and early twentieth centuries, progress in research was moving rapidly. Antibiotics began to be developed in response to the discovery of the bacterial origin of many diseases, with penicillin and streptomycin two outstanding examples (though their development took until the 1940s and 1950s). The systematic screening of compounds for medicinal value, the modification of the molecular structure of existing drugs, and the often serendipitous drugs that have been discovered in the side effects of research on other drugs all pushed the research along.[3] By the 1970s the creation of new drugs related to the molecular biology of the human organism was under way, slowly at first but by the 1990s in full bloom as the new biotechnology industry emerged. That latter industry, which began with Genentech in 1976 and then Amgen and Chiron, initiated a development that was not only important in its own right but by the 1990s was influential as well for the pharmaceutical industry.

It is doubtful that the scientific development would have come about so quickly and richly had it not been for the managerial and marketing skills of the drug companies.[4] The work of the H. K. Mulford Company in Philadelphia in the nineteenth century was a harbinger of the spread of those skills, in part borrowed from the German model but eventually having its own American flavor. The ideology of scientific progress, long a part of American culture, had by the early twentieth century pervaded the pharmaceutical industry. Together with the emergence of a large market for drugs, a result of population growth and urbanization, the development of industry-foundation-university-state public health networks fostered research creativity and manufacturing skills.

When the federal government entered this research world with the rapid development of the National Institutes of Health after World War II, the networking took on added weight. The pharmaceutical industry has shown exceptional creativity over recent decades, strong on research, creative in crossing the boundaries of the private and governmental worlds, and ingenious in its ability to translate research findings into clinical and pharmaceutical applications. Targeted biochemical research, stronger coordination between research and marketing, and the seeking of strategic alliances to broaden its research base all flourished in the work of the Merck, Sharpe & Dohme Research Laboratories in the 1970s and were to serve as a model for other companies.[5]

THE PRESENT INDUSTRY

Money has been its reward, lots of it. With a profit margin of 18 percent industrywide in recent years, and much higher for the largest companies, it is the most lucrative of all industries (with investment banking second).[6] Anyone with an interest in the stock market knows that it has been a consistent winner, facing down recessions and bear markets in a way that the dot-coms can only envy. Health sells, and the pharmaceutical industry knows how to squeeze all that it can out of an already fat cash cow. That is not a fact advertised by the industry. The 2000–2001 annual report of the Pharmaceutical Research and Manufacturers of America (PhRMA), its trade organization, says on its cover that it is "leading the way in the search for cures." It includes not a word on industry sales or profit but many pages about the money to be spent on research and development (R & D) and how the medicine it produces "will reduce overall health care costs."[7] Wisely enough, it does not say just *when* that happy day will arrive. Total international sales for 2000 are estimated at $317 billion, an increase of 10 percent over 1999, with $152 billion (48 percent) coming from North American sales (a 14 percent increase).[8]

The biotechnology industry, using biological information to develop clinical applications, and still young, now has some 1,300 companies and over 150,000 employees. Those companies spent some $9.9 billion on R & D in 1998. While profit has been slow in coming, some two dozen publicly traded companies were in the black in 1999, and investor optimism remains high, encouraged by the new frontier of genomics. Because it has so far turned such a small profit it has not been subject to the criticism of the pharmaceutical industry, though some of its early products are highly expensive. No doubt following the lead of the pharmaceutical companies (but with more modesty in its rhetoric), the biotechnology industry could boast in 2000 that it was adding $47 billion in additional revenue to the country, providing directly and indirectly 434,470 U.S. jobs, $10 billion in tax revenues, and $11 billion in R & D spending. As an industry, it already ranks ahead of toys and sporting goods, periodicals, and dairy products, and not too far behind cable and other pay TV companies.[9]

Perhaps the most important long-term development for both industries is the wave of mergers that has taken place in recent years. There have been some thirty mergers within the pharmaceutical industry, with that between Glaxo Wellcome and SmithKline Beecham, and that between Pfizer and Warner-Lambert, among the most important. The aim of the mergers has been to increase market share and to strengthen R & D capacity. The latter is taken to be necessary to meet the challenge of new drug targets emerging from genomic advances, which are expected to be expensive and eventually to raise the cost of drugs.[10]

At the same time as the drug companies were merging with each other, they were also buying up or developing relationships with the biotech companies. Those companies had shown that they could crash the walls of the pharmaceutical industry and sell drug candidates for research to the pharmaceutical companies (thus saving themselves the need to do so); by concentrating on molecular biology rather than traditional chemistry, they gave drug research a new direction.[11] In practical terms, the biotech advances have opened the way for large-scale production of scarce existing substances (such as human growth hormone), development of novel medicines and chemically synthesized drugs with greater potency and specificity, and elimination of contamination risks from infectious pathogens. The very smallness of most of the biotech companies, their close link with academic science, and their heavy focus on innovative drug-related research, make them attractive partners for the large drug companies (with some 712 strategic alliances recorded in 1998).[12] Biotech firms such as Millennium may in time also become competitors as more of them gradually enter the pharmaceutical arena on their own.[13] An important part of the race between biotech and pharmaceutical companies is to find and patent key disease-related genes.

Historically, the pharmaceutical industry has benefited enormously from the basic research supported by the NIH. Though there is usually a long time period between publicly funded research and the clinical development of a new drug, ten to fifteen years, one study found that publicly funded research made the majority of "upstream" studies critical to drug development.[14] That kind of support has provided a research base that the pharmaceutical industry has not attempted to build itself (less than 1 percent of its R & D money goes to basic research). The industry must of course spend large amounts of money on the translational research necessary to turn basic knowledge into clinical application, but government-supported research has given it a vital leg up, so much so that proposals are afoot to bring some of the profit back to the NIH. (One reason for the massive campaign to get embryonic stem cell research supported by the NIH is that the research will be difficult and too much of a gamble for the private sector.)

Tax breaks for the drug companies offer a bonus, as do various strategies to extend patent duration and directly produce generics.[15] Generic drugs, which in 1984 had only 18.6 percent of the market (prescription units), had 47.1 percent by 1999.[16] The importance of government for the industry—from the regulatory front to tax breaks to the future of Medicare drug coverage—may be gauged by the fact that it spent $235.7 million to lobby Congress and the executive branch between 1997 and 1999 and had spent $42.9 million by the first half of 2000.[17] Not taking any chances, it added to that amount a contribution of $1.7 million toward President Bush's inauguration ceremony, about 10 percent of the estimated $17 million cost of the event.[18]

THE COST OF R & D: WHAT DOES IT MEAN?

The public relations decision of the pharmaceutical industry in the late 1990s to emphasize its commitment to research, evident in its advertisements and other public relations activity, suggests two observations. One of them, historically important, is that research is the key to the ongoing financial success and clinical benefits of its work. If nothing else, patent protections run out and new products must take their place. "What have you done lately?" is a question the industry must always take seriously. Another is that an invocation of the research imperative, the saving of lives and the relief of suffering, is popular and persuasive, one of those global imperatives that hardly anyone sees fit to criticize. It makes for good advertising copy, embodying a high moral claim, and has been so used, again and again, and then again some. Faced with calls for price controls and Medicare drug coverage (with attendant governmental buying clout), the industry invokes the research imperative as its best possible defense against proposed price controls.

The main vehicle for making this case has been the industry's R & D expenditures. As the PhRMA brochure copy indicates, that money is meant to demonstrate its good faith, its seriousness of purpose.[19] That is not a bad tactical move: R & D is an expensive item for the companies, a necessity for their survival, and an attractive public relations move. The expense comes from the great attrition rate of drug candidates together with the need to meet regulatory standards for safety and efficacy. A 1979 study suggested that for every ten thousand drug candidates synthesized at the discovery phase, only about one thousand will make it to preclinical animal testing, then only ten to clinical trials, and finally only one to market as a new product. More recent data show some improvement, a one in four thousand chance to make it.[20] PhRMA said that $26.6 billion would be spent by the industry in 2000 for R & D, and the long-standing estimate is an expenditure of $500 million to bring a new drug to market (recently increased to $800 million). Because the drug companies do not release specific data on such costs, critics repeatedly challenge such figures.[21]

In recent years as those costs have increased, the trend is commonly attributed to increased regulation, more elaborate clinical trials, and the shift of research to chronic medical conditions (requiring long-term testing and greater investment in the discovery process). Even when a new drug is introduced, it was estimated in the early 1990s that there was only a one in sixty thousand chance of that product becoming highly successful. Another estimate, in the mid-1990s, was that only 4 percent of marketed new chemical entities would achieve international sales over $200 million.[22] With all these barriers to hurdle—and an effective patent life in the United States of ten to twenty years together with competition from generics—it can be difficult, the companies say, to return a profit on R & D. Too little discussed, however, is the relative efficiency of developing and marketing drugs. There is no available basis for making such a judgment, comparative or otherwise. The interest of a relatively new biotechnology company now moving into pharmaceuticals, Millennium, in showing its achievement of much greater efficiency, and thus lower costs, is telling.

Moreover, while the industry's public relations material lays the greatest emphasis on its research work, companies spend three times as much on marketing and general administrative costs. More money goes into sales than science: 70,000 sales representatives in the United States at a cost of $7 billion. The industry invested an estimated $2.5 billion on consumer advertising in 2000, bringing perhaps a $5 to $6 return for every dollar spent.[23]

The industry's self-promotion material does not mention such figures. Listening to its insistence on the need for high prices to support research, the public might marvel at its altruism and wonder how it can stay solvent, but in 2000 it had a net profit of 24 percent before taxes.[24] Moreover, while the NIH budget has increased rapidly in recent years, its share of total health (research) expenditures has dropped from 35 percent in the mid-1980s to 29 percent in 2000; industry's share during the same period increased from 34 to 43 percent (though it includes market research as well).[25]

New drug productivity, however, has remained more or less static over the years. Why, then, do the companies do so well? What seems to do the job is a heavy reliance on established products, extension of existing product lines to new applications and effective defense strategies against generics as their key drugs come off patent for some companies—and, to be sure, some periodic big winners.[26] The ability of drug companies to raise their prices with ease (and much public muttering but no serious obstacles) does not hurt either. In 1999, the average cost of a prescription drug increased by 9.6 percent (with a 14 percent increase for those over age seventy), well ahead of the 3 percent general inflation rate; and the total increase in drug expenditures for that year was 17.4 percent, meaning that 50 percent of that increase is traceable to higher drug prices, not to increased usage.[27]

The pharmaceutical industry has also benefited from the sharp increase in drug utilization. That increase—a 20 percent sales jump in 2000—can be traced not simply to new drugs being put on the market but to a greater use of drugs already on the market, driven by an older population, to changes in physicians' prescribing habits (including a willingness to prescribe drugs that patients see advertised in the lay media), and most generally to an intensified use of drugs.[28] "Direct-to-consumer" advertising, some $2.5 billion in 2000, and rising at a rate of 45 percent since 1994, accounted for 15.7 percent of the industry drug promotion expenditures in 2000.[29] Complaints about the price of drugs and the inability of an estimated 20 percent of the elderly to pay for those prescribed for them have not dampened their use. Quite apart from the old law of supply and demand, long favorable to the industry, medicine is gradually moving away from surgical interventions and hospitalization to a greater dependence on drugs. For all its troubles in keeping up with the earlier fast pace of developing new drugs, it is a healthy and highly profitable industry and should remain that way for the indefinite future. The volatility of the industry is a reality, but it is also a reality that the large companies, usually old even with mergers, learned long ago how to live with that flux, smoothing out the deepest valleys and surviving the sharpest downturns to live another day (or century, as the case may be).*

---

* I completed this section during the late winter of 2001. In April 2002, a number of news stories began to appear noting that the pharmaceutical industry was suddenly in financial trouble. As a *Wall Street Journal* story put it, "After nearly a decade of double-digit growth, highflying stocks, and some of the world's loftiest profit margins, one big company after another is taking a beating. Analysts estimate that combined profits of the nation's top nine drug makers grew by less than 1% in the first quarter of 2002" (Gardiner Harris, "For Drug Makers, Good Times Yield to a New Profit Crunch," *Wall Street Journal*, 18 April 2002, A-1). While there were perhaps some earlier hints of such a downturn, I did not see it coming. Whether there will be

CRITICISMS OF THE INDUSTRY: WHAT'S FAIR?

I want now to confront the major criticisms leveled at the industry and examine its response to them. I think it useful, however, to distinguish between two types of problems: those that stem from the industry acting alone, without the help of others (such as its pricing policies), and those that require the active participation of others outside the industry (such as biased research results from academic researchers who have agreed to work with the companies).

The industry has argued that it is precisely its market-driven, market-affirming values that explain its contributions to health. The editorial pages of the *Wall Street Journal* have time and again picked up on that rallying cry in the struggle against price controls—even though its news stories about the pharmaceutical industry offer the best possible antidote to its editorials. It is never easy to measure claims of civic virtue with for-profit enterprises. Is the good they do an accidental, unintended by-product of their business aims? Is it a goal given equal value to the drive for profit? Or is it important, but of secondary value, to be jettisoned or minimized if profits are threatened? The pharmaceutical industry does not, in its public relations advertising, mention profit at all, only the health benefits of its work, implying that altruism is the principal motive for the industry's existence. Those of us on the outside have no way, other than its visible behavior, to make any final determination of the mix of motives at work in the industry. But let me at least raise some speculative questions that seem pertinent for making any judgment about its motives and priorities.

Is the industry willing to sacrifice some significant profit to carry out its altruistic mission? Are its executives prepared to sacrifice some salary to help that mission? How does its altruistic mission affect its research priorities? If pressed, could it produce some data to indicate how its altruistic aims actually affect its profits? Are some high-level executives outside the public relations division charged with assessing its altruistic possibilities and pro-

---

an upturn soon remains unclear, and whether what I have written above on pharmaceutical industry profits will hold for the future is no less uncertain. During this most recent period it can also be noted that the pressure on the drug companies to lower their prices, by assorted state legislation in particular, and public opinion more generally, reached a new intensity; and the companies were forced to make a number of unprecedented accommodations to the pressures. A sharp decline in new drugs coming on the market, however, particularly those that the FDA considers "priority," and new molecular entities different from those already available, may well be the hardest blow afflicting the industry.

posing strategies for achieving them? I have no decisive answer to those questions one way or the other, but keep them in mind as I assess a variety of the industry's practices. Its pricing policies offer a good place to start.

The Pricing of Drugs

Complaints about the prices of drugs and the profits of those who make them are nothing new. In *The Wealth of Nations* in 1776, Adam Smith wrote, "Apothecaries' profit is a bye-word, denoting something uncommonly extravagant."[30] Nor is it anything new for the industry to develop a vigorous defense against its critics, even if that does not work so well in many countries. In most of Europe, though not Switzerland, governments have the clout to hold down drug prices by using their centralized buying power. They can and do say to the drug manufacturers, take it or leave it. That is not so easy to do in a market-loving America. Our political culture constrains government's power to act the way other governments do and, besides, making a good profit is something thought worthy of congratulation, not stigmatization.

There are a variety of ways to describe the relation between pricing and profit.[31] One way is simply to say that, so great have been the past and present benefits of drugs, and even greater the all-but-inevitable future benefits, that the industry needs no defense. Its good works speak for themselves, self-evidently negating complaints about profits. As the subhead of one article summed it up, centering on their contribution to health, "The drug companies—so easy to defend."[32] Another way is to say that, yes, profits are high but that there are plausible ways of interpreting the figures to show that they are not as high as generally thought.[33] Still another way is to argue that the industry is volatile, heavily dependent on innovation, and not fully able to have assured profits year after year. Then there is the way I argue the issue: the prices are generally too high, the industry is more financially stable than given credit for, and the profit margins higher than necessary to make good drugs and to continue innovative research. But first I must step back a bit.

There is no doubt that the industry requires innovation. That is its future. But it is also true that much innovation is for "me-too" drugs, and for new drugs that provide only marginal benefits over old drugs, slightly changed but of no great value to the improvement of health. The large pharmaceutical companies, moreover, are part of corporations that are in the chemical and consumer product business more generally. Their long-term financial viability is influenced by, but not entirely dependent on, their drug products.[34] The long-standing product lines, and consumer loyalty to older drugs, give the industry much more stability than the riskiness of its R & D investment would suggest. Those investments are chancy, no doubt about that, but that is not the whole story. As Stephen Hall crisply put it, in an analysis of the history of the antihistamine Claritin—a virtual me-too drug, and efficacious with at best 50 percent of those who use it but worth over $2 billion a year in profit to Schering-Plough (and recently approved by the FDA as an over-the-counter product)—"it is not always about innovation but rather about finding little edges here and there and then marketing the hell out of them."[35]

The high profitability of the drug companies over the years surely makes clear that risk will not cause their financial undoing. Large companies spread the risk over a number of drugs in the pipeline, playing the odds against the unlikely failure of every one.[36] Industry risk taking rests on a foundation of successful marketing and research strategies and on the cushion of older products that often continue selling well even after their patents run out. Despite the industry's defense of patent protection as a basic necessity for its existence, several critics plausibly question that assumption. Patent protection may lead both to higher prices and to drugs less valuable for improving health.[37]

"We cannot know," John E. Calfee has written in defense of high profits, "what new drug therapies will become available, how well they will work, or what populations will benefit from new or existing therapies."[38] But a large drug company does not need to know that, nor do its investors. As long as it is pursuing many leads simultaneously, history shows that a few will pay off; the statistical odds are in their favor. That a company cannot know in advance which ones they will be is in general irrelevant for its shareholders (even though a promising research report, or an FDA approval of a new drug, will drive the price of its stock up). The real payoff for the investor is in the long-term track record of the industry, and the successful companies in it, not this or that discrete new drug idea.

The rise of the biotechnology industry has increased, and promises to increase, competition with the drug industry. But to the average consumers, the drug industry still looks like a classic oligopoly, with few players. Even if there is meaningful competition among them, it is hard for the average consumers to appreciate that. All they can see is that it has not led to any absolute reduction in drug prices, which continue to rise at rates well above the index of consumer prices. The best that might be said is that the prices might be even higher but for the competition. Yet new pressures against high prices brought about by HMOs and drug contracting organizations have had some effect, and are one reason for the variable pricing of drugs in the United States.

The Wharton School economist Patricia Danzon has argued, in fact, that once the price of generics is factored in, U.S drug prices fall in the middle range of developed countries, below those in Germany and Switzerland, higher than those in France, Italy, and Great Britain. As for variations in the domestic price of the same drugs, she concedes that considerable discounting takes place (in HMOs, for instance) but contends that this increases the total quantity of drugs used and also helps cover the fixed R & D costs.[39] But that misses the point of observations about the differentials: that companies can charge some customers less and still make money.

While it may happen, as Danzon predicts, that the large number of start-up companies will force more competitive pricing, there is no hint it will do so in the near future. More competitive pricing, in any case, hardly guarantees lower costs. The drugs can all be competitive, but at a high level, much like the competition between BMW, Mercedes-Benz, and Lexus. Great cars, great competition, great value for the money—but most of us can't play in that game. The new genetic drugs, thought to be the future of the industry, are expensive to manufacture, as is the case with the arthritis drug Enbrel, which costs $12,000 a year per patient.[40] Competition has increased in recent years, in great part because of the generic drug industry. The Congressional Budget Office estimated that by substituting generic for brand-name drugs, purchasers saved about $8–$10 billion in 1994.[41]

The industry has not been much forced to adapt to complaints. It is, after all, an old hand at living with them, and no less at living profitably with R & D risks. As for the claim that regulation hampers the companies, that is no doubt correct. Yet they seem to weather that obstacle just fine. It is a gnat on the back of an elephant that bestrides the industrial profit mountain.

Even so, one standard way of determining profits may make those of the industry appear higher than they actually are. What has been called the "accounting rate" of determining profit fails to take adequate account of the much longer time companies in the drug industry may need—up to fifteen years—to bring a product to market and advertising costs to sell it. That rate thus significantly overstates industry profit.[42] The so-called economic rate of return better takes those factors into account, with the result that, while the industry remains ahead of all others in profit, claims that the profit is inexcusable and outrageous (to cite some common complaints) are harder to make. That much said, even if that alternative calculation is correct, it still remains a highly profitable industry. The economist Uwe Reinhardt has reckoned that if, in 1999, all drug profits were rebated to the public, that would amount to only about $50 per person, an insignificant amount.[43] But if it was rebated only to the elderly, and the uninsured, it would be a much larger amount.

One of the most careful, fair, and level-headed analysts has concluded about prices and profits, "while it is safe to say pharmaceutical industry profits have been consistently higher than industry averages, there is no real evidence that such profits have been unjustifiably higher."[44] The word "evidence" gives the impression that the issue is somehow empirical, solvable one way or the other with some kind of data. That is not so, since the word "unjustifiably" implies a moral judgment (as does another common word about profits, "excessive"). Clearly, the drug industry and its market-oriented supporters do not take the profits to be unjustifiable or excessive—even the average 30 percent profit margin of the top ten companies—and, however high the profits, they are unlikely to do so.

For those whose only test of an acceptable profit is that the product serves some useful purpose, and that people are willing to pay high prices for it, the very notion of "unjustifiable" or "excessive" profit is thus meaningless. Within a market model, acceptable language speaks of a good or bad return on investment. It surely would set no limits on what level of profit a good investment ought to bring. Supply and demand, moreover, plays itself out in the pharmaceutical industry: people are eager to get drugs and are willing to pay high prices for them. Dialysis and organ transplantation are expensive also, and they are available. The fact that government heavily supports them, but not pharmaceuticals, is a reflection of American health policy rather than a failure of the pharmaceutical industry.

Yet if we judge an industry by the benefits it brings or the desires it satisfies, we miss the reason why high drug prices grate in a way most other products' prices do not, or why industry apologists refuse to allow into the discussion any moral judgment about what ought to count as justifiable profit. The industry's characteristic response rules the critics of its profits out of order. But by virtue of its own altruistic practices—the contributions of free drugs in some circumstances, the lowering of prices for charitable purposes in others—which of course have some impact on profit, it tacitly admits the importance of its product for people's lives in ways that go beyond simple market calculations. It says it recognizes that some of those who need the drugs cannot pay for them and that, if they don't get them, then the results may be disastrous. It has in effect conceded the limitation of a pure market stance. A simple supply and demand model is far less defensible in an industry whose products are necessities of life for millions of people. They *must* choose to use those products; and their need creates a seller's market.

Even so, by resting the case on the benefit of the product, and on the self-proclaimed research imperative to do good, the industry leaves itself open to an obvious question: given your proclaimed values and high goals, how can you justify pricing your products so high that many cannot afford them (many elderly in this country and millions of people in poor countries)? Even if the argument from the financial riskiness of R & D is valid—and it makes sense—how does that justify setting prices at a level, and accepting the profits thereof, that deal many people out of the benefits? The industry brushes aside the fact that it engages in a wide range of pricing patterns, suggesting it can get by with less when forced by competition or governmental pressure to do so.

That just shows, its supporters say, that the industry is hardly the monolithic monster it is made out to be, reacting only to market forces. What matters, the industry holds, is that it needs the high prices in those countries that can and will pay them (notably the United States and Switzerland) to support the industry as a whole, to keep its research drive rolling, and to allow price sensitivity in those places that cannot or will not pay the full freight. But of course that response does in effect concede that the industry is sensitive to pressure, and that it can live with the pressure. Precisely that insight is pertinent in the case of the growing gap in the United States between elderly with drug coverage and those not so fortunate; that is a situation ripe for changes in purchasing practices favorable to the latter group.[45]

Is there evidence, then, that *only* the highest profits of all industries can sustain the industry and its innovation? Very little. The computer and software industries, with smaller profits, have had no shortage of innovation—or any trouble attracting investors (at least as long as they see promise of some profit). Is there evidence that *only* a profit margin of 20 percent plus is tolerable for the pharmaceutical industry to keep its R & D going? Or that *only* such a margin can justify the R & D risks, even though reasonably run pharmaceutical companies live with risk for decades and still do quite well? Just what exactly would be lost if the profit margin was not low, just lower, making the industry, say, only the fourth or fifth most profitable?

If prices were lower, and more people could take advantage of the drugs, would that outcome not better manifest the altruistic goals of the industry, which it has not been loath to broadcast far and wide? How can an industry justify a level of profit that will deny its product to many of those who need it—the elderly in the United States or those afflicted with AIDS in Africa? How can it justify a denial in the name of a research imperative that aims to save future lives and relieve future suffering? Are the lives of those future beneficiaries more important than the lives of those who now, by virtue of current drug prices, cannot hope to save *their* lives or reduce *their* suffering?

That last question is surely implicit in the struggle to find a way to include drug coverage as a part of the Medicare program.[46] With pharmaceutical costs a growing portion of elderly citizens' out-of-pocket health care costs, and many unable to pay for drugs at all, the nasty stick of price controls has been raised as a threat.[47] The industry has howled at the very idea. Price controls—principally used in times of war and national emergencies—are politically unlikely, but the use of governmental purchasing and taxation power to control costs is possible. Complaints against the industry are once again on the rise. If the companies do not find better ways to respond, they can expect if not the price controls they dread, then other unpleasant methods to cool public hostility. The debate over Medicare and prescription drugs may well show which way future winds will blow.[48]

Drugs for Poor Countries

Those questions take on even greater urgency in the context of poor countries. The practices of the pharmaceutical companies, which are international, affect rich and poor countries alike. In the United States some people cannot afford the drugs they need—in poor countries most people cannot afford them. The industry is well aware of this, and by 2001 it was the target of a great international outcry occasioned by its failure to provide, at affordable costs, the drugs necessary to treat those afflicted with HIV/AIDS in Africa. It was not that companies had done nothing to deal with AIDS. In 2000 Bristol-Myers Squibb announced it would contribute $100 million to an AIDS initiative in Africa, emphasizing medical research and the education of health care workers. Merck would later offer in 2001 to sell two of its AIDS drugs at cost, $600 for the protease inhibitor Crixivan and $500 for Sustiva, an antiretroviral.[49] Hoffman LaRoche announced it had developed a preferential pricing list for African countries, while GlaxoSmithKline offered discounts up to 90 percent to some twelve countries. Beyond those efforts the European pharmaceutical trade group was able to compile a thirty-page listing of various efforts worldwide covering a broad range of health problems in developing nations.[50]

Those efforts did not win the companies much praise. Even sharply discounted, the offers to cut prices still left the cost of AIDS treatment well above what the poorer countries can afford. There was also a strong suspicion that what dictated some of the response was not simply public and governmental criticism, but an attempt to ward off competition from Cipla, an

Indian company manufacturing generic drugs, which was prepared to sell an AIDS regimen of three drugs for $350 per patient a year.[51] The threat that some African nations, particularly South Africa, would develop their own generic drug industry was not a welcome thought either. The decision of the United States not to come to the aid of a number of drug companies fighting an effort in South Africa to have the courts there declare an emergency, forcing the companies to license their drugs to be sold at a low price, suggested an important turning of the tide against the industry. As a *Wall Street Journal* headline put it, "AIDS Epidemic Traps Drug Firms in a Vise: Treatments vs. Profits."[52]

Whether the AIDS crisis will force a general change in the pricing practices of the pharmaceutical companies for AIDS drugs or any others in developing countries is far from clear. The companies have a great deal at stake in maintaining their present practices. While 8 to 10 percent of health care budgets in developed countries are spent on drugs, the figure can reach 25 percent or more in developing countries. They are the largest expenditure item within the public health sector in developing countries, constituting 40 to 60 percent of all costs.[53]

There is both more and less to those figures than meets the eye. The "more" is that the international drug industry has a real stake in the drug market in poor countries. It does not want competition and has over the years worked against the development of an indigenous drug industry in those countries. The "less" is that the vast majority of people in poor countries do not get anywhere near the drugs they need. By the mid-1980s the average consumption of drugs in developed countries was 11.5 times as much per person as in developing countries, and by the mid-1990s North America and Europe accounted for 64 percent of the world pharmaceutical market.[54]

The drug companies are right in pointing out that they alone should not be held responsible for the plight of poor countries. Even much lower prices would not make up for great obstacles in infrastructure and distribution.[55] Most poor countries have terrible distribution systems, inefficient and often corrupt. When drugs are not stolen they are often dispensed by poorly trained personnel. Lacking poor regulatory structures, many countries have the kind of market practices that are a libertarian's dream, no regulation or control whatever. As a result, expired drugs are common, self-medication with prescription drugs is widespread, and little or no information on appropriate dosages is available. Caveat emptor is the rule, but that is an empty phrase for poorly educated people. And the international drug firms make their own contribution to the problem. They often use misleading promotion efforts in poor countries, market inappropriate drugs, and overpromote brands and trademarks. Lacking their own drug industry, which the multinational companies have resisted, the poorcountries remain dependent on them and in a poor position to fight back.[56] The 1977 effort of the World Health Organization to promote a program of essential drugs has met with mixed success over the years: many useless and inappropriate drugs continue to be marketed, not only consuming scarce health care funds but of no value to desperate patients.

In its less defensive moments, the industry has not denied the validity of many of the charges against it, but has defended its practices as a matter of prudence and necessity. Yes, drugs are too often misused, out of date, and inappropriate; but the consuming countries are more at fault than the companies that made and sold the drugs. Yes, there has not been nearly enough research on tropical diseases, such as malaria, that are major killers in the third world; but drugs for those diseases are expensive to develop and market in countries that could not pay enough to return even a small profit and, in any case, local companies might copy and sell them without licenses from their originators. Yes, the absence of drugs widely available in developed countries is harmful to the health of millions of poor people—but why should the drug companies be held solely responsible for that situation, which calls for a joint effort by the governments of developed countries, private foundations, and international aid agencies? There is some truth in those responses. The pharmaceutical companies can hardly do it alone, but their role is important. If they don't do their part, then the demand on other potential partners may be excessive.

A change may be coming. The announcement by Bristol-Myers Squibb in March 2000 that it would stop attempting to prohibit generic drug makers from selling low-cost versions of one of its HIV drugs in Africa, following the earlier concession by Merck & Co., agreeing to sell its two HIV drugs at cost, was an important development. Political pressure and public opinion brought the change about, but the important point is that more and more companies recognize that business as usual is no longer possible. To be sure, they are asking for further trouble in giving in to the pressure: if they can do that for Africans with AIDS, why can't they do it for poor Americans with different but no less deadly problems? Altruism has its own slippery slope though not necessarily a bad one.

The Industry and the Universities

In chapter 2 I surveyed the threats to good science and to the integrity of scientists. Among them was that of conflict of interest, which can deflect scientists from the norms of good science and harm its public reputation. There is nothing good to be said for that situation. Far more complex is the relationship of universities as institutions to the pharmaceutical and biotechnology industries. There is nothing new about commercial and research bonds between industry and higher education, notably in engineering, agriculture, and chemistry. The 1862 Morrill Act, establishing the land-grant colleges, aimed at helping the states support colleges of agriculture and the mechanical arts, and the late-nineteenth-century push for improved research added a powerful new impetus. By the early part of the twentieth century, both industry and universities increasingly sought closer contact. Industry needed the research talents of universities, and universities sought to strengthen their reputation for producing good research.[57] For the first three decades of the century the presidents of the Massachusetts Institute of Technology urged the faculty to have strong industry ties, and their efforts established trends that continue into the present. Income for the university was no doubt a factor in their interest, but not the dominant note. Service to industry, improved teaching, and a stronger role in public life were more important motives.

The entry point for my discussion of the pharmaceutical industry–university relationship is the 1970s and early 1980s. That era saw three important developments. The first was the emergence of the biotechnology industry, stimulated by the development of recombinant DNA technology, monoclonal antibody technologies, gene sequencing, and gene synthesis. Unlike the pattern in much industrial development, its initial entrepreneurs were university faculty members in the life sciences. They saw the possibility of making large amounts of money and went for it. Some left the university altogether but most kept a foot in each camp. Either through mergers or working relationships the companies they founded gradually came to be part of the pharmaceutical industry.

The second development was the sharp rise in the number of clinical trials necessary for drug testing and marketing. For a time universities led the way in carrying out those trials, but some erosion set in, particularly challenges by for-profit contract research organizations. The past few years have seen a renewed effort by academic medical centers to recapture that lucrative market; they have been hurting financially and its profits would help.

The third development involved Congress and the Supreme Court. The passage of the 1980 Bayh-Dole Act allowed universities to gain ownership of intellectual property stemming from federal research support and academic researchers to share in the profit from commercialization of their research results. The 1980 Supreme Court ruling in *Diamond v. Chakrabarty* that new life forms resulting from biotechnological techniques could be patented meant that universities could gain patent protection from research carried out under academic-industry relationships. American universities now own more patents than the twenty-five largest pharmaceutical firms and the biotechnology companies put together.

At the midpoint of this era and verging on the Reagan years, grant money from the NIH was relatively static and the proportionate share of federal research funds for university-based research was beginning to decline. American universities were suffering from financial strain in 1980, with faculty salaries falling behind, and capital construction for laboratories, dormitories, and classrooms deferred. The Bayh-Dole Act opened the door to an entirely new source of income, eagerly seized on by university administrations acting in an entrepreneurial way and no less sought by faculty members caught up in the market spirit of the Reagan years.

Almost overnight, the onetime scorn of university life science researchers for the life of commerce became a puritanical fossil for many, economically untenable at a time of rising research costs, and, in any event, financially naive (if we don't take the money, others will). By the 1990s the shift from government-funded to industry-funded research was well under way, even though by the late 1990s the budget of the NIH began once again to grow by leaps and bounds. Starved during the 1970s and 1980s, universities came into good times by the 1990s, able to raise tuition well beyond the increase of the cost-of-living index, to engage in massive capital expenditures, and to pick up more than a little money from their industry ties. Only academic medical centers suffered, deprived of infrastructure and teaching support, and they too looked eagerly to industry to get them out of the red.

In addition to spawning many of the individual conflict-of-interest and other abuses cited in chapter 2, the ties with industry threaten the independence of higher education.[58] At one level industry's commercialization and market practices affect the university, whether in athletic departments (large moneymakers for many schools), the declining humanities (no money there), or salary-driven competition for visibly prominent professors (useful PR, attractive to well-heeled alumni). At another level, particularly in the life sciences, dual loyalties tear at faculty members and universities seeking to turn their academic research roles into profit centers, aiming at a balance that will do justice to the legitimate demands of both.

Once again, then, a balancing issue is at stake, as is the case with many instances of controverted research discussed in the previous chapter: can universities maintain their integrity and central educational mission while they feast off the money and other benefits that industry can make available? Can they maintain academic integrity when they have an equity interest in companies whose products their faculties are studying? Can they maintain their integrity when companies design the research, retain the data, analyze the studies, write the papers, and decide whether the results will be published at all? Even the federal government is not immune. Drug companies now fund half the drug evaluation unit of the FDA, making it dependent on the industry it regulates.

Three problems are immediately apparent in any attempt to find an appropriate balance. The first is that many if not most of the benefits and risks of academic-university relationships are matters of degree, leaving considerable room for disagreement about what is too much or too little. The second is that, while a voluntary regulatory approach—such as university rules—is the principal means advocated to deal with the relationships' potential harms, that approach has little chance of success in the absence of a willing self-imposed individual adherence to the norms of good science and socially responsible science. A failure to report required conflicts of interest is already common. The third problem is that a culturally powerful value sees no inherent conflict between doing good and doing well, or even any serious tension—indeed, it understands the market itself as a valuable moral force, with profit and a good living the just rewards for those who work hard enough.

When one of the most careful analysts of academic-university relationships over the years, David Blumenthal, calls for more data on their effects, it is not altogether clear just what kind of data, put in the context of what principles, would provide a clear pathway for the future.[59] If the university is a place that must always keep its distance from commerce, with the burden of proof resting with those who would promote a relationship, any data it generates will differ sharply from those that emerge from a campus where there is nothing considered wrong if universities economically gain and can avoid abuses.

When the University of California at Berkeley agreed in 1998 to take $25 million from Novartis to support basic research in the Department of Plant and Microbial Biology there was a faculty outcry. The agreement gave Novartis the right to license upward of 30 percent of the department's research discoveries, including research that had been funded by federal and state money as well; and two of the five seats on the department's research committee were given to company representatives.[60] But the faculty protest was hardly unanimous: 41 percent of the faculty supported the agreement, while 50 percent felt it was a mistake, a threat to academic freedom. The department did not back down. Just what kind of data, from what ideological perspective, would help decide which group was right, particularly if the department profits, the abuses are of a minor kind, and the faculty grows passive with the (new) status quo?

Or what might be said about the all-too-shrewd comment of a Stanford administrator who, combating resistance to an office devoted to commercializing faculty research discoveries and managing its patent portfolio, said, "So how do you offset that? You make them stakeholders—you make them beneficiaries." What kind of data might have persuaded them not to become stakeholders, to resist the dollar signs put into their heads, and the university not to push the commercial opportunities open to it and its faculty? I say this not to deny Blumenthal's call for more data, but simply to underscore the reality that, at bottom, the issue is one of university values, and like all such matters deeply influenced by culture and ideology. "What is striking," two commentators have noted, "is that universities themselves are beginning to look and behave like for-profit companies."[61] How far should that trend go, and how will we know when it has gone too far, particularly if it becomes harder and harder to turn back?

Even without clarity about those values to frame and evaluate any available data, perhaps repugnance at really horrendous findings will overwhelm us. It was once said of pornography, "I can't define it but I know it when I see it." Maybe that will happen in this case—the balance collapsing before our eyes—but the past few decades have seen a remarkable change, overturning long-established academic values; and yet, like invisible carbon monoxide it creeps in day by day. We would do far better to have a clearer framework in mind, beginning with the purpose of the university and its necessary sustaining ethos. The practice now seems to be to encourage universities to make up their values as they go along, with the economic advantage going to those who swallow their doubts when the old puritanical uneasiness arises. That Stanford administrator did indeed know what to do when the uneasiness started.

In speaking about industry-university relationships it is important to distinguish among a variety of different arrangements.[62] There can be direct grants or the awarding of contracts for research, consulting arrangements, the sale or licensing of university-held patents to companies, the founding of new companies, and academy-industry training programs. These arrangements can bring many benefits to universities: money ($1.5 billion and 6,000 life science projects for research universities); enhanced academic productivity and faculty promotion advantages; increases in commercial opportunities for both university and industry; less bureaucracy than with governmental grant programs.

For industry, the greatest benefit is access to ideas and research talent. That faculty members with industry ties tend to be more productive than their colleagues (as long as those ties do not command most of their time) while keeping up comparable teaching and committee activities is surely in their favor. University offices designed to manage the industry-university connections, and to help faculty members pursue useful working bonds with interested companies, or to develop their own companies, explain the proliferation of such university-industry ties.

With these benefits in mind, the emergence of a money-minded and entrepreneurial group of faculty members in the life sciences during the past few decades is not hard to understand. Nor is universities' decision to run with a ball they saw floating in the air, ready to be intercepted. But the potential harms this new partnership can cause in university communities are not hard to discover either, some of them mentioned in earlier discussions of conflict of interest. They encompass the exercise of proprietary secrecy, in direct conflict with the traditional scientific ethic of the open exchange of information (Merton's communalism); delay of publication and pressures on occasion to suppress commercially harmful research findings; pressures and lures away from basic research; negative educational and training impact; and a loss or dilution of scientific objectivity.

The effort to pursue the benefits and minimize the possible harms has, as one might guess, created a struggle between those who want as little restriction as possible in developing commercial ties and those who look for tighter regulation and oversight. David Blumenthal, whose work I have drawn on, concluded in 2000 that the "risks seem not to present a clear and present danger . . . [but that] it would seem prudent for academic institutions to avoid excessive dependence on industrial relationships for research support."[63] Marcia Angell, a former editor of the *New England Journal of Medicine*, took a tougher line in an article entitled "Is Academic Medicine for Sale?"—its title makes clear her worry. She does not quite say it is for sale, but enough is happening to leave that impression. She later called for an institutional policy that would require researchers receiving grant support from private industry to have no other financial connections with the company providing the grant.[64]

Yet if federal support declines as private research support rises and academic medical centers continue to face grave economic problems, it is hard to see how academia can avoid Blumenthal's "excessive dependence." Only if Dr. Joseph Martin, dean of the Harvard Medical School—which has set firm limits on consultation time, company ownership, and consultation fees—is successful in persuading other institutions to adopt common and tough rules, is Marcia Angell's anxiety about academic medicine likely to ease. The Howard Hughes Medical Institute (a leader in private foundation research, not a university) has put in place a strict rule for its researchers, requiring prior review and approval for agreements with outside companies. That is what's needed. Despite many useful reform proposals, the auguries are not favorable.[65] As the history of collegiate athletics shows, universities are not notable for their resistance to making money where they can; and resistance grows even harder when the faculty wants to get its cut as well.

Research and Health Care Costs

Up until a few years ago, the NIH annually published the *NIH Data Book*, putting in one place considerable information about its grants. At the very beginning of the book each year was a graph that showed the rise year by year in "total health cost," next to "health R & D" expenditures. What caught my eye when I first looked at the book, in 1985, was the almost perfect parallel between the two tracks going back to 1975, moving upward together. That apparently lock-step pattern persisted into the 1990s until the chart disappeared; and it continues today.[66] There was no commentary on the phenomenon in the book, and I rigorously reminded myself every year that even the tightest correlation does not prove causation. But the persistence of the correlation was, to use a phrase from *Alice in Wonderland,* "curiouser and curiouser," particularly since research had been promoted for decades as one of the best ways to control or reduce costs.

Though the NIH has from time to time made the same claim, it is the pharmaceutical industry that has really run with that argument. The surest way to reduce health care costs, it says, is to constantly improve the drugs available to cure or control disease. "Prescription drugs," PhRMA has said, "will continue to play an important role in containing costs, even as overall health care expenditures increase."[67] That statement is curiouser and curiouser also. It comes at a time when the evidence solidly in hand shows that the main force driving up health care costs is technological innovation—a research result—and intensified use, with pharmaceuticals at or near the top of the list. Is this simply rhetoric warring with contrary empirical evidence, or is there some way to make them compatible?

To answer that question, a good starting point is the emergence once again of double-digit inflation, with health insurance premiums in 2001 rising from 10 to 20 percent, over three times greater than the increase in the consumer price index. That was not supposed to happen. With the surge of managed care in the 1990s, stimulated by the failure of the Clinton reform initiative, costs were brought under some control for a few years in the mid-

1990s, exactly as its promoters promised. It was a short pause. By 1999, costs were rising once again, with no sign of a new plateau in sight. That increase was not happening because the HMOs and health insurers had become lax about controlling costs. That has always been a high, necessary, priority. Indeed, they had abuse heaped on them for the various (sensible, I think) methods they used to do so: gate keeping by primary care physicians, tougher use of evidence-based medicine, and reduction of hospital stays.

It wasn't enough. What the HMOs could not control was the constant introduction of new technologies and the increased use of older ones. Along with many other agencies watching the technology trend, the Health Insurance Association of America in 2000 predicted that double-digit inflation for prescription drugs would continue for five years, with forty cents of each drug dollar to be spent on drugs currently in development. Based on the findings of a study of the impact of drugs in the pipeline, the insurance association expected total prescription drug expenditures in the United States to double between 1999 and 2004, from $105 billion to $212 billion.[68] Then, in 2001, another study concluded that one-third of projected health care spending over the next five years will come from technology.[69] Other analysts came to similar conclusions. The economist David M. Cutler, looking at six different factors affecting health care costs, determined that 50 percent of them come from technology (including pharmaceuticals), a finding consistent with a number of earlier studies.[70]

How can this be? It seems to fly in the face of common sense. After all, the claim that research and related technological innovation will reduce costs has a reassuring air about it. If, the industry says, we could get rid of or reduce the impact of the costly diseases that kill and disable people, keep the sick out of hospitals by the use of drugs (much cheaper than hospital stays by comparison), and find inexpensive alternatives to costly surgical invasions of the body, expenditures would surely drop. Anyone should be able to see that, right? Wrong, or at least not quite right.

There is another no less commonsensical set of considerations about the effect of technology on health care costs. New technologies often make possible the treatment of earlier untreatable conditions, adding fresh expenditures to the system. Many technologies, such as those that screen for disease, can themselves be expensive when used with large populations. Even though unit costs of individual technologies may decrease over time, that outcome usually results in a larger number of people using them, increasing the aggregate costs. Many drugs do not save or avert disability but improve the quality of life by reducing pain or discomfort. They still cost money.

Improved versions at higher costs of many drugs (and there are almost always supposedly improved versions) will not do much good to costs either.

That many of these technologies are what are commonly known as halfway technologies, neither curing nor preventing, is only part of the story here. The biological reality behind that story is that most of the chronic diseases of aging societies have so far seemed amenable only to mitigation, and expensive mitigation, not to cure. Half-way technologies happen to be what the pharmaceutical industry is best at, and they turn out to offer the most profitable kinds of technology. Long-term treatment of a chronic condition costs more than a cheap vaccine, which is why Claritin brings in so much money.[71]

Despite these background considerations, both the NIH and the pharmaceutical industry like to point to supposed cost savings that stem from research. The NIH examined thirty-four instances of health care advances resulting from research it had supported between 1989 and 1992. They included a two-stage diagnosis-treatment of breast cancer, improved diagnosis of malignant melanoma, development of an antenatal steroid therapy to prevent neonatal respiratory distress syndrome, and formulation of the hepatitis B vaccine. They estimated that the thirty-four examples they examined had saved a total, at the lowest, of $9.3 billion and, at the highest, $13.5 billion in the cost of illness.[72]

The pharmaceutical industry has its own matching figures. It reported in 2000 that H2 agonists for ulcer therapy had, by 1987, reduced the incidence of surgical treatment from 97,000 cases a year to 19,000. For congestive heart failure it could show a 78 percent decrease in hospital costs (compared with a 60 percent increase in pharmacy costs for the same condition), and an AIDS combination therapy cost of $10,000 to $16,000 a year compared with an estimated hospitalization cost of $100,000 a year.[73] A Battelle Institute study, commissioned by Schering-Plough, looked at five disease categories: cardiovascular disease, cancer, arthritis, Alzheimer's, and HIV. It estimated that over the next twenty-five years, "if advances in biomedical technology are made *as expected*" (emphasis added), there would be a saving of $407 billion in indirect costs (principally productivity losses), and $77.7 billion in direct costs. Some 5.4 million lives would be saved and millions more cases of illness avoided.[74]

Not all estimates of research benefits have come from NIH or the drug companies. The research advocacy organization Funding First flatly states, "research ultimately lowers health care costs."[75] A distinguished group of biomedical scientists contended in a *Science* article in 1999 that the demographic shift occasioned by the aging of the "baby boom" population would create enormous financial and health care needs. To lower the expected costs and improve health will require a central role for biotechnology and new paradigms of disease as its interventions change outcomes. The group listed seven factors working together to improve the situation: declining disability among the elderly, changing paradigms of medicine (fewer invasive procedures), the paradoxical effects of longevity (less expensive deaths at the end of longer, healthier lives), revolution in pharmaceutical R & D methods (notably improved methods of compound screening), a better educated elderly population, labor productivity as a function of improved health, and the impact of biomedical technology on the economy (enhancing U.S. economic growth and improving global competitiveness). But it is a change in the "medical paradigm" that seems to them most important, one that "could lower costs for many diseases."[76] "Costly (and often clinically inadequate) interventions could be replaced by genetically engineered pharmaceuticals and other treatments (such as gene therapy)," they wrote. "We must," the authors conclude, "increase investment heavily in biomedical research to realize benefits in time to control the impact of Medicare costs."[77]

Studies that show the effect of biomedical research on the health of the elderly reinforce the authors' last point. Kenneth Manton and his colleagues at Duke University have focused much work over the years on the decline in disability among the elderly, a crucial element in health care costs. Between 1982 and 1994, for instance, the prevalence rate of disability declined by 15 percent, which translates into 1.2 million fewer elderly persons with chronic disabilities. The rate of institutionalization was 19.2 percent smaller in 1994 than would have been expected if 1982 rates had remained the same.[78] Before 1994, the authors judge, the major health changes came from improved socioeconomic conditions and changes in health-related behavior. After that point, biomedical innovations played an increasingly important role, from preventive efforts through improved therapies. Surgical innovations have meant that the elderly now receive care of a kind unimaginable even two or three decades ago, adding to the impact of advances in the prevention and treatment of circulatory diseases. Though more statistically controversial, improvements in cancer therapies have apparently made a great difference as well.

Though it does not specifically focus on the elderly, a recent study sponsored by the Mary Woodard Lasker Charitable Trust, *Exceptional Returns: The Economic Value of America's Investment in Medical Research*, pursues just what its title suggests. Its broadest claim is that there is hardly any better research investment than biomedical research and that almost any plausible combination of research efforts would have an enormous economic payoff. Increases in life expectancy in the 1970s and 1980s, heavily even if not solely attributable to pharmaceuticals, were worth $57 trillion, and the gain associated with the treatment of cardiovascular disease alone was $31 trillion. Medical research that reduced cancer deaths by 20 percent would be worth $10 trillion, double the national debt.[79] David Cutler and his colleagues have shown that while there has been a rapid increase in the cost of care for heart attack victims in recent decades—the result of changes in acute treatment, such as beta-blockers, thrombolytic drugs, and invasive procedures—that cost has been far more offset by a sharp reduction in mortality, by improvements in the care of those who have had heart attacks, and particularly by the economic value of the lives saved. Changes in medical treatment account for about 55 percent of the mortality reduction, with about 50 percent of it coming from pharmaceuticals.[80]

WRONG AND MISLEADING CLAIMS

Just about every common claim about the relationship between research and costs warrants a challenge. The economist Frank R. Lichtenberg, for instance, in a study supported by Pfizer, presents data to show how more and better drugs significantly reduce hospital stays. "An increase of 100 prescriptions is associated with 19.3 hospital days."[81] In the case of AIDS, however, hospital stays of one year were not common between 1985 and 1995, death intervening; and the cost of the AIDS combination drugs, necessary for the rest of a patient's life, now equals the earlier hospitalization costs— and the drug cost recurs each year, while the earlier hospital costs were for once only (since the patients died). Of course it is a great benefit that patients now lived who once died, but it is important not to confuse that benefit with the cost of its achievement by the use of drugs.

Lichtenberg's optimism does not look so good up close. But what are we to make of such widespread optimism about the economic benefits of medical research, fed by the NIH, the drug industry, and many (though hardly all) economic analysts? It contradicts most previous studies of the impact of medical advances on health care costs, and it obviously contradicts the data before our eyes over that past few years, that those advances are a major reason for rising costs.[82] Something or other must be missing here. It might be, simply enough, that some advances increase costs, others are neutral, and some lower costs. This argument surfaces from time to time, but no one seems to have done the detailed, difficult, and perhaps impossible research necessary to sort out *all* the advances and technological innovations; and sampling alone would not do the job, since extrapolations cannot easily be made from one technology to another. Nor have there been any concerted efforts to define exactly what advances would lower costs once and for all, with no residual health care expenditures, other than the oft-repeated claim that inexpensive disease prevention programs could do so.

Alternatively, perhaps research advances did in the past push up costs, but things are different now: some corner has been turned, the new drugs and other technologies coming on-line at present are more cost controlling than those in the past. I have not heard anyone make that argument, though (and the genomic drugs gradually appearing hardly seem likely candidates for the honor). Kenneth Manton and his colleagues have wisely noted that we lack "a systematic empirical base from which to monitor the long-term benefits for the entire clinical interventions generated from biomedical research."[83]

In the meantime, before that "empirical base" is in place—hardly imminent—some judgments need to be made. Just how valid are the claims of the NIH and the drug industry that research will control or reduce costs? It is impossible to begin making such a judgment without noting some critical and frequent ambiguities in the language used to describe the research benefits. Sometimes the benefits are described as "saving" money, which Manton and his colleagues see as possible with a reduction in cholesterol levels; or which the NIH and the pharmaceutical industry see happening with the illnesses averted by research-driven technologies; or which Lichtenberg says happens when drug therapies substitute for hospital stays.

But sometimes "saving" money means not a direct reduction in costs but costs lower than they might have been without the technology. The phrase "containing" costs, often used, is also ambiguous. It can mean stopping an increase in costs, or keeping the cost increase below what it might have been, or bringing costs down. A very different way of specifying benefits is to push cost issues to one side and focus instead on social and economic gains to society. By that standard, a good research investment will be one that produces good medical and economic benefits; their cost is another matter and not part of the calculation.

My aim here will be twofold: to show how misleading many of the claims of the economic benefits of research are, and to propose a few ways of thinking about the problem. I begin by suggesting some definitions, which might bring initial clarity to the subject.

- cost saving: an absolute reduction in costs, both direct and indirect—for example, a drug cures a disease and allows a patient to return to a fully active life with no further related medical costs—(pneumonia treated with a relatively inexpensive antibiotic on an outpatient basis rather than in a hospital)

- cost control: a counterbalance to a steady rise in costs (the cost of a particular illness is rising steadily, but a new drug or combination of drugs significantly reduces the cost increase or allows it to plateau)

- economic benefit: a benefit that is unrelated to cost considerations in gaining the benefit (the saving of a valued life), or one that represents, on balance, a favorable benefit-cost ratio

- quality-of-life benefit: a benefit that averts or reduces pain and suffering in patients and unrelated to cost consideration of achieving the reduction (relief of arthritis pain)

- aggregate accounting: the lifetime cost implications of an otherwise successful medical intervention (the cost of saving a life at time x + y [the potential long-term or follow-up costs associated with saving that life] and z [the entailed costs of treating the person for other diseases at later times]—for instance, a person saved from a heart attack in middle age only to contract treatable cancer at sixty-five and then to die of Alzheimer's at eighty-five)

- cost transfer: the cost of shifting patient care from one modality to another (treating with drugs someone who would earlier have been hospitalized)

With these definitions in mind, consider the claim pressed by the Lasker Charitable Trust in its *Exceptional Returns* report. Its contention is that, because there has been a great decline in death rates from cardiovascular disease, heavily due to research and the resulting technologies, this shows the economic benefit of research-driven health gains. The benefit flows directly from the economic value of the life saved (using accepted economic techniques for valuing life). Those whose lives are saved and would otherwise have been lost have an important economic value to society. "The often-ignored economic value of increases in life expectancy," the report asserts, "must count as the single largest gains in living standards in our time."[84] This point was made in the 1970s in a fine study by the late economist Selma Mushkin, who argued that for the period 1900–1975 the net benefit economically of biomedical research was "ten to sixteen times the opportunity costs of the research."[85] Like contemporary commentators, however,

she said it was not known what the research benefits for a reduction in morbidity were—and she did not comment at all on the follow-up medical costs
of the lives saved.

Her conclusion is consistent with what David Cutler and his colleagues
have argued: "that receiving more in improved health than we pay in treatment costs implies that medical care is a more productive investment than
the average use of our funds outside the medical sector."[86] Cutler's analysis
of the decline in mortality from heart attacks shows both that technological
developments have increased the costs of treating those attacks and that,
balanced against the economic value of the life saved, they achieve a
tremendous economic gain. Using this mode of analysis—which is that of
the Lasker report—the economic benefits of research can run into the trillions of dollars, which become *"the true economic value of our national investment in medical research"* (report's original emphasis).[87]

Even if we agree that this is a valid mode of economic analysis in some
general way, it is full of problems. For one thing, those saved from heart attacks will ordinarily remain under medical treatment, at high cost, for the
rest of their lives; treatment in the aftermath of heart attacks is expensive
and lifelong. For another, many of those who have suffered heart attacks
will not return to the workforce, brought down by chronic heart disease. For
still another, by an aggregate mode of accounting, noted above, the true cost
of saving their lives must also include the costs of whatever other illnesses
they incur over the remainder of their lifetime, which death from heart attacks would have foreclosed; these are the aggregate longitudinal costs of
the research outcomes. As the economists Kevin M. Murphy and Robert
Topel have noted, using disease-specific data "assumes that increased survival from one disease leaves the risks from other diseases unchanged . . . if
the incidence of disease is correlated across diseases at the individual level
this will not be true."[88]

Those points are meant simply to indicate that the cost of treating a heart
attack has many follow-up expenses, direct and indirect. In part they reflect
medical sequelae to heart attacks, usually of a lifelong duration, and aggregate accounting's assessment of the costs of further diseases. Even if we acknowledge that economic reality, the Lasker report argues that an overall
enormous economic benefit means it is *worth it* to society: people live
longer and they make a contribution to society. But that mode of calculation
does not answer a nagging question: how are we as a society to pay for those
economic benefits and their sequelae?

Unless we understand what that nagging question implies, we cannot appreciate the grand paradox of our situation. Analysis assures us that many

advances worth trillions of dollars have come along in recent years and—referring to long lists of the kind the NIH has prepared—that numerous technologies are cutting costs and drugs are keeping people out of expensive hospitals. Meanwhile, a prime source of overall cost increases is technological innovations, with drugs leading the pack. We are back to the contradiction I noted at the beginning of this section: the more we spend on research, the more we spend on medical care; it's not supposed to be that way.

It is appropriate here to look closely at two features of the present situation. The first is that the argument from economic benefits—the *worth it* argument—fails to take sufficient account of the cost of *paying* for the benefits and their medical sequelae, which can be considerable, the latter as much as the former.[89] The economic benefits are shared by the society as a whole, but the direct medical costs of those benefits are paid for by the health care system. It is those costs that increase annual health care expenditures; the aggregate social benefits of the research do not do so. "Technological change is bad," David M. Cutler and Mark McClellan have written, "only if the cost increases are greater than the benefits."[90] But if those costs affect some groups more than others, and if the costs of the health care system as a whole become hazardous, then there remains a serious problem, casting *worth it* into a different light. There has been a sharp decline in mortality rates from heart disease, but it has not led to any notable decrease in the costs of caring for its victims, who will need treatment for their ongoing, lifelong cardiac morbidity, which can run into well over a $1,000 a year for each person's drugs alone (for instance, diuretics, beta-blockers). More generally, a large proportion of those suffering from chronic conditions would have died earlier in previous eras; and the medical costs of that survival are enormous (even if socially well worth it).[91]

This is simply a variant on an old story, that of the price of success. A heart attack is a temporary crisis within the context of heart disease, which is a chronic condition; and it is that latter circumstance that really runs up the costs. The American Heart Association estimated the direct cost of cardiovascular disease and stroke as $181.8 billion for 2001, of which the costs of drugs and other durables came to $27.1 billion. In 1998, "there were 13.9 million people alive who had a history of heart disease, angina pectoris . . . or both."[92] It might have added that most of these people still receive medical care and continue to use drugs. Between 1979 and 1998 the number of Americans discharged from short-stay hospitals with diagnosed cardiovascular disease (CVD) increased by 28 percent—and that of course at the same time the mortality rate from CVD was decreasing.

The perception that research progress against heart disease has a paradoxical quality appears well based: declining mortality, increasing morbidity, and steadily rising costs. There is great benefit in this kind of progress, for the length of life and quality of life. But it does not get directly translated into the dollars necessary to protect the health care system from once again experiencing double-digit inflation. The social benefit brings no benefit to the control of costs.

In many ways, that seems to be the main story behind the relationship of research and health care costs: great benefits combined with increased costs to pay for those benefits—at the front end in expensive research, and at the back end in increased health care costs to deal with the medical consequences of the research, successful though it may be. It is possible to imagine forms of research progress that would not leave higher costs in their wake: successful prevention of disease in the first place, or full cures for chronic illness, those not succeeded by other diseases and followed by inexpensive, quick deaths (the compression of morbidity ideal). Right now, however, here and there are drugs, and other technologies, that cut or contain costs, but they are self-evidently in the minority. Otherwise technology would be unlikely to remain the primary driving force in rising health care costs—even if we factor in the patterns of distribution of technology and the incentives for its use. At the least, the pharmaceutical industry's claim of past and present triumphs in saving money is a fairy tale.

If my conclusion is that research tends (even if not always) to push up health care costs, is there a way out? Not easily, but four possibilities are worth considering. I have already alluded to one of them: the use of governmental pressure and buying power to hold down the price of pharmaceuticals. That can be done and is already being done here and there. The second is to work harder to develop drugs and other medical technologies that will be less expensive and oriented more toward disease prevention than cure or mitigation. Anti-hypertension and cholesterol-lowering drugs provide a model for moving in that direction. Efforts to improve patient compliance with drug regimens can be effective by using such low-technology methods as patient education and telephone reminder campaigns. They allow us to continue using older treatments rather than more expensive new ones (some of which have been developed to improve their convenience rather than their efficacy).[93] The third is to emphasize other forms of research and to put more money in them: cost-effectiveness, health service delivery, socioeconomic determinants of health, and evidence-based medicine, for instance.

The fourth, as urged by the economists Kevin M. Murphy and Robert Topel, is to be alert to the influence of third-party payers and their incentives to place the emphasis on the increased value of life rather than the economic costs of treatment. "This [combination] will," they conclude, "skew innovations toward those that are cost increasing. This is aggravated by the fact that cost-increasing innovations often involve new equipment or drugs that allow at least limited ability to collect the value produced. Funding criteria for medical research should be conscious of these incentives, and perhaps lean toward development of cost-reducing innovations."[94]

Rationales and Rationalizations

In this chapter I took on two important features of the research imperative as commonly deployed in the United States. Neither of them bears on a misuse of research imperative arguments to justify the pursuit of wrongful ends (e.g., reproductive cloning), to legitimate debased means (e.g., the use of research subjects without informed consent), or to justify controversial research (e.g., embryonic stem-cell research). These deployments of the research imperative are of a different order. One of them is the use by the pharmaceutical industry of the research imperative as a rationalization for high prices and high profits. The other is the contention that research not only does reduce or stabilize health care costs, but that its economic benefits are enormous, worth trillions of dollars.

Both of them might be termed an instrumental use of the research imperative, that of helping make the case for high drug costs and for the social benefits of research. As such, they raise both empirical and ethical questions. The empirical questions are straightforward enough: can a case be made for the high price for drugs charged in the United States? I think not, but I could be wrong about that. And can a case be made that the economic benefits of research are such that, even if hardly helpful to an affordable health care system, they are still worth it in terms of the values of lives saved and improved? I am not convinced by those arguments, but I could be wrong about that too.

In both cases, however, there are some important normative issues at stake, and of the kind that will influence the way empirical information is interpreted. The ethical bias I bring to the debate about health care costs is that it is the duty of everyone connected with the delivery of medicine and health care, including the pharmaceutical industry, to discharge its moral obligations to those who will be affected by their activities. The pharmaceutical industry, I believe, has as great an obligation to those whose drugs it serves as to its stockholders. Most industries do not have comparable obligations. Few of us can avoid the use of drugs to preserve our health; there are no alternatives in most cases. This means that the pharmaceutical industry must be judged by other than ordinary market standards. My objection to that industry is not simply that it charges excessively high prices. It is that it could do otherwise and, if it did so, it could better serve the cause of health in a way more consistent with its own self-advertising.

In the instance of the economic benefits of research, my distress is occasioned by more than my doubts about the validity of the economic arguments. My main worry is that the country is now caught up once again in escalating health care costs. Can research do something about that? Some research defenders deny that the problem of costs should be laid at their feet: too much of that problem comes from the way the health care system is organized, not something the research community can do much about (or be charged to do something about). They have a good case for their reluctance to assume blame for problems beyond their control. Even so, I believe it fair to ask the research community to be willing to admit that there are some problems that it might be able to take on, that of working for a research imperative that takes the costs of the products of that research seriously. There is, in the end, something disconcerting about claims that the health benefits are worth trillions of dollars while, at ground level, more and more people—and more and more governmental programs, here and abroad—are finding it hard to pay for its blessings.

What should the national health priorities be, and where should the money be spent? Those are the questions that emerge from this chapter, and the next chapter explores the way the federal research priorities are set and might better be set. It is clear enough that the private research sector sets its priorities based on the likelihood of a market for its products; and it makes sure, by its advertising and other campaigns, to help create that market. Sometimes that results in meeting national needs, and sometimes not: the outcomes are arbitrary. Often enough people want to buy what is necessary for their health, and the drug companies are there to respond. But equally often there are products people desire that will not do much for their health; they just want them—and the industry is ready to respond also. The federal government, however, must have different standards much more consciously focused on health needs. How it sets priorities makes a great deal of difference, especially with the congressional commitment to a strong NIH budget.

9   Advocacy and Priorities for Research

Although federal support for medical research has had its peaks and valleys, few governmental programs have been as enduringly popular. The crown jewel of that research is the National Institutes of Health, and of late the enthusiasm for its work has had uncommon bipartisan support in Congress. At the same time, the private sector's pharmaceutical and biotechnology industries have benefited from strong sales, generating increased research enthusiasm as well, so much so that they now spend more on research than the government.

Though few available public opinion surveys directly ask about research priorities, a recent survey on health priorities comes close and allows some reasonable extrapolations.[1] Cancer, particularly breast cancer, HIV/AIDS, and heart disease were at the top of the list of "very serious" problems. Chronic disease generically turned up in the middle of the extremes. Among Americans' health care priorities the survey showed the costs of health care (their personal costs, not national costs) at the top of the list followed by a lack of or inadequate health insurance coverage. Most strikingly, the researchers concluded, "The public had little sense of urgency about any of the health or health care issues currently before Congress."[2] In any case, public opinion surveys have not been a driving force in setting research priorities. One determinant of research directions is the proclivities and passions of researchers themselves, from both the public and the private sector. A second determinant draws on congressional interest, advocacy groups, and informally discerned patient preferences; and this most directly expresses itself in the budget of the NIH. The third reflects the force of the market, with the public's willingness to pay for various health products heavily determining the direction of pharmaceutical and biotechnological research.

If the ability to gain large amounts of money is one sign of high prestige in the United States, the research imperative is alive and well. It has rarely done better. Less clear, however, is whether the money is being well spent, and just how great its contribution to health has been. Of considerable importance in that respect is the way priorities for research are set. How are health needs understood? How is a determination made of the comparative needs of the country and the setting of research priorities?

LASKERISM AND THE POLITICS OF ADVOCACY

The NIH is at once a great institution and a great tribute to the power of political advocacy. If the art of advocacy is the trademark of American politics, the career of Mary Lasker (see page 21) stands as an almost perfect model of how to get what you want and, along the way, do much good. The rise of the NIH immediately after the World War II and well into the 1960s owed much of its success to the efforts of this wealthy woman who used her intelligence, money, and connections in a single-minded way to promote biomedical research. I coined the term Laskerism to capture the critical ingredients of her method: rounding up support among the rich and powerful, cultivating presidents and congressmen, enlisting the help of prominent scientists and physicians, learning how to gain media attention, and using the stories of desperately sick people to make the research point.

It became a well-used formula, though no lay figure since then has achieved her status or power. What she did with her skills was to address a basic problem: how to increase federal support of research and promote the NIH as the vehicle to lead the way. Up to the late 1920s the government provided little significant research money. As one historian noted, the support for medical research in the 1920s was not much better than in the 1880s. That was "partly because of the nature of medical science prior to 1885 and partly because human research brought no direct financial return. Hogs did."[3] Then in 1928 the first bill ever passed in Congress for research on cancer marked a significant shift by appropriating $10 million for research on human, as distinguished from animal, diseases. Where private foundations and universities had earlier taken the research lead, the government moved in not only to provide much more money for research but also to take on a leadership role. It was not until the 1990s that the pharmaceutical industry overshadowed its research role—at least in terms of money, though hardly of prestige.

Despite the 1928 bill, cancer research commanded little governmental support, and even the leading group advocating greater attention to cancer, the American Society for the Control of Cancer, spent its money on every aspect of cancer other than research into its causes.[4] In the 1940s Mary Lasker helped change that group, getting research on its agenda, and Laskerism helped put other diseases on the list as well. It also became clear that success in advocacy required paid lobbyists, the ready testimony of doctors and important laypeople, the recruitment of celebrities with some personal connection to a lethal disease, and highly organized efforts to promote funds for the various NIH institutes. Those institutes that could not enlist the help of professional associations or "citizen witnesses" often found their budgets cut.

Not all the successes of the leadership of the advocacy groups, with Mary Lasker as its queen, drew praise. Elizabeth Brenner Drew, in a 1968 *Atlantic Monthly* article entitled "The Health Syndicate: Washington's Noble Conspirators," noted their "tendency to attempt to translate personal experience and concerns into national health policy." Between 1948 and 1968, when the standing joke was that Congress supported research on those diseases that killed old men, just like those in Congress—and Congress raised each of the president's annual budget requests for the NIH—Drew picked up on that theme, noting that most resources "go into the research and treatment of diseases that affect primarily the elderly . . . [even though] the United States has an infant mortality rate that is worse than that in fourteen countries." She said of the efforts of the "health syndicate" that "the resulting distortions in federal health policy cannot be blinked aside."[5]

By the end of the 1960s, complaints of this kind, and even more about the lack of actual research success on the part of the NIH, were leading many to wonder, as Elizabeth Drew did, whether in "buying health services we have bought health." It was a rhetorical question: her implied answer was no. That kind of skepticism did not last long. Though the late 1960s marked the end of an era, and a temporary low point for the fortunes of the NIH, it was not the end of Laskerism and hardly the end of rising NIH budgets. The politics of advocacy, especially of the disease-oriented kind, would continue unabated, growing even stronger in the 1990s and into the new millennium. Between 1948 and 1968, twenty of the annual budget requests by the president were rejected in favor of even higher budgets, and ever since then no proposal to reduce the NIH budget has been brought before Congress.

A search through congressional hearings on the NIH budget since the late 1940s reveals a remarkable fact. To say, loosely, that the NIH has bipartisan support does not catch the full flavor of that support. There has simply been no congressional opposition whatever to the annual budget increases or to the more recent push to double the NIH budget. Here and there can be found complaints that other federal research agencies, notably the National Science Foundation and the Centers for Disease Control and Prevention (CDC), have not kept pace with the NIH and, as we will shortly see, mutterings about NIH research priorities, but that is all. No other federal agency has lived such a charmed life.

Why is that? A number of reasons seem likely: disease affects everyone; most people have had some personal or family experience with a disease; beneficiaries of federal grants are scattered throughout the country; there is a great confidence that a research investment will pay off; and the lobbying on behalf of NIH has been remarkably productive. If a large portion of Americans apparently know nothing at all about the NIH, they nonetheless have heard of the benefits of research and overwhelmingly support it.

Recent congressional advocates for the NIH, notably former Congressman John Porter and Senator Arlen Specter, have been uncommonly effective in the legislative efforts. Senator Specter has on occasion been open about the NIH dominance. In a 1998 appropriation hearing he said that "when we take money for NIH, candidly, we are shorting education in some phase, or worker safety."[6] That acknowledgment did not stop him, or anyone else, from voting for an increased NIH budget. There has been a mystique for medical research never matched by public health research or anything quite so pedestrian as worker safety. Adequate rest breaks for workers, or immunization drives, do not command the attention of the six o'clock TV news.

ADVOCACY: STRENGTHS AND LIMITS

The main research struggles have not, then, been at the level of finding money for the NIH. That has been relatively easy. The real struggles have turned on how best to spend the money, and how to get more money for various special purposes, most notably research on particular diseases. There are a large number of research advocacy groups. Some are simply devoted to promoting medical research in general. These include organizations such as Research!America, Funding First, and the Ad Hoc Group for Medical Research Funding. Others are particularly interested in gaining funds for academic research, and particularly for infrastructure support (buildings, laboratories, and equipment, salary subsidies and fellowships). These include the Federation of American Societies for Experimental Biology, the Association of American Medical Colleges, and the American Association of Universities. By far the largest number of groups are dedicated to gaining disease research support, and many of their names are now well known to the public (the American Heart Association, the Juvenile Diabetes Foundation, and the Alzheimer's Association, for instance). Many other smaller groups—such as Consider Alexander, pushing for research on Sudden Infant Death Syndrome, which my wife and I work for—are almost unknown.

The greatest political problems have come from those disease-oriented groups, which in recent years have become more effective in getting their voices heard but have also been criticized for the narrowness of their interests, particularly failing to take into account the nation's health needs other than their own. Over the years there has been a constant tension between money given to the NIH for its own discretionary purposes, most notably for basic research, and money earmarked for research on specific diseases or for the creation of new institutes. The advocacy efforts in behalf of disease research make full use of the Lasker techniques. Yet even advocacy groups will admit that earmarked research is not necessarily the best policy but that, without it, they would have less research money than they need. Members of Congress who say they oppose earmarked funds are still likely to support them on occasion. At an abstract level earmarked funds are easy to dislike but hard to give up as a tried and true way to gain an increased research budget.

It is useful to take a look at the various tactics used by advocacy groups, to ask what is reasonable and fair, and what oversteps the advocacy line. Advocacy for AIDS research, beginning in the mid-1990s, was particularly aggressive, aiming to get research money quickly and in large amounts— and, at the same time, to reduce the stigmatization of the disease. The American Diabetes Association is noted for its aggressive, even "hard-ball," tactics in going after increased NIH funds, while the Juvenile Diabetes Foundation has worked in a more peaceful way, not challenging the grant system.[7] The various breast cancer organizations, and the National Alliance for Breast Cancer Organizations, have stressed the particular health needs of women, tying their pursuit of research funds to the broader needs of women in American society. The National Alliance for Aging Research has of course promoted its area of interest but has also been active in ad hoc causes that do not directly deal with aging, most notably in pushing for stem-cell research.

Though there are faint signs of late that the hazards of the in-fighting for research funds among the advocacy organizations serve to alienate members of Congress, advocacy can serve valuable purposes.[8] Those organizations bring neglected issues to the attention of Congress and the public (as was earlier the case with breast cancer), they educate public officials, they unearth possibly unjust patterns of grant distribution, and they offer those suffering from various diseases a strong sense that their interests are being looked after. Women and minority groups have made considerable gains in recent years because of special efforts made in their behalf, some of it focused on particular health needs and some on their general health status. There can be drawbacks to disease advocacy as well, most notably the possibility that some groups' more effective lobbying efforts or greater financial resources may create unacceptable research disparities. Advocacy groups may proclaim exaggerated returns from research that far exceed reasonable expectations—misleading both Congress and, even worse, those suffering from the disease.

The legal scholar Rebecca Dresser has suggested ethical guidelines for research advocates.[9] They should be realistic, particularly avoiding inflated optimism; appreciative of the diversity of their own constituency's needs and levels of education; willing to reject parochialism in advocacy to take on the full range of their constituency's needs, not simply research benefits; and open to inclusiveness, recognizing the need for the different research advocacy groups to work together and no less recognizing that their own constituents may have many different health needs.

Are these realistic principles? They are surely reasonable enough and would do much good, but the politics of advocacy seems to offer the most success to the single-minded. Until that reality changes, those otherwise fine guidelines may have to wait. But if Michael J. Fox would speak up on behalf of heart research, and Michael Milken on Parkinson's disease, and Christopher Reeve on Alzheimer's—well, that would be the day.

SETTING PRIORITIES

While research advocacy and its politics have played a central role in the allocation of research money, some higher standards can be envisioned. Medical research ought also to reflect some vision, some long-range picture of what a society reflectively desires in the name of greater biological knowledge and improved health. Setting priorities is one way of working out what we want to count as good health, what we believe our society most needs to improve its physical and psychological well-being by means of improved health, and what we judge to count as significant medical progress.

At a more pedestrian level, down where actual policy is made, the questions are different, but no less hard: how to determine the amount of money to invest in research or to cope with the private agenda of varying interests (and self-interests), and how to cull out the most promising scientific leads.

Prodded by Congress, the NIH has had to grapple with those issues in recent years. Internationally, in a parallel development, the International Society on Priorities in Health Care was formed to promote priority setting for health care delivery. That organization has flourished but no comparable international group for priorities in research has emerged.

Not everyone in science welcomes the idea of setting priorities. Since we cannot predict the future of science, the skeptics ask, how can we set priorities? Is it not the essence of good science and creative innovation to be open to future possibilities we cannot foresee? Yet as Floyd E. Bloom, a former editor of *Science,* has argued in favor of setting priorities, "Does it make sense to be scientific about everything in our universe except the future course of science?"[10]

Remarkably enough, there is little theoretical literature on priority setting for research. By that I mean an effort to conceptualize long-term medical goals, to determine their relative importance, and then to devise sophisticated models of priority setting that are sensitive to ethical, economic, and political values. By contrast, there is a substantial literature and a worldwide movement in health care delivery.[11] They offer many suggestive ideas for medical research, which I will draw on in what follows.

What are the similarities and differences between priority setting for health care delivery and for biomedical research? Both require a reasonable way of dealing with scarce budgetary resources, determining what seems comparatively more or less important. Both need to allocate resources in an equitable manner, both for researchers seeking funds and for the health needs of the public. The differences are that health care delivery priorities use available resources to deal with immediate health care needs, making use of existing knowledge and skills. Research priorities focus on gaining new knowledge and skills, for the sake of the knowledge itself and to meet existing or projected health care needs. Considerably more uncertainty marks the impact of research outlays than of health care resource allocations.

Priority setting is not an easy exercise, beginning with the problem of defining the idea. I will specify some definitions, categorize the various priority-setting schemes in practice and the literature, look at the NIH debate for what can be learned about the politics of priority setting, and offer my version of a model process for government-supported research.

Types of Priority Setting

To begin at the beginning: what is a "priority"? The most pertinent dictionary definition (*Webster's*) is that of a "preferential rating." I understand that notion to be a ranking of goals or purposes in the order of their perceived importance. Strictly speaking, then, institutional or other goals should be understood as prioritized only when they are ranked or rated on a scale of most important to less or least important. Yet whether priority setting should aim for such a precise rating or remain a looser concept can itself be seen as part of the problem. Just how much precision is possible or desirable?

Drawing mainly on the health-policy debates and literature, I present possible four ways to set priorities along a continuum, from the most informal to the most formal (and, putatively, the most scientific at the latter end of the spectrum). With each I briefly note what seem to be their strengths and weaknesses.

Identification of needs and unranked criteria. Perhaps the most frequent forms of setting priorities encompass need identification and the use of unranked criteria. Need identification is simply the specification of perceived needs, collectively or individually, with the emphasis on large-scale shifts in policy direction. Speaking, for instance, of a forthcoming European intergovernmental conference on health care in 1997, two critics of the planned agenda argued, "Rather than [a] disease based strategy, we need greater focus on risk factors associated with diseases and determinants of health."[12] The phrase "greater focus" is a common one, representing the most informal approach to priority setting. There is no specificity about what "greater focus" means, in money or other resources.

More common is the use of a list of criteria for setting priorities with no attempt to rank them. That is the method used by the NIH (see below). The Commission on Health Research for Development urged in 1990 that research priorities for developing countries should include work on acute respiratory infections, tuberculosis, and research on reproductive health, among other needs.[13] The report contended that mortality alone is not a sufficient standard for ranking diseases in terms of importance. Given international mental health data, it said, a greater emphasis on morbidity would be appropriate. A similar approach—urging that more attention be paid to chronic and degenerative diseases of aging societies—can be found in a 1993 World Bank report on priority setting for disease control in developing countries.[14] A comparable approach was taken in a 1996 World Health Organization report.[15] In none of these cases were the priorities rank-ordered. A somewhat more formal approach was employed in a recent proposal to set priorities for research and development in the British National

Health Service pertinent to the relationship between primary and secondary care. It specified no less than twenty-one different "priority areas."[16]

There are both advantages and limitations in using need specification and unranked criteria. Their main advantage is to underscore the importance of prudential judgment and political flexibility. Their principal disadvantage is to set up a decision-making procedure—a kind of "this is what we think about when we decide" standard—rather than priorities. And being unranked, the criteria offer no way to distinguish "more important" from "less important" or to reconcile conflicts among them.

Ranking of general criteria. This method, proposed in Sweden and Norway for health care delivery, develops a set of general criteria and ranks medical conditions within them from more important to less important.[17] The Swedish model distinguishes between priority setting at the political and administrative level, and at the clinical level. The former gives the highest priority to the treatment of acute illnesses that will lead to permanent disability or premature death, the care of the chronically ill, and palliative care at the end of life. Preventive measures and physical therapy have a lower priority, while the treatment of less severe acute and chronic diseases has a still lower priority. Though the political/administrative and the clinical levels roughly correspond, the latter assigns a higher place to rehabilitation. The Norwegian model, which does not distinguish between the clinical and administrative levels, generally corresponds to its Swedish equivalent but is noteworthy for its inclusion of emergency psychiatry and childbirth complications among the highest priorities. The Danish Council of Ethics, reflecting on the Swedish and Norwegian proposals, rejected both of them, arguing that they were too general to be useful at the clinical level, opting instead for a list of unranked general criteria.[18]

The advantage of ranking general criteria is that the ranking process is easy to understand, operates flexibly, and tends to be acceptable to medical professionals. The principal disadvantage is that there is plenty of room for disagreement with specific complicated cases, such as infertility treatment, as well as problems in determining the economic impact of the general categories.

Numerical ranking within general criteria. This method goes a step further than simply ranking by degrees of importance. It devises a base of categories, as was done in Sweden and Norway, but then numerically ranks the various medical conditions within each one. Oregon used this method in setting its spending priorities for the state's Medicaid program.[19] There are more than seven hundred medical conditions in the overall ranking. Its general criteria are "essential," which includes "acute fatal" conditions, maternity care, and reproductive services; "very important," which encompasses acute and chronic nonfatal conditions; and "valuable to certain individuals"—the lowest category—which includes infertility services and medical therapy for viral warts. The criteria and rankings were put in place by a special commission following statewide public meetings.

Though the Oregon plan did not move on to provide universal coverage for all citizens, as originally planned, I judge the priority-setting process a success.[20] The prosperity of Oregon in recent years (at least until 2001), which has allowed coverage of most conditions in the overall list, has surely contributed to that result. But the success of that method in Oregon—a culturally and ethnically rather homogeneous state—does not prove it can work elsewhere. No other states have followed Oregon's lead, though many have considered it, perhaps because they fear it would be politically difficult to institute and sustain.

Ranking by economic techniques. For well over three decades, a number of economists and policy analysts have been trying to develop a quantitative formula for allocating resources. The aim has been to bring objectivity and higher rationality to political and policy processes thought to lack those features. In assessing research priorities based on burden-of-illness studies, the formula would take a significant variable—cost, or mortality, or disability, for instance—and use it to either set policy or be an important determinant of policy.[21] A comparison on the basis of QALYs, or quality-adjusted life years, is one method proposed for health care delivery that would develop an index number for determining which types of treatments to receive priority in situations of scarcity. A procedure that produced a relatively low quality of life for a few years (such as kidney dialysis for elderly patients) would rank lower than one that produced a high quality for a longer life (such as childhood immunization).[22] Or analysis of DALYs, disability-adjusted life years, would enable ministries of health in developing countries to determine comparatively their most pressing health needs. In comparison with QALYS, disability may well be a more validly measurable variable than quality of life.[23]

For all their attractiveness and purported objectivity, all these methods (and others have been proposed as well) have notable liabilities. It is difficult to assign quantitative values to the key variables, to assign a proper decision-making place to such values in shaping health care systems, and to come up with results that do not put various groups in the population at special risk. Any formula that takes the number of life-years remaining seriously, for instance, almost automatically situates the elderly as poorer prospects for health care than younger people. The "quality" of a life can be very much a function of individual values: what some persons would consider an unacceptable quality, others can live with (and prefer to being dead). One person's life-shattering disability is another person's acceptable challenge. Oregon's first cut at priority setting, using quantifiable criteria, produced such bizarre results that the state promptly abandoned all such efforts.[24]

I dwelled on the variety of ways to set priorities in health care because the systematic models used there are for the most part, though not entirely, transferable to the setting of research priorities. With that background in mind, I turn now to the NIH and its priority-setting system.

RESEARCH PRIORITIES AT THE NIH

In the late 1990s there was pressure on the NIH to explain and justify its methods for setting priorities. The pressure came from various disease advocacy groups, claiming their particular disease was not getting a fair share, and from Congress, which not only listened to those pleas and complaints but had some questions of its own. Some disease advocacy groups, in particular, made much of the discrepancy among the various diseases in the amount of research money spent on one disease versus another. In the late 1990s, for example, HIV/AIDS research got $1,069 per afflicted patient, while heart disease got only $93 per patient, and Parkinson's disease still less, at $26 per afflicted patient.[25] The congressional pressure has not been harsh, but it has been persistent, particularly as the NIH budget has grown. At least some observers believe that the recent large increases in the NIH budget, which should please NIH, will be matched by an increase in pressure to justify the way it allocates its funds, which may not please it. In response to the various pressures to explain itself better, the NIH in 1997 issued a white paper, "Setting Research Priorities at the National Institutes of Health."[26] That paper set forth the complexity of the NIH mission, criteria used to set priorities, the process used in deploying the criteria, and a response to various proposals to use a more objective burden of illness standard in setting priorities.

The complexity of its mission, the paper noted, stems from its aim to simultaneously carry out basic research—which can cut across a number of its institutes and often lead to unexpected practical results in the treatment of various diseases—and to do research on specific diseases. But even the latter kind of research is not confined to a specific institute. Accordingly, the paper contends, "There is, consequently, no 'right' amount of money, percentage of the budget, or number of projects for any one disease." At the same time, the NIH also has the obligation to provide infrastructure support to the entire biomedical research enterprise in the United States.

The criteria used by the NIH to set priorities are

- public health needs
- scientific quality of the research
- potential for scientific progress
- portfolio diversification across the broad and expanding frontiers of research
- adequate support of infrastructure (human capital, equipment and instrumentation, and facilities)[27]

The process for deploying these criteria is mixed. Congress from time to time mandates particular lines of research, leaving NIH less room to articulate its own criteria. Internally, each institute sets its own priorities using (presumably) these criteria; and the director of the NIH uses them as well, taking into account lay opinion, scientific advice, and internal discussion. The white paper describes the process of decision making in a general way but does not indicate how formal and systematic it actually is.

Of particular interest is the way the white paper responds to proposals over the years to use some form of a burden-of-illness standard to set priorities. It notes that the NIH could distribute research funds based on

- the number of people who have a disease
- the number of deaths caused by a disease
- the degree of disability produced by a disease
- the degree to which a disease cuts short a normal, productive, comfortable lifetime
- the economic and social costs of a disease
- the need to act rapidly to control the spread of a disease

While it does not refer to debates about QALYs and DALYs, any observer familiar with the international priority-setting literature in health care can find their echoes in that list. Americans will promptly recall the arguments about funding AIDS and cancer research, squabbles about the recent increases in the budget for Parkinson's disease and diabetes, and complaints of shortchanging diseases that bring severe disability but not death (such as arthritis) in the competition for funds.

The NIH white paper decisively rejects the use of any one of those possible standards as the sole determinant for priority setting. To use the number of people affected by a disease as the standard could come to emphasize less serious medical conditions (such as the common cold) and have a limited impact on population health. To focus on the number of deaths would neglect nonlethal chronic disease and disability and their high human and societal costs. Yet to focus exclusively on disability or economic costs would raise difficult questions about the feasibility of quantifying them and of calculating both direct and indirect costs. To use economic costs as a sole standard would neglect short illnesses and rapid death (for instance, Sudden Infant Death Syndrome). To base funding solely on immediate dangers to public health could take funds away from areas of greater long-term impact.

As it turned out, a 1999 study reported that there has been a significant relation between NIH research funding and measures of the burden of disease, although no particular association between the prevalence and incidence of a disease and research funding. Even if that was not the aim of the funding, it was surely not a bad outcome.[28] A 1997 NIH paper on the relationship of research priorities and cost of illness studies had reached no very specific conclusion. It noted that the difficulty in gaining accurate cost information, and relating costs to burden of illness, precludes hard judgments, offering at best rough orders of magnitude, useful as background information but of limited value for priority setting.[29]

Drawbacks of the NIH's Use of Criteria

As its principal guidelines in setting priorities the NIH uses unranked criteria and deploys them informally. The drawbacks of the use of unranked criteria are not hard to discern. With no distinction among them, is the criterion of public health really no more important than infrastructure support? With no hint of how to adjudicate conflicts among criteria, what if in fact the greatest scientific opportunities lie in combating the common cold? The criteria themselves are, moreover, radically dissimilar. How can anyone strike a balance between the need of institutions for new equipment and the possibility of progress in understanding Alzheimer' disease? The white paper simply does not address problems of that kind.

To make matters worse, the deployment of those criteria, described in a vague way only—and in the end heavily dependent on essentially black-box

decisions taken by NIH leadership—provides no clues about how such conflicts and dilemmas are handled. The NIH argument that no single standard—economic or medical—should be used to set priorities does not confront the obvious point that it might meaningfully combine two or three or
more of the standards it rejected for single use. The white paper's hinted implication (but only that) of combining them in some fashion is less than illuminating.

It is hard to avoid an unsettling conclusion: despite what NIH says, it really has no settled priority-setting procedure at all. If a priority is "a preferential rating," a definition consistent with other dictionaries, then there
is none. The lack of a preferential rating or ranking of the criteria it em-
ploys deprives the NIH system of the minimal elements necessary to set
priorities in a systematic fashion. It may be a method of decision making,
or a method of "this-is-what-we-think-about-as-we-make-our-choice-of-
research-allocation-possibilities," but it is not a priority-setting *method*,
lacking the necessary ingredients to make it so. Without ranking, there are
no priorities. To say this is not to deny that, when the final decisions are
made, some things will get more money than others and thus that de facto
priorities will be observable. It is only to say that the NIH does not have a
priority-setting method in the strict sense of the term.

The NIH's way of setting priorities has not gone unchallenged. Congress
was sufficiently concerned to ask the National Academy of Sciences'
Institute of Medicine (IOM) to conduct a study of the way the NIH set priorities. Chaired by a leading and thoughtful scientist and former dean of the
Yale Medical School, Dr. Leon Rosenberg, and working with a tight dead-
line in the first half of 1998, the committee interviewed key NIH staff
members, invited comments from various disease advocacy groups, and
sought the judgment of many scientists and their professional organizations.[30]

While the IOM committee had a number of recommendations to make,
two were of special importance. One of them was that the NIH should have
better procedures in place to allow the public to make its views known, and
specifically known within the director's office (by establishing an office of
public liaison), a recommendation immediately seized on.[31] The other was
that the NIH should work more diligently to gain knowledge about the
burden of illness within the United States, arguing that the NIH needs a
better data base for its priority decisions. Additionally the IOM committee
recommended greater clarity on the part of NIH in implementing its priorities.

If It Ain't Broke, Don't Fix It

What stands out in the IOM report is that it expressed no basic dissatisfaction with the way the NIH sets its priorities. In a variant on "if it ain't broke, don't fix it," the report's very first "recommendation" is a broad endorsement of the NIH procedures: "The committee generally supports the criteria that NIH uses for priority setting and recommends that NIH continue to use these criteria in a balanced way to cover the full spectrum of research related to human health." Since the mere existence of unranked criteria offers no guidance on what counts as a "balanced way" of setting priorities, the committee in effect overlooked or sidestepped the theoretical difficulties of working with nonpreferential, unranked criteria. Nor did it make clear just how a greater public input would facilitate hard decision making—many scientists claim there is more than enough public influence already—or what difference better and more extensive burden-of-illness data would make either. Congress has not demanded more data and might not want different priorities even if it had them. The data might, however, add useful information to the budget debates, at least serving as a corrective to poorly based claims and complaints.

In light of the serious substantive problems that can readily be unearthed in the NIH priority-setting criteria and processes, what are we to make of the IOM report? A facile answer is that the IOM committee would have profited from a close examination of the international priority-setting literature even though it is mainly focused on health care delivery. That would at least have made evident some of the more subtle problems of priority setting.

A more pertinent answer is probably that the committee's composition (heavily weighted with scientists) and its report reflected a broad and deep consensus within the American medical research and clinical community. It is that the NIH is a vital, effective, and well-run organization and was blessed then with a particularly distinguished and effective leader in Dr. Harold Varmus. Even if by some more rigorous standards the IOM report did not go very deeply into priority setting, it was in effect saying, we like what the NIH is doing, we trust its leadership to make good priority decisions, and we see no good reason to shake the faith of Congress or the general public about the way NIH goes about carrying out its mission. That was a reasonable and fair conclusion, reflecting the fact that the IOM study uncovered no egregiously irrational or unfair practices.

Now if that judgment is correct, it nonetheless raises an additional question. If in the end a basic trust in NIH and its leadership rests as the final standard of the way the NIH sets priorities, what would happen with bad leadership? Isn't one point of having a well-defined, organized scheme for setting priorities to allow an institution (or health care system, as the case may be) not only to judge the ways resources are allocated by some higher standards, but also to control the way administrators and others in power actually do so? Of course that has always been the attraction of some formal, scientifically grounded, putatively objective way of setting priorities. That is why the economic techniques of QALYs, DALYs, and the like have attracted at least academic attention (and a bit more than that in the case of DALYs, officially embraced by the World Bank). And it is surely why another, less noticed, critique of the NIH procedures places its emphasis almost entirely on burden-of-illness studies as the way NIH should set its priorities (giving the health of the public a clearly higher priority than other NIH goals).[32]

SCIENCE, POLITICS, AND RATIONALITY

Often enough, the economic and other formal methods of priority setting are called "rational," such as the use of QALYs and DALYs. The implication is that any other method is less than rational, probably irrational. But the IOM committee—the evidence of the report suggests—tacitly adopted a different standard in making its assessment, one that might be called political and pragmatic. It judged the past and present results of the work of NIH to be important and exemplary, however it managed to achieve them. It concluded that its leadership is responsible and sensible and that it can work perfectly well with somewhat vague and potentially contradictory priority-setting criteria. It almost surely made the political judgment that little good for the future of NIH would come by holding it up to some supposedly higher, more theoretical, standard of methodological rationality.

That can be a perfectly sound conclusion. It also suggests to me why politicians and administrators are far less drawn to the more elaborate kinds of priority setting their advocates might expect and hope for. Politicians are more trustful of politics and pragmatic common sense to deal with the complexity of priority setting than they are of more formal schemes, whether those of economists or health-policy analysts. It is probably no accident that Oregon is the only state to have adopted an explicit priority-setting formula. Nor is it probably mere chance that most of the countries that have put together commissions to propose better means of setting priorities for health care allocation have not succeeded in getting their legislators or health care administrators to share their enthusiasm.

For all its faults, inequities, and irrationalities, what I have called the political method of setting priorities still seems attractive. It is familiar, messy, and yet comparatively simple in its operation: people argue, struggle, and lobby to get what they want, and there are winners and losers—but also another chance on another day for the losers to turn the tables. By contrast, the more technically sophisticated a priority-setting scheme, the more difficult its advocates' job in gaining support for actual implementation. Burden-of-illness studies, for all their elegance, are almost always mired in technical disputes among competing experts, but also difficult to carry out even if a consensus on methodology can be reached.

I am not arguing against the search for good methods of setting priorities. I was an early and enthusiastic supporter of the Oregon Medicaid effort to set priorities and of the broader international effort now under way to develop good strategies and methods for priority setting in health care delivery. Better ideas for setting research priorities are in particular short supply. Nonetheless, if the international priority-setting movement is to get anywhere in the long run, it will have to accomplish two tasks. The most evident one is to generate good, and politically persuasive, ideas about how best to set priorities, in terms of both substance and process. Can it overcome the bias toward messy, but familiar, politics? The less explored, but to my mind no less important, task is to assess the political and administrative attractiveness of the kind of informal model used at the NIH. It reflects, I am convinced, a way of working with priorities and difficult decisions that might have appeal in other countries as well. Congress wanted to know how NIH sets its priorities, but it did not ask for or seem to expect anything too precise or too scientific; and the IOM committee did not look for, much less demand, that either. The IOM report recommended modest changes perfectly consistent with what NIH is already doing (as NIH defenders said, "but we're already doing that!" and, to some extent, that is true).

A PROPOSAL FOR REFORM

Sympathetic though I am to the political mode of priority setting—informality has its (unsung) virtues—in the long run the NIH needs to develop more explicit and refined means of setting priorities. It may not always have good leadership or such a sympathetic and permissive Congress. While there seems at present to be no significant pressure to reform the NIH priority-setting method, and no urgent need to do so, it is far from ideal. It rests on no clearly articulated view of the long-range health needs of the nation. It engages in piecemeal warfare against illness and disease, aiming to take enemy territory and to win whatever battles that can be won. While indefinite increases in the NIH budget are conceivable, Congress may not fix them at the rate of 10 percent a year. Prosperous times and generous legislatures can take the sting out of priority setting, as both the Oregon Medicaid program and NIH can testify. The real test will come when and if the good times disappear, forcing steady-state or declining budgets.

On the assumption that greater knowledge is an infinite good, and better health always worth pursuing, then the present pattern makes considerable sense. But once it is recognized that there are other social goods, many of which can make a more direct contribution to health than medicine (such as education or decent jobs), then a more nuanced approach to medical research will be needed. And in resetting our research priorities, we must start to take serious account of the fact that much, even if not all, research increases health care costs with only a marginal gain to population health; that day of reckoning will someday come. Most generally, the more public money we invest in research, the higher the standards for determining how best to spend it.

Culling useful ideas from priority setting in biomedical research and in health care delivery, and from the various approaches sketched above, I offer an outline for an enriched approach to priority setting for biomedical research. It has five ingredients, two bearing on research substance and three on process.

Creating the baseline: the goals of medicine.   Early in this book I contended that the research agenda needs to embody the proper and appropriate goals of medicine as its starting points. The priority for each goal should not be fixed but should shift at different points in time according to those health needs discerned to be most pressing. Any attempt to specify research priorities should, then, begin by attempting to discern what those needs are at present and likely to linger into the future and those that are likely to appear in the future. At present, for instance, the de facto research priorities displayed by the NIH budget give a primacy to lethal diseases and a lesser place to disabling but not necessarily lethal conditions.

Does that priority still make sense as chronic disease becomes more dominant? My answer is yes, but I will not develop that point. I want instead to take a step back and simply list here the leading categories of health care goals in an effort to determine which seem, at any given point in time, to require the most attention, and which can comparatively receive less attention. To make these goals more usable for policy purposes, I present them here in a somewhat different way than I did in chapter 4. It is important to understand that my order of listing does not try to suggest what at present the appropriate priorities ought to be. Nor does it urge my list's adoption: what is important as the first step in any priority-setting discussion is to develop and publicly debate its categories.

Foundational goals of research. A plausible set of goals, for instance, would be

the cure of diseases likely to cause a premature death among a large portion of the population, with the highest priority within this category given to those diseases that are infectious and capable of rapid spread to younger age groups

the promotion of health and the prevention of disease

the reduction of disability, physical and mental, to the degree that it ceases to be a significant social and economic burden

the rehabilitation of the disabled

the relief of pain and suffering to the level that the majority of those burdened by them are able to function effectively as persons, family members, workers, and citizens

the compression of morbidity and a disability-reduced old age

palliative care for those with serious pain and suffering and at the end of life

Special needs and priorities. Special needs and opportunities are always likely to be present and they will and should affect priority setting:

imperative social considerations (such as redressing past discrimination; issues of race, gender, and aging)

disease stigma and public fear (e.g., cancer and Alzheimer's disease)

promising research opportunities (e.g., genomics)

preserving and strengthening scientific infrastructure (laboratories, fellowships)

An optimal model for priority setting. By optimal I mean a system of priority setting that responds to the weaknesses and problems of the present methods and selects from those available their most positive features. I propose, then, that any method of choosing priorities for government-sponsored research should have the following specifications:

the collection and use of appropriate scientific and economic information (e.g., as recommended by the IOM study and the Progressive Policy Institute)

a *method* for establishing priorities, that is, for rank-ordering its aims

considerable discretionary leeway for those who administer governmental programs, but within a broad framework of rank-ordering

the use of a reasonable and feasible political process, drawing on public and professional opinion in a methodical and balanced way

A model political process. An effort should be made to develop a good political process for priority setting, one that goes beyond lay advisory committees. A more direct and determinative public role would require

systematic and extended public education on the goals of medicine and national health care needs, together with a corresponding explication of research options and the possibilities of achieving them

carefully developed public opinion surveys on research priorities

a parallel discussion of the same issues by biomedical and other health professionals, with opinion surveys taken

establishment of a permanent commission, with rotating membership, to collect and evaluate the results of the public and professional discussions and results of the opinion surveys, to take testimony from scientific, academic, and other advocacy groups

periodic recommendations by the commission to Congress (e.g., every three to four years) of a set of research priorities

The emphasis of this process should be to set broad priorities, not to micromanage research. It should seek a balance between the aims and needs of the scientific community and of the general public that is paying for the research. One model for the commission I have in mind is that of the Council of Economic Advisers, established in 1946 to advise the president on national economic policy, but whose recommendations are influential within Congress as well. As an advisory group that council's recommendations are not binding but nonetheless have been important over the years. Alternatively, Congress could establish a joint committee on medical research priorities, composed of members from both houses of Congress and modeled on the Joint Economic Committee. The advantage of the latter is that it is Congress that determines the actual NIH budget each year, and it is likely to be more responsive to a congressional committee than to the executive branch. The crucial point is that a mechanism is needed to evaluate national health care needs, and to do so based on good information.

Criteria for evaluating the setting of priorities. Whatever the method of priority setting that is chosen, it should meet the following standards:

- simplicity (understandable to the public)
- transparency (open and clear in its procedures)
- reformability (easily modified and adaptable to changing circumstances)
- equity (fair to researchers and to the health needs of all groups in the population)
- participatory (reflects scientific and public influence)

As a process, priority setting in medical research should seek to blend long-term health goals, social and moral values, and an open political process. If it confines itself to an acceptable political process only, procedural only in its focus, simply negotiating the desires of various interest groups, it is likely to neglect the hard work of devising a plausible and attractive picture of future directions for human health that will collectively serve the entire community. If it sticks to the scientific venture only, then it is likely to scant the moral and social meaning of research directions. As with any good recipe, it is not the ingredients alone that make it nourishing and tasty, but skill in assembling and blending them. Priority setting is not much different.

Setting Priorities in Health Care and Scientific Research

As with most other aspects of federally supported research of all kinds, the government's various health-related research interests and programs exist without coordination or any formal prioritizing of funds allocated to them. The government's allocation of science research in general does not prioritize or coordinate that research.[33] In addition to the NIH, there are also the CDC, the Agency for Healthcare Research and Quality, as well as assorted other health-related research programs in various governmental agencies, such as the Department of Defense.

Though medical research dominates other forms of health-related research, it does so unsystematically. It had the historical momentum of the generally successful campaign to eradicate infectious disease from the late nineteenth century onward, the advent of antibiotics in the 1930s, and the organized efforts to improve health during World War II. The medical route made great sense and still does. But there are a number of important research directions now, and a systematic comparison of their various contributions is now needed. Among the most important dimensions of research are

medical research

health service research

technology assessment, especially related to evidence-based medicine

public health research for health promotion and disease prevention, including epidemiological research

socioeconomic research on the background determinants of health

information research, especially on the storage and retrieval of patients' histories, and readily accessible treatment information for physicians

For well over a century our medical motto has been that the key to better health is better biological knowledge and the application of that knowledge to the development of various technologies to cure disease. Yet it has been known for decades now that public health and socioeconomic status are comparatively more determinative of health status than the availability of medical care. Why is it, then, that public health and behavioral research still lag behind medical research? Part of the answer is doubtless the historical momentum of medicine mentioned above, the better play medical research gets in the media, the excitement of its heavy focus on the cure of particular diseases, and very active lobbying for medical research funds.

There has never been a Mary Lasker fighting for public health research or health service research. Neither is ever likely to produce notable spin-offs or exportable products for pharmaceutical or other companies. The few companies devoted to behavioral change, usually selling their service to HMOs and corporate health plans, are nowhere near the top of the biomedical hill in sales or profit. With the exception of the NIH, none of the other agencies has the kind of congressional support or legislative advocacy it needs to command significantly higher budgets. What should be an integrated health research policy is fragmented. The failure here lies not so much in the de facto budgetary dominance of the NIH but in the total absence of a forum to assess and compare the various health research budgets.

This lack is not a trivial omission. The aim of a national health care system and policy is to improve health, whether by preventing disease or treating it once it has appeared. There are many ways of doing this. It would then seem reasonable to lay the various means of accomplishing those aims side by side to see what, at any given historical moment, is likely to make the greatest comparative contribution, and what will make lesser contributions. The working assumption at present is that medical research belongs at the top, but there has never been a serious public or congressional debate about this, much less a debate that would see the various claimants going head-to-head in public forums and congressional hearings. The debate should not simply be between different research budgets, though we need that too, but also between spending money on research to improve future health and spending less on that and more money instead to equitably and fully distribute what is already available.

The fragmentation of medical and other forms of health-related research is replicated within scientific research more broadly. Former Representative Porter, the House leader in promoting the doubling of the NIH budget in the late 1990s, spoke tellingly in a speech commemorating the twenty-fifth anniversary of the White House Office of Science and Technology Policy.[34] That office had been created in 1976 to provide the president with timely scientific information and to act as a formal liaison agency between the executive branch and the scientific community. Porter noted that, many months after President Bush had taken office, no director of that agency had been appointed. He also noted that science and technology portfolios are distributed in at least nine departments and four major agencies of the federal government—and no less distributed among many different committees of Congress. To add to the confusion, no more than 2 to 3 percent of the members of Congress have a scientific background. Ironically, he observed, "while science and technology are ascendant in Congress, they are not so ascendant within the White House."

Porter's observation helps make sense of the otherwise crazy-quilt pattern of federal research budgets. For the fiscal year 2003, the Bush administration requested $2.1 trillion for scientific research (compared with $379 billion for the Department of Defense), broken down into some of the following categories.[35]

National Institutes of Health, $27.3 billion, an increase of 17 percent

National Science Foundation, $5.0 billion, an increase of 5 percent

Energy (Office of Science), $3.2 billion, the same as in 2001

Defense R & D, $45.1 billion, an increase of 9 percent

NASA, $15.0 billion, an increase of 1 percent

Environmental Protection Agency (Office of Research and Development), $697 million, an increase of 6 percent

The NIH increase will complete in 2003 the five-year drive to double its budget, though half of that increase was slated for bioterrorism and cancer research. Out of the overall science budget of $2.1 trillion, two-thirds of the government's spending on basic research will go to the NIH. The CDC has finally seen, in the past few years, a decent increase in its budget, if not up to that won by the NIH at least beginning to approach it. Its $4.3 billion budget for 2002 represented an 11 percent increase for its regular activities (though additional large increases for bioterrorism and emergency activities brought the full total to $7.5 billion). Though the complaint of a advocate for the American Physical Society that the president's budget gave "short shrift to everything except the life sciences" seems exaggerated, the amount devoted to health is surely striking. There is no need to begrudge the money given to the NIH, money well spent, but there is something strange about a science budget that sees only minor increases in other areas, particularly energy, climate, and the environment (with only a 6 percent increase for the Environmental Protection Agency). Quite apart from the value of research in many non–life science areas for improving the country's economic strength, the budget cuts for welfare programs in recent years ignore the enormous impact of socioeconomic factors on health status.[36] The California energy crisis of 2001, eventually brought under control, nonetheless foreshadows similar crises projected to occur across the country in the near future. Yet the 2003 budget for basic research on energy is slated for only a 2 percent increase.

John Porter wryly noted that for well over a hundred years a federal department of science has been proposed, a good idea, but that it is unlikely ever to be created. If so, that is a shame. It could provide the vehicle for a careful comparison of health, social, economic, and environmental needs and a place for debate on reasonable research priorities. Perhaps our military and health needs are the most important of all and need the most research money—or perhaps they are just the most politically appealing ways to spend research money. But this country has never had a serious and extended debate on scientific research priorities.

10 Research and the Public Interest

The aim of medical research is to better understand the human body and mind, and to make use of that knowledge to improve human health. My argument has been that the very importance of that research, its power to attract good scientists, to excite the public, to reduce pain and suffering, to turn a profit, and to offer tantalizing possibilities of human enhancement, opens the door to hazardous possibilities. Those possibilities coexist with the good that research brings. An intense commitment to research has its own problems. It falls into that category of human life where the good and the bad often intermingle, where the desire to do good can be potent enough to invite the temptation to go too far, thus undermining itself, and where the benefits of research appear so self-evident that they need no defense.

Some threats to the integrity of research come from within the research community, when for various reasons researchers manipulate scientific data or risk conflict of interest and degradation of the value of scientific communalism to gain financial benefits and corporate ties. The misuse of human subjects has come partly from within—often when a noble research goal overshadows the risk to its subjects—and partly from the outside, where pressures for money, prestige, and academic promotion often put researchers in a vise.

The deepest conflicts and the greatest threat to scientific integrity come from old-fashioned hubris, a prideful conviction of our ability to transform the human condition, whether in overcoming aging and death or making use of genetic and other knowledge to enhance human nature and its traits. To be sure, in the struggle against fatalism, medical research has made many important contributions—bringing both hope and genuine progress—but it has not found ways of determining where to set limits or what, in the end, truly contributes to human happiness. When the research imperative acts as a moral bludgeon—turning a moral good into a moral obligation and then into a call to arms—to level other values in the name of reducing suffering, it goes too far. Hubris does not dominate medical research, but it is there and growing, worthy of our scrutiny. It is a function of the public dreams and expectations of research, supported by Congress with few questions asked; the mixing of monetary and melioristic motives that industry brings with it; and the hard fact that we human beings always seem to want more than we have, however much we have—and perfect health is a good we do not have, at least not for long in our lives.

That last fact perhaps best explains the steady rise in the National Institutes of Health budget, one of the few federal budgets in recent years to get large annual increases. How otherwise can it be that, as the nation's health steadily improves, and mortality rates drop for every age group, the budget to fight disease gets larger and not smaller? Should it not be the other way around—as, say, happened with the Defense Department budget with the end of the Cold War? One argument, commonly offered when more, not less, money is sought, is that the research opportunities have never been greater. That has been said before, and many times, over the life span of the NIH, but not so effectively. The increasingly salient pharmaceutical and biotechnology industries, which also proclaim the research message, have worked in tandem with the NIH to advance their case. In the selling of stocks and bonds the advertising rule stipulated by the Security and Exchange Commission is this: past performance is no guarantee of similar future performance. No such rule obtains in the drive for research funds, where it is precisely past success that underwrites the guarantee of still more success in the future; and often enough that is a valid claim.

There is another possible explanation for the attraction of medical research. At some point in recent years our ideas about medicine and health crossed a great divide. Health *was* a necessity of life, but a time-limited necessity. We would eventually get sick and die, maybe as children, maybe as adults. No one could know when. Our human nature held us within the boundaries that nature had given us, and those boundaries had some flexibility, but not much. That belief has eroded in recent decades. For most people it is anachronistic to speak of a "natural" life span or to oppose lines of research on the grounds that they aim for what is "unnatural" or to question advertised possibilities of a longer and better life we are told research will bring us.

Health and good medicine to make it possible were once seen as necessities of life, but not themselves the source of a good life—that we drew from our family life, our society, our religious and philosophical traditions. Now we assume that research can eventually rid us of our mortality and our aging bodies; well, maybe not quite, we concede at more sober moments, but close enough. It can no less assist us in devising a higher quality of life, transforming and expanding our choices. The meaning of the enhancement drive is not just the once-fanciful desires it may satisfy, but the perfectly acceptable, not even futuristic, possibilities for changing ourselves or our children into something more attractive.

Am I not, however, confusing the enthusiasm of outlandish research advocates or hyperventilating media with reality? A bit, but not much. Increasingly what were once thought of as utopian hopes are being presented as likely outcomes, needing only more time and research money to bring them to fruition. Hope and reality have fused. Medical miracles are expected by those who will be patients, predicted by those seeking research funds, and profitably marketed by those who manufacture them. The budget of the NIH rises because the dreams of health grow ever larger. The healthier we get, the healthier still we want to become. If we can live to eighty, why not to one hundred? If cosmetic surgery can make our noses look better, reproductive biology can make our children look better. What the biologist René Dubos some decades spoke of as "the mirage of health"— a perfection that never comes—is no longer taken to be a mirage, but solidly out there on the horizon, already foreshadowed in, say, the Human Genome Project or embryonic stem cell research.

RESEARCH AND OTHER HUMAN PRIORITIES

A significant part of the new outlook is the belief that research will lead to knowledge that will *always* improve the human condition. The shadow of nuclear weapons, which made it difficult to hold such a vast view of science just after World War II, has now passed. Medical research is now treated as if it is an independent actor, with its own force and momentum for the good. Historically speaking, that may well have been true for much of its early history. By leading to improved health, it brilliantly dealt with a critical variable in the wealth and welfare of society. In many parts of the world that is still a valid perspective, and a lightening of the burden of disease and disability will make a huge difference.

But most of the world's medical research goes on in developed countries, and most of its hoped-for benefits aim at those countries; and it is in those countries that the greatest push for still more research has come. Yet for all the research possibilities, health progress in developed countries will no longer dramatically improve their overall welfare. Health care costs are a great problems in all countries, but I know of none that blame the general burden of illness for whatever other economic or social problems they may have. Burden-of-illness studies may show that a reduction of illness would be of economic value to a country, and surely desired by most people. But that is not the same as showing grave harm to the country, competitively or otherwise, from the burden of its population's poor health. No developed country could make that claim and none do. Subgroups within those countries need to have their health improved—blacks and Native Americans in the United States most notably—but typically they need a fairer and better distribution of available resources, not necessarily more medical research (though here and there that could help, particularly public health and socioeconomic research), but also research on various ethnic propensities to various maladies.

While it surely neither will nor should happen, consider—as an imaginative exercise—what we would get if there was no progress at all from this point forward, and medicine remained restricted to what is now available. The rich countries would remain rich. Most of their citizens would make it to old age in reasonably good health. There would continue to be incremental gains in mortality and morbidity, the fruit of improved social, economic, and educational conditions, and improvements in the evaluation and use of present therapies. No prosperous country would sink from the lack of medical advances.

If that judgment seems extreme, consider the difference between rich and poor countries. No rich country faces a situation as desperate as AIDS in many African nations, which not only kills tens of thousands of people but also destroys the infrastructure of society by depriving it of teachers, government administrators, family leaders, and health care workers. But then no rich country is forced to deny its citizens the available AIDS therapies, which can now keep people alive. No developed country has an epidemic equivalent to that of HIV disease in sub-Saharan Africa. We can go on, but those other countries cannot, at least not at a humane level of civic life. Most of all, they need the research that will lead to an inexpensive and efficacious vaccine. They need it for their sheer survival as functioning nations. The developed countries in contrast need it to reduce premature deaths and economic and social burdens. That is an important difference, even though both developed and developing countries need the vaccine; it is the urgency and priority that are different.

Medical research for the benefit of affluent countries raises their already high quality of life to one that is still higher. Medical research that benefited poor countries would, in contrast, allow them for the first time to have something that could even be called a quality of life. If American health is not the best in the world, and it is not—ranking fifteenth according to a WHO study—that is a distribution failure, not a research failure.[1] Our "efficiency" ranking is thirty-seven, about the worst of any developed nation. Another study found that the relative U.S. performance in providing health care is, by most indicators, declining.[2] Even so, we spend ever more money on research, and more on the provision of health care—an unsettling situation. It is not the United States that *needs* medical research for its survival and flourishing, though it certainly welcomes it. The poor countries, still facing a long list of lethal diseases, with malaria, tuberculosis, and assorted tropical diseases as outstanding examples, do need it.

The point of pushing the difference between rich and poor countries is to bring two neglected questions to the foreground. What is an appropriate research agenda for countries that *already* have a high level of health, general well-being, and social viability? What are sensible health care priorities for a country that leads the world in medical research, technological application, and the highest per capita health care spending—but still does not get the best outcomes and has over forty million uninsured, erratically able at best to gain the benefits of the latest technological advances made possible by research?

I will get at those questions by employing the category of basic human needs, in part the needs of different age groups in society, and in part individual and population needs. I take this approach for two reasons. The first is that, if the agenda of research is simply and utterly to vanquish death and disease, pain and suffering, that is unrealistic, even if the excitement of research possibilities leads some to talk that way. The test I want to propose is whether research helps manage them in the way that a society functions effectively in supporting its crucial institutions, which include the family, government, education, voluntary organizations, and economic entities. The second reason is that I hope the research medicine of the future will remain a medicine of health, to be judged by common standards for the public good, and not a medicine of personal desire and private enhancement, much less one driven and determined by the market.

RESEARCH AND HUMAN NEED

In chapter 9, I set out a possible approach to priority setting. Its starting point was the need to understand what constituted the most important and less important health needs at any given moment in history. Not everything that would have been a priority a century ago should be a priority now. I now extend that idea by proposing that a fruitful way to assess health needs is to look to the life cycle, and the health needs of people at different stages of life. Three stages offer a sufficiently clear set of categories: childhood and adolescence, the adult years of work and family, and old age.

Childhood and Adolescence

There was a time when the primary threat to childhood was a high infant mortality rate, with infectious diseases such as scarlet fever, measles, diphtheria, and smallpox putting young children at special risk. Older cemeteries in the United States and Europe are filled with the graves of children, strikingly different from the pattern to be observed in more modern cemeteries. With the now-available immunizations, healthier living conditions, and good prenatal care, hardly any child in a developed country needs to die young.

Most of the leading childhood health problems that remain are the result of harmful social and economic conditions, not the kind of diseases that medical research goes after. While there remain a formidable number of genetic diseases affecting children, perfect targets for research, their contribution to the poor health of children is statistically minimal, even if terrible for the children and their parents. The United States lags behind other developed countries in its indicators for child and maternal health because of social and economic ills, not because of diseases not yet cured or prevented by a lack of research. Heart disease killed 214 children between the ages of one and four in 1998, while homicide killed 399. In that same year 1,000 children between five and fourteen died of cancer, while 777 were murdered or committed suicide.[3]

I am hardly denying the value of research on, say, childhood cancer or the control of childhood asthma and juvenile diabetes—and the latter two have disturbingly become more common. Or research on Sudden Infant Death Syndrome that took the life of an infant son of mine at six weeks. For children in developing countries there are still many diseases where research is required, but if the present medical and preventive advantages now routinely available in the United States were available there, the drop in infant mortality rates would be striking. The larger question I am raising, for the developed countries, is this: when can it be said in general that the health of an age group has improved to an extent that the greatest need lies with other age groups?

Though childhood is the clearest case I can think of where medical research that aims to cure disease has comparatively less (but still much) to offer to improve the welfare of children in developed countries in comparison with other age groups, there is still a great deal that other kinds of research bearing on childhood health can offer. Social science and economic research can help us better understand how poverty affects the health of children (for instance, in understanding the recent increase in asthma among poor children), while behavioral research may provide insight into the failure of many parents to seek available, and free, immunization for their children. Many of the great health threats to children are not medical in the usual sense at all: murder, violence, substance abuse, sexually transmitted disease, teenage pregnancy, and suicide. They require various forms of research, most of it social rather than medical. To be sure, medicine will have a role to play in dealing with harms of that kind, but they are harms that are not biological in origin, and medicine's role will be that of helping repair social harms, not eliminate them, which is beyond its power.

The Adult Years

By "the adult years," I mean that time of life between, roughly, ages eighteen and seventy. It is a time of higher education and job entry at one end of the age spectrum, and of the formation of families, of finding meaningful work, of taking an active community role; and, at the other end of the spectrum, of seeing children off into their own lives, of winding down the occupational part of life, of giving thought to old age. It is also a period when the incidence of premature death, illness, and disability begin to rise and continue upward as age advances. The role of medicine increases in importance during these years. In addition to its lifetime role of helping people deal with the failing of their bodies and minds, medicine becomes particularly important because of the need of people during this period to function well. They need good health to get and keep a job, to have children and raise them, to take an active political and social role in society. If disability threatens the discharge of the important social and familial roles they—not yet old and no longer young—take on, its impact is huge.

Hence three health issues are of special importance during this stage of life. The first is that of premature death, now most likely to come not in childhood but during these adult years. The avoidance of a premature death becomes particularly important for research initiatives, particularly death from cancer, heart disease, diabetes, and the other notorious killers. This effort also requires understanding that it is not death that is the enemy, but death at the wrong time, for the wrong reason, and for those who have not had the chance to live out a full life cycle. Hardly less important is the necessity to combat those mental health conditions that can have almost the same effect as a premature death, that of a premature social death, of a kind that severe schizophrenia and depression can bring with them.

The second issue is that of reproductive medicine and the health of women. The control of reproduction by safe and effective contraception is an appropriate and much-pursued research area. Infertility relief is of importance as well, but here (as noted in chapter 7) more research on infertility as a public health problem rather than as a medical problem is clearly in order. That should include behavioral research working to persuade women not to delay childbearing until their late thirties or early forties (and social research and occupational changes to make that more easily possible in light of job and career demands). Infertility can be, for the individual woman, a serious crisis; procreation is an important part of life. But it is not, for developed societies, a serious social problem, threatening their very structure. Nor is it a problem for the world as a whole, suffering no population shortage. Nonetheless, research on infertility needs to proceed, but in such a way that the results do not continue the present pattern of high-cost treatments with relatively poor outcomes, available primarily to the affluent. Late procreation and sexually transmitted disease, major causes of infertility, are not problems to be left to medical research as the solution.

The third issue of special importance is that of health promotion and disease prevention. The middle years of life, often full of stress because of work and family demands, are a particularly important time for health promotion and disease prevention efforts. Here the recent and welcome initiatives of Research!America, of the CDC, and of the American Heart Association to promote greater research on health promotion have a special relevance. The vast amounts of money spent on the Human Genome Project should be matched by equally large amounts to be spent on behavioral research. The estimate that 50 percent of all deaths in the United States can be traced to behavioral causes, with smoking at the top of the list, make self-evident the value of such research, more so even than genetic research. The possibility of a more equitable way to improve health, independent of the pharmaceutical and biotechnology industries, ought to be an important attraction also. American health care for those in their adult years is lavish and expensive, at least if they have adequate health insurance. Even so, the outcome in comparison with other countries is not something worth boasting about. That is not a research failure, only an equity, efficiency, and distribution failure.

Old Age

The compression of mortality, as I contended in chapter 3, is a wholly suitable, even ideal research goal for that final, decisive stage of life known as old age. Death itself is not an appropriate, or even sensible, target for medicine. Nor is aging in and of itself an appropriate target. There is no known social benefit that a radically increased life expectancy would bring, but many plausibly envisioned harms. But it is within the range of research to improve the health of the aged, mentally and physically. A long life, followed by a relatively quick death—the ideal of the compression of morbidity theory—is now within the realm of plausibility; that it is already happening to some considerable extent is an encouraging note. A wholly defensible ideal is an old age marked by vigor (though not the unrealistic, and unneeded, vigor of a twenty-year-old), by physical mobility, by independence, by sociability, and by a continuing interest in life and the world in which one lives. It would be remiss not to add that, while the idea of a compression of morbidity offers an ideal research goal for the well-being of the elderly, it must ideally begin at a much earlier age with healthier lifestyles, not when aging itself has already taken place (though better late than never); but research aiming for that final result can appropriately be best thought of as aging research.

The main threat to this possibility is that medical research is far more likely to develop expensive means of easing the conditions of aging than of curing or otherwise eliminating them. As with the existing drugs to slow the progress of Alzheimer's disease, such as Aricept, they are expensive and often not covered by health care plans. Neither prevention of Alzheimer's nor its clean cure is on the immediate horizon, only more drugs to slow it down. What is true of the dementias of old age will be true of most other conditions of aging, where the principal threat to health will be chronic and degenerative diseases. All of them are associated with aging and all of them pose difficult research problems. Heart disease, as mentioned earlier in the book, shows all those problems: mortality is down from heart disease, but morbidity and costs are up; and it is the old who are the beneficiaries (they are still alive), but also the victims (still sick and expensively so).

GOOD RESEARCH, GOOD SOCIETY

On the surface at least, medical research oriented toward children in developed countries would seem to have the weakest claim to any kind of priority. They are, statistically, the healthiest of all age groups. Even the failure of many thousands of children to receive ordinary immunization in the United States is not the source of many deaths. Yet since children are the main resource of a society for its future good, health care must be a central part of an integrated approach to their well-being—and that would include the health of their parents. Since many of the health threats to children are the result of poverty and family breakdown, and those in turn a contributor to poor education, medical research is not the decisive answer. It might help individual children here and there, but not the continuing emergence of new generations of children similarly afflicted, each of whom must run an old, tragically old, gauntlet of possible social threats to make it to adulthood. Health programs for children must, then, be well integrated with other social programs, each reinforcing the others.

At the other end of the life cycle, health and social services need no less tight integration. Coping with chronic disease in the aged requires social as well as medical resources, and the purchase of needed drugs requires good insurance coverage (not now provided under Medicare). Drugs that are unaffordable to many are the fruit of research efforts with an inevitably inequitable distribution pattern. That in turn increases the social welfare needs, which will have to cope with poorer health. During the adult years, a similar phenomenon can manifest itself: the sickness of a family breadwinner, or the presence of chronic schizophrenia in a family, can mean its destruction. Good, affordable medicine is an obvious first line of defense. Unaffordable drugs—or those that are affordable only with the sacrifice of other family needs—will only worsen the situation, exacerbating the mental and emotional turmoil that poverty brings. Even affordable drugs (say in the case of schizophrenia) will not achieve their full potential apart from good medical supervision and social help for what is likely to be a demoralized family.

In relation to the needs of various age groups, two drawbacks of the present research enterprise stand out, both unavoidable to some extent, but neither of them closed to reform. One of them is the lack of a good fit between the reigning research imperative and the provision of health care. The second is that the research enterprise itself has aims other than improving health.

Research policy and health policy: the great divide.   Critics of health care and research in the United States make the oft-repeated charge that there is no system. Pressures from disease and patient advocacy groups, and assorted political interests, have helped shape the NIH over the years, and it has worked to put its priorities in some plausible order. Moreover, as the NIH has reasonably held over the years, good research depends on available research opportunities; neither more money alone nor a better political system of priority setting can guarantee those opportunities (though the money, if available, will be spent). The successful lobbying of scientists to leave a large space for basic and untargeted research has also shaped the research enterprise.

Neither influence can fairly be described as harmful. Both serve legitimate political and scientific purposes. But as elements in a research mix that includes the now-dominant pharmaceutical and biotechnology industries—dedicated to making a handsome profit from the translation of research into merchandisable profit—they merge with other interests to make the research system look like little more than a grab bag. Some of those interests are good, some are bad, and some a little of both.

Taken together they show a sharp divide between research aims and the delivery of good health care. Those interested in research policy show little interest in health care policy. Conversely, programs in health policy rarely offer courses focused on research policy, and journals that identify their interest as "health policy" rarely publish articles on research policy. When discussed at all, the relationship between research expenditures and health outcomes is too heavily dominated at the moment by the efforts of research advocates to show the economic benefits of research, and those efforts in my view fail or at least should prompt some serious skepticism. A shotgun approach covers health care needs, scattering research pellets far and wide hoping, and expecting, that most of them will do good somewhere and somehow. No doubt repeated shots in all directions will eventually hit something.

Yet in the process of discharging the research shotgun, the research enterprise leaves a number of important ideals by the wayside, where at best they have effect only by accident. Nothing in that approach promotes an equitable and sustainable health care system. Medical research has never tried to promote it. The research enterprise proceeds with almost total indifference to what the translation of the research into usable technologies will cost, or who technologies will go to, and there are at least some who think that even to introduce cost implications into research analysis is dangerous.[4] That problem lands, by default, in the hands of politicians and health care administrators, subject to politics and the play of the market. The research enterprise's net economic result, through its costly even if often beneficial innovations, is a health care system becoming rapidly unaffordable, at least unaffordable as a system that hopes for (even if it fails to organize for) equitable access. A quirk of the present historical moment may explain the reappearance of double-digit inflation of health care costs since 2000, heavily fueled by the cost of new and more intensively used technologies and pharmaceuticals, but there is good reason to doubt such an explanation.[5] If research and technological innovation are indifferent to cost implications, why express surprise when they show up, unwelcome and un-invited, on our doorstep? The rarely voiced worry that the genetic developments will simply exacerbate that problem is not misplaced.

In a comment not picked up by the media, much less featured by research advocacy groups, Harold Varmus, the distinguished former director of the NIH, spoke more bluntly on this problem shortly before leaving office in 2000 than anyone in his position ever has:

> We have a problem in this country in that there is nothing people place a higher value on than a healthy life, but I'm concerned about two things—the number we allocate to health becoming just too great to sustain even for people who are relatively well to do, but more troubling is the idea that we're going to cut a very significant portion of our population out of the benefits of certain kinds of approaches to health that were paid for by public money and ought to be publicly accessible.[6]

People like myself who say such things run the risk of being called Luddites, but that charge cannot be leveled at Varmus. The message, at least implicit, is that it is possible (an idea often denied) to think of research in ways that will be equitable and cost-effective in their outcomes, and that perhaps we are worrying too much about health (which no earlier director of the NIH ever said). A parallel observation is pertinent: "the vast majority of research funding from the National Institutes of Health is aimed at learning to cure diseases that historically have been incurable. Much less is spent on learning how to provide health care that most of us need most of the time in a way that is simpler, more convenient, and less costly."[7]

However difficult, the possibility of affordable health care will diminish until we learn how to develop affordable technologies and to scale back the deployment of those that are expensive. Though the process will surely bring howls of displeasure and anguish from parts of the research community and its advocacy groups, we must assess new research directions for their likely impact on costs and patient affordability, screen new technologies prior to their distribution for their cost implications, and exert government and health provider leverage to refuse to pay for unaffordable research products.

With the prospect of even more expensive biotechnology products in the pipeline, especially coming out of genomics, now is the time to start down that road. It may well be an austere road for researchers but is our only hope to avoid an even more austere road for patients, faced with a growing array of research triumphs that more and more of them or their insurers cannot afford. Even with governmental purchasing muscle, the cost of pharmaceuticals alone appears to be out of control; and, meanwhile, we are almost daily being told of the new, even more promising drugs on the way, not one of them advertised as inexpensive. It is no doubt true that Americans are unwilling to accept limits on medical technologies. In comparison with other countries, we are lovers of technology, with uncommon proclivities toward medical discoveries. But those proclivities no longer fit economic realities.[8]

Serving too many masters. Many foreign observers of the American scene are puzzled by the fact that we spend more money per capita on health care than citizens of any other country in the world but, despite all the money, that the United States ranks well down the list of national health indicators and outcomes. Many reasons are given to explain this puzzle, but the one that catches my eye is little mentioned: the United States allows, even encourages, the health care system to play many roles other than improver of health. We equally often bemoan hospital closings, or a reduction of hospital beds, for the loss of local jobs as for possible health harms to the community. If the loss of jobs happens to minority groups, the complaint is all the greater. The economic value of health care to communities even apart from jobs comes in for comment: the benefits to local subcontractors of food, laundry services, and assorted other service industries.[9] While they have their ups and downs, but mainly ups, health care stocks remain one of the best financial sectors, a mainstay of personal, institutional, and retirement investments. No one complains about the good returns on those investments, the fine living made by investment banking in the health care sector, or the rewards of venture capital firms in raising money for research. As the title of an article in the *New York Times* suggested—"Health Care as Main Engine: Is That So Bad?"—what we might otherwise treat as a problem turns to triumph: "the health care industry may be the only driver of [economic] growth in the near term . . . the health care sector is likely to expand faster than most industries in the years ahead."[10]

What gets overlooked in this cornucopia of side benefits from the health market—which rise and fall not in relationship to improvements or declines in health, but only as market prospects—is that they are one of the reasons for the high costs of health care. One person's profit and job is another person's expense. The pharmaceutical industry is the great exemplar of this phenomenon. Its public relations literature gives almost equal billing to its national financial benefits and the good it does for health. While the pharmaceutical and biotechnology industries are more than a little shy about revealing profit margins and actual costs, they readily disclose the large number of employees they have or their economic contributions to the communities, and the nations, in which they operate. Frequently cited in congressional hearings is the enormous export value of pharmaceuticals, as well as the proud (or is it defensive?) claim that the high price of drugs in the United States subsidizes research for the rest of the world.

There are surely many economic benefits showered on the world from the pharmaceutical industry, but those benefits are of little help to poor countries or, for that matter, to poor Americans. A stark conclusion seems evident: the economic benefits of the industry to society have no effect on equitable access to either its products or health care—and too little effect on its population's health status. Even more evident is the corollary: when the industry's profits become someone else's costs, those benefits have nothing to do with promoting an affordable and sustainable medicine, a goal that is receding from sight even in many affluent countries at the same time as they celebrate the glories of research.

Far from a health care system that is resistant to market forces, ours is one now dominated by them. While those forces alone are not responsible for the failures of the American health care system—or the pressures it is putting on European systems and Canada as well—they play a critical role. When the market and the research imperative merge, they make a formidable pair, hostile to equity, hostile to affordability, hostile to sustainability. There can never be a plausible scheme for universal health care in the United States as long as health care costs keep rising at a rapid rate. No legislator will go near that kind of a fiscal black hole. Meanwhile those costs will continue to go up in an unsustainable way as long as research does its unwitting, and usually indifferent, part to push them up.

If much of the basic research behind pharmaceutical development in the United States comes from the NIH, and if that development is the first step down the primrose path that Dr. Varmus identifies, then can the NIH avoid making our health care system even more expensive, more unaffordable? I am not sure of the answer to those questions, since I presume that the clinical applications of much basic research are not known at the time it is going on. The NIH cannot be held responsible for the pharmaceutical industry's use of its research in developing drugs that may make little additional contribution to health beyond those already available and add to the cost of health care. Some recent congressional proposals to have a certain portion of the drug profits returned to the NIH make some sense in dealing with the high private profits derived from its publicly supported work. The proposals would produce additional funds for the NIH but ignore the impact those same profits have on the provision of health care.

My point here is not to condemn individual researchers, or the NIH— nor did Varmus—for seeming indifference to the impact of research initiatives and outcomes on the cost of the health care system. The very logic of the research system sharply distinguishes between research benefits and the cost of distributing them. Congress has never raised the issue, perhaps because of its sole focus on the evils of diseases to be eradicated; the constantly fueled (though false) optimism that research is the long-term key to controlling costs has made it seem irrelevant. Researchers themselves have no training in cost-conscious research, and while every major disease no doubt has researchers interested in finding an inexpensive vaccine (or disease-prevention) solution, no one has figured out how to design research approaches that can incorporate a cost-control perspective. And surely, as expensive as it is (up to $30,000 a year), the present "AIDS cocktail" solution to AIDS (AZT and protease inhibitors), which keeps people alive without curing them, is better than no solution at all.

But this kind of solution, extended to the more common diseases of aging—costly heart defibrillators and implantable artificial hearts—will be devastating in its aggregate economic impact. The earlier complaints against halfway technologies were lodged during an era, the 1960s and 1970s, when their cost was not a major consideration; and they were typically used with infectious diseases, of a kind where an eventual vaccine could be envisioned. Since then, halfway technologies have proliferated, decisive vaccines are not appearing, and the costs have come to matter. These are, in any event, considerations that Congress needs to take into account as it debates the annual budget of the NIH.

INDIVIDUALS AND COMMUNITIES

The approach to medical research I have been urging in this final chapter comes to this: it is focused on a population's health needs, subdivided into the needs of different age groups, and requires an effort to coordinate socioeconomic research and social programs to be fully efficacious. That approach is far from the present pattern of disease-constituency research policy, matched by hodgepodge health care provisions. The NIH pioneered this policy when it established the National Cancer Institute as its first institute and went on from there to create institutes that have been, for the most part, organized along disease lines and have had behind them powerful professional and lay advocates. Distributing the fruits of research has always been someone else's problems. The private sector, whose motives are different, has more or less emulated that pattern.

Is that a sensible way to organize research, focusing on research gains, not the distribution of those gains? Since the NIH seeks public money, it is surely a politically effective way to get it. Celebrity advocates, whose number is increasing and whose use as a money-raising strategy is being exploited, are almost always disease oriented, whether for research on prostate cancer (Michael Milken) or Parkinson's disease (Morton Kondracke). Yet while the NIH has gone down that path—usually at the behest of Congress—its own literature and congressional wooing have stressed the way research ideally crosses disease lines, how serendipity has a large role to play (research on one disease turns out to be helpful to understanding others), and how the fruits of basic research can provide insight into a variety of diseases. Over the years the NIH itself has opposed the disease orientation, but it has always worked in a political culture that puts up money for results and direct social benefits. A disease orientation does not do that nearly as well as its proponents seem to believe, and nothing could be more beneficial for the future of research than to get those proponents to listen more to the research community and the scientists at the NIH. The case for funding curiosity is as strong as, if not stronger, than an assault on disease.[11] At the same time, as A. L. Cochrane noted some years ago, commenting on the British National Health Service, more scientific research on medical effectiveness and efficiency would help control cost inflation, a source of the gap between the "cure" and "care" sectors of health care.[12]

So far, neither common sense nor curiosity has been enough to overcome a disease focus. This focus lends itself well to media deployment, particularly the visualization of the effects of specific diseases and their impact on individual lives. It also fits well with the individualism of American culture and its market values. Behind it lies the assumption that what interests most people is not health problems of various age groups but particular diseases that have harmed their friends and family members and that may harm them. Yet my impression is that, while many people are disease oriented in the way they think about health (particularly if they have a family history of a particular disease), most of us worry more that something or other will get us rather than that some specific foreseeable disease will bring us down. We simply don't know what that "something" will be. Advocates against specific diseases, in contrast, argue forcefully from the perspective of people who either have the disease themselves, are at special risk for it, or have a family member who has been harmed by it.

Can an approach to research policy that looks at populations rather than individuals and favors increased basic research over (but does not banish) disease-oriented research do justice to individual needs? I believe the answer to that question to be yes, but only if we better coordinate research policy with social and health policy. The lack of universal health care and affordable and sustainable medicine that would make it economically feasible is our greatest failure in meeting individual health needs. The excessive free play of the market, both its growing force in research and its already strong place in health care more generally, only compounds that failure.

The lack of universal health care already bespeaks an excessive emphasis on individual health: those who have decent access to good care tend to worry more about their health than those without such access. Not for us, unhappily, the value of solidarity and community that have been the marks of the Canadian and Western European health care systems. The play of the market, which directly focuses on individual desires, only worsens the American situation, helping create an expensive kind of medicine that provides a poor foundation for universal health care. It provides no foundation at all for a health care system that gives a leading place to health promotion and disease prevention, particularly of the kind that looks to behavioral change and not medical screening as its main thrust.

The ancient perception is still true: we must face the prospect of illness, and the eventuality of death, in the privacy of our individual lives. No one can do that for us. Yet we can ask for a community that seeks, through its research, to help us through the various stages of life in good health, free of mental illness, able to use our bodies as we need to use them to take up our place in society, and to go into old age and death as little burdened with disability and dementia as possible. That requires a vigorous and continuing research effort. There is a long way to go. It also requires a health care system that does not depend on medical research to solve problems that could be solved by better social programs and healthier modes of living a life.[13] But it does not require a research agenda (mainly from the private sector) that plays to personal fantasies: the perfect baby, the optimal body, the full head of hair, and the youthful old age.

As citizens within the larger world community, we do not require, even though we enjoy, a research imperative that directs too much of its effort to making the healthy even healthier, that ignores those hundreds of millions of people who have a need for research to deal with those diseases that still kill them, and for health care programs that can give them research benefits now available to us but not to them.

But wait, a harried consumer might ask, surely in a prosperous country there is nothing wrong with looking at health care expenditures as a reasonable way of spending discretionary money, as useful as better wines, faster cars, and foreign cruises. What difference does it make anyway if the health care portion of the gross domestic product rises beyond the present 14 to 16 percent, even 20 percent? The difference is this: it bespeaks a narrow, stunted view of the human good, an excessive emphasis on health, an invitation to inefficiency and waste, an insult to the poor (who have no guarantee in the United States, much less in developing countries, of a place at that health-laden table), and an inefficient allocation of resource expenditures, bound to shortchange education and environmental protection, among other losses.

The research imperative in medicine is now a permanent part of our culture. It will make its best contribution if it (along with its zealous advocates) understands that it is not necessarily any more valuable than the other sciences, that health is only one among the necessary elements of human life, and that if it unwittingly contributes to a medicine that is unaffordable and unsustainable and falls prey to the temptation to push aside moral constraints in the name of future health, it will do as much harm as good.

It need not be that way. The research imperative draws on the best of human instincts and, far more often than not, does honor to them. It can do even better and surely should not allow itself to do any worse. If that imperative comes to encompass an increase in public health and epidemiological research, technology assessment and evidence-based medicine research, and health care quality research, then we can close the gap between research and health care delivery We would then be in a much better position to devise and support research that looked to its outcomes: to its impact on health care costs, equitable access, and sustainability. The health of each and every one of us would be the better for it.

Notes

INTRODUCTION

1. Langdon Winner, *The Whale and the Reactor: A Search for Limits in an Age of High Technology* (Chicago: University of California Press, 1986), 13.

2. Daniel S. Greenberg, *Science, Money, and Politics: Political Triumph and Ethical Erosion* (Chicago: University of Chicago Press, 2001), 3.

3. Paul Ramsey, "The Enforcement of Morals: Nontherapeutic Research on Children," *Hastings Center Report* 6, no. 4 (1976): 2.

4. Eric J. Cassell, "The Sorcerer's Broom: Medicine's Rampant Technology," *Hastings Center Report* 23, no. 6 (1993): 33.

1. EMERGENCE AND GROWTH

1. Gerald Holton, *Science and Antiscience* (Cambridge, Mass.: Harvard University Press, 1932), 112, 114–15.

2. Benjamin Franklin, "Letter to Joseph Priestly, Passy, France, February 8, 1780," in *The Private Correspondence of Benjamin Franklin*, ed. William Temple Franklin (London: Henry Colborn, 1817), 52.

3. Antoine-Nicolas de Condorcet, *Sketch for a Historical Picture of the Progress of the Human Mind*, trans. June Berraclough (New York: Library of Ideas, 1955).

4. Benjamin Rush, "Observations on the Duty of a Physician," *Medical Inquiries and Observations* 1 (1815): 251–64, and quoted in *The Codification of Medical Morality*, vol. 2, ed. Dorothy Porter, Robert Baker, and Roy Porter (Dordrecht: Kluwer Academic University Publishers, 1993).

5. Joyce Appleby, quoted in Gordon S. Wood, "Early American Get Up and Go," *New York Review of Books*, 29 June 2000, 52.

6. Richard H. Shryock, *American Medical Research Past and Present* (New York: Commonwealth Fund, 1947), 8–77.

7. Robert V. Bruce, *The Launching of Modern American Science, 1846–1876* (New York: Alfred A. Knopf, 1987).

8. Shryock, *Medical Research Past and Present*, 47.

9. Quoted in Kenneth M. Ludmerer, *Learning to Heal: The Development of American Medical Education* (New York: Basic Books, 1985), 103.

10. John Ettling, *The Germ of Laziness: Rockefeller Philanthropy and Public Health in the New South* (Cambridge, Mass.: Harvard University Press, 1981), 77.

11. Quoted in E. Richard Brown, *Rockefeller Medicine Men* (Berkeley: University of California Press, 1979), 106.

12. Harry M. Marks, *The Progress of Experiment: Science and Therapeutic Reform in the United States, 1900–1990* (New York: Cambridge University Press, 1997), 2, 3, 39.

13. Ettling, *Germ of Laziness*.

14. Jack D. Pressman, "Human Understanding: Psychosomatic Medicine and the Mission of the Rockefeller Foundation," in *Greater Than the Parts: Holism in Biomedicine, 1920–1950*, ed. Christopher Lawrence and George Weisz (New York: Oxford University Press, 1998), 190.

15. Sinclair Lewis, *Arrowsmith* (New York: Grosset and Dunlap, 1925); and Charles E. Rosenberg, *No Other Gods: On Science and American Social Thought*, rev. ed. (Baltimore: Johns Hopkins University Press, 1997), 122–31.

16. Daniel M. Fox, *Health Policies, Health Politics: The British and American Experience 1911–1965* (Princeton: Princeton University Press, 1986), x.

17. Ludmerer, *Learning to Heal*, 202.

18. Henry Pritchett, "The Medical School and the State," *Journal of the American Medical Association* 63 (1914): 28.

19. Quoted in Brown, *Rockefeller Medicine Men*, 251.

20. General Education Board, *Annual Report (1919–1920)*, 1920, 28.

21. Frederick T. Gates, *Chapters in My Life* (New York: Free Press, 1977), 188.

22. Victoria A. Harden, *Inventing the NIH: Federal Biomedical Research Policy, 1887–1937* (Baltimore: Johns Hopkins University Press, 1986), 4.

23. Ibid., 21.

24. Editorial, *Journal of the American Medical Association* 109 (1937): 16.

25. Quoted in Stephen P. Strickland, *Politics, Science, and Dread Disease* (Cambridge, Mass.: Harvard University Press, 1972), 14.

26. Vannevar Bush, *Science: The Endless Frontier* (Washington, D.C.: Office of Scientific Research and Development, 1945); see also Nathan Reingold, "Vannevar Bush's New Deal for Research: The Triumph of the Old Order," *Historical Studies in the Physical and Biological Sciences* 17 (1987): 299–328.

27. John R. Steelman, *The Nation's Medical Research*, vol. 5 of *Science and Public Policy: A Report to the President* (Washington, D.C.: Government Printing Office, 1947).

28. Elizabeth Brenner Drew, "The Health Syndicate: Washington's Noble Conspirators," *Atlantic Monthly*, December 1967, 84.

29. James Fallows, "The Political Scientist," *New Yorker*, 7 June 1999, 68.

30. Kelly Moore, "Organizing Integrity: American Science and the Creation of Public Interest Organizations, 1955–1975," *American Journal of Sociology* 101 (1996): 1601; and Susan Wright, *Molecular Politics: Developing American and British Policy for Genetic Engineering, 1972–1982* (Chicago: University of Chicago Press, 1994), 36–49.

31. Henry K. Beecher, "Ethics and Clinical Research," *New England Journal of Medicine* 274 (1966): 1354–60.

32. M. H. Pappworth, *Human Guinea Pigs: Experimentation with Man* (Boston: Beacon Press, 1967).

33. "The Nuremberg Code," *Journal of the American Medical Association* 276 (1997): 1691.

34. Willard Gaylin, "We Have the Awful Knowledge to Make Exact Copies of Human Beings," *New York Times Magazine*, 5 March 1972.

35. Peter Singer, *Animal Liberation*, 2d ed. (New York: New York Review of Books and Random House, 1990).

36. News and Comments, *Science* 185 (1974): 332.

37. James D. Watson, *The Double Helix: A Personal Account of the Discovery of the Structure of DNA* (London: Weidenfeld and Nicolson, 1968).

38. Deborah Fitzgerald, *The Business of Breeding: Hybrid Corn in Illinois, 1890–1940* (Ithaca: Cornell University Press, 1990); and Rosenberg, *No Other Gods*, 185–99.

39. Mary Warnock, *Report of the Committee of Inquiry into Human Fertilisation and Embryology* (London: HMSO, 1984).

40. U.S. National Institutes of Health, Human Embryo Research Panel (ad hoc group of consultants to the advisory committee to the director, NIH, 1994).

41. See 29 July 1997 hearing on HR 922, p. 20; see also proposed 1998 Senate bills S.1574, 368, 1599, 1601, and 1602.

42. Shryock, *Medical Research Past and Present*.

43. Pharmaceutical Research and Manufacturers of America, *Pharmaceutical Industry Profile* (Washington, D.C., 2000).

44. Research!America, "Public Opinion Polls" (1998); see also "American Views of S & T [science and technology], National Science and Technology Medals Foundation" (Washington, D.C., 1996; last accessed at 7/7/00 at http://asee.org/ustmf/html/avst.html); see also Dinah Kim, Robert J. Blendon, and John M. Benson, "How Interested Are Americans in New Medical Technology? A Multicountry Comparison," *Health Affairs* 20, no. 5 (2001): 194–201.

45. National Science Foundation, *American Views* (Washington, D.C., 1996).

46. Arthur Barsky, *Worried Sick: Our Troubled Quest for Wellness* (Boston: Little, Brown, 1998), 184, 214.

2. PROTECTING THE INTEGRITY OF SCIENCE

1. Robert K. Merton, "Science and Democratic Social Structure," in *Social Theory and Social Structure* (New York: Free Press, 1957), 553.

2. Ibid., 556.

3. Ibid., 559. David Baltimore pointed to this value when he wrote in praise of the completion of the Human Genome Project, "It reflects the scientific community at its best: working collaboratively, pooling its resources and skills, keeping its focus on the goal, and making its results available to all as they were acquired" ("Our Genome Unveiled," *Nature* 409 [2001]: 814–16).

4. Merton, "Science and Social Structure," 560.

5. Alexander Kohn, "Making and Breaking the Rules of Science," in *The Ethical Dimensions of the Biological Sciences*, ed. Ruth Ellen Bulger, Elizabeth Heitman, and Stanley Joel Reiser (New York: Cambridge University Press, 1993), 56; and Sigma Xi, the Scientific Research Society, *The Responsible Researcher: Paths and Pitfalls* (Research Triangle Park, N.C., 1998).

6. I. I. Mitroff, *The Subjective Side of Science* (Amsterdam: Elsevier, 1974).

7. Michael J. Mulkay, *Sociology of Medicine* (Bloomington: Indiana University Press, 1991).

8. Daniel S. Greenberg, *The Politics of American Science* (Harmondsworth: Penguin Books, 1969); and R. C. Tobey, *The American Ideology of National Science* (Pittsburgh: University of Pittsburgh Press, 1971).

9. Kelly Moore, "Organizing Integrity: American Science and the Creation of Public Interest Organizations, 1975–1995," *American Journal of Sociology* 101 (1996): 1592–1627.

10. Bentley Glass, "The Ethical Basis of Science," in *Ethical Dimensions of the Biological Sciences*, 43–55; see also Carl Mitcham and Rene von Schomberg, "The Ethic of Scientists and Engineers: From Occupational Role Responsibility to Public Co-Responsibility," in *Research in Philosophy and Technology*, vol. 2, ed. Peter Kroes and Anthony Meijers (Amsterdam: JAI Press, 2000).

11. Ibid., 53.

12. Ibid., 54.

13. Ibid. See also Gerald Holton, "Scientific Optimism and Social Concerns," *Hastings Center Report* 5, no. 6 (1975): 39–47; though over twenty-five years old this article does not date easily: much of what Holton discovered about societal concerns of scientists—not a great deal for most—has a still familiar ring about it; Terry Ann Krolwich and Paul J. Friedman, "Integrity in the Education of Researchers," *Academic Medicine* 68, s.s. (1993): 514–18; see also Philip Kitcher, *Science, Truth, and Democracy* (New York: Oxford University Press, 2001), 193–97.

14. Daniel J. Kevles, *The Baltimore Case: A Trial of Politics, Science and Character* (New York: Wiley, 1998).

15. Office of Science and Technology Policy, " Proposed Federal Policy on Research Misconduct to Protect the Integrity of the Research Record," *Federal Register* 64, no. 198 (1999): 55722–25.

16. C. K. Gunsalus, "Institutional Structure to Ensure Research Integrity," *Academic Medicine* 68, s.s. (1993): 533–38; Donald F. Klein, "Should the Government Assure Scientific Integrity?" *Academic Medicine* 68, s.s. (1993): 556–59; and Leon C. Goe, Adriana M. Herrera, and William R. Mower,

"Misrepresentation of Research Citations among Medical School Faculty Applicants," *Academic Medicine* 73 (1998): 1183–86.

17. Douglas L. Weed, "Preventing Scientific Misconduct," *American Journal of Public Health* 88 (1998): 125–29; and Ruth Ellen Bulger and Stanley Joel Reiser, "Studying Science in the Context of Ethics," *Academic Medicine* 68, s.s. (1993): 55–59.

18. John Maddox, "Valediction from an Old Hand," *Nature* 378 (1995): 521–23; Kay L. Fields and Alan R. Price, "Problems in Research Integrity Arising from Misconceptions about the Ownership of Research," *Academic Medicine* 68 (1993): 560–64; see William P. Whitley, Drummond Rennie, and Arthur W. Hafner, "The Scientific Community's Response to Evidence of Fraudulent Publication," *Journal of the American Medical Association* 272 (1994): 170–73.

19. Pamela Luft and Robert L. Sprague, "Scientific Misconduct: Individual Deviance or Systemic Complacency?" *Journal of Information Ethics* 5 (1996): 72–81.

20. Alison Abbott, "Science Comes to Terms with Lessons of Fraud," *Nature* 398 (1999): 13–17.

21. Goe et al., "Misrepresentation of Research Citations."

22. Drummond Rennie, "Fair Conduct and Fair Reporting of Clinical Trials," *Journal of the American Medical Association* 282 (1999): 1766–68; see also Mark Hochauser, "Conflict of Interest Can Result in Research Bias," *Applied Clinical Trials* 10, no. 6 (2001): 58–64.

23. Marilyn Larkin, "Whose Article Is It Anyway?" *Lancet* 354 (1999): 136; and Eugene Tarnow, "When Extra Authors Get in on the Act," *Nature* 398 (1999): 657.

24. Abbott, "Science Comes to Terms"; see also Rebecca Dresser, "Defining Research Misconduct: Will We Know It When We See It?" *Hastings Center Report* 31, no. 3 (2001): 31.

25. Paolo del Guercio, "Tougher Crack Down on Fraud Needed," *Nature* 394 (1998): 823.

26. Paul E. Kalb and Kristen Graham Koehler, "Legal Issues in Scientific Research," *Journal of the American Medical Association* 287 (2002): 85–91.

27. Guercio, "Tougher Crack Down on Fraud Needed"; Weed, "Preventing Scientific Misconduct"; Tarnow, "When Extra Authors Get In"; Rennie, "Fair Conduct and Fair Reporting"; and Niteesh K. Choudry, Henry Thomas Stelfox, and Allan S. Detsky, "Relationships between Author of Clinical Practice Guidelines and the Pharmaceutical Industry," *Journal of the American Medical Association* 287 (2002): 612–17.

28. Richard A. Deyo, Bruce M. Psaty, Gregory Simon, Edward H. Wagner, and Gilbert S. Omenn, "The Messenger under Attack—Intimidation of Researchers by Special Interest Groups," *New England Journal of Medicine* 336 (1997): 1176–80.

29. R. A. Deyo, D. C. Cherkin, J. D. Loeser, S. J. Bigos, and M. A. Ciol, "Morbidity and Morality Associated with Operations on the Lumbar Spine: The

Influence of Age, Diagnosis, and Procedure," *Journal of Bone and Joint Surgery, American Edition* 24 (1992): 536–43; and R. A. Deyo, D. C. Cherkin, J. D. Loeser, S. J. Bigos, and M. A. Ciol, "Lumbar Spinal Fusion: A Cohort Study of Complications, Re-Operations, and Resource Use in the Medicare Population," *Spine* 18 (1993): 1463–70.

30. Deyo et al., "Messenger under Attack."

31. B. M. Psaty et al., "The Risk of Incipient Myocardial Infarction Associated with Anti-Hypertensive Drug Therapies," *Journal of the American Medical Association* 274 (1995): 620–25.

32. Deyo et al., "Messenger under Attack," 1178.

33. J. P. Swann, *Academic Scientists and the Pharmaceutical Industry: The Formation of the American Pharmaceutical Industry* (Baltimore: Johns Hopkins University Press, 1988).

34. Thomas Bodenheimer, "Uneasy Alliance—Clinical Investigators and the Pharmaceutical Industry," *New England Journal of Medicine* 342 (2000): 1539–44; Jonathan Moreno, "Ethical Considerations of Industry-Sponsored Research: The Use of Human Subjects," *Journal of the American College of Nutrition* 15 (1996): 35S–40S; Michael S. Pritchard, "Conflicts of Interest: Conceptual and Narrative Issues," *Academic Medicine* 71(1996): 1305–13; and Erica Rose, "Financial Conflicts of Interest: How Are We Managing?" *Widener Law Symposium Journal* 8 (2001): 1–29.

35. Andrew Webster and Henry Etzkowitz, "Toward a Theoretical Analysis of Academic-Industry Collaboration," in *Capitalizing Knowledge: New Intersections of Industry and Academia*, ed. Henry Etzkowitz, Andrew Webster, and Peter Healey (Albany: State University of New York Press, 1998).

36. M. K. Cho, R. Shohara, A. Schissel, and D. Rennie, "Policies on Faculty Conflicts of Interest at US Universities," *Journal of the American Medical Association* 284 (2000): 2203–8; Elizabeth Boyd and Lisa A. Bero,"Assessing Faculty Financial Relationships with Industry," *Journal of the American Medical Association* 284 (2000): 1621–26; and Karen Seashore Louis and Melissa S. Anderson, "The Changing Context of Science and University-Industry Relations," in *Capitalizing Knowledge: New Intersections of Industry and Academia*, ed. Henry Etzkowitz, Andrew Webster, and Peter Healey (Albany: State University of New York Press, 1998).

37. Bernard Lo, Leslie E. Wolf, and Abiona Berkeley, "Conflict of Interest Policies for Investigators in Clinical Trials," *New England Journal of Medicine* 343 (2000): 1616–20.

38. Stuart E. Lind, "Financial Issues and Incentives Related to Clinical Research and Innovative Therapies," in *The Ethics of Research Involving Human Subjects: Facing the 21st Century*, ed. Harold Y. Vanderpool (Frederick, Md.: University Publishing Group, 1996), 199.

39. Lo et al., "Conflict of Interest Policies."

40. "Strength in Numbers," *Science* 295 (2002): 1969.

41. Eliot Marshall, "Publishing Sensitive Data: Who Calls the Shots?" *Science* 276 (1997): 523–24.

42. "A Duty to Publish," *Nature Medicine* 4 (1998): 1089.

43. David Blumenthal, Eric G. Campbell, Nancyanne Causino, and Karen Seashore Louis, "Participation of Life Science Faculty in Research Relationships with Industry: Extent and Effects," *New England Journal of Medicine* 335 (1996): 1734–39; and David Blumenthal, Nancyanne Causino, Eric G. Campbell, and Karen Seashore Louis, "Relationships between Academic Institutions and Industry: An Industry Survey," *New England Journal of Medicine* 334 (1996): 368–72.

44. Lisa A. Bero, Alison Galbraith, and Drummond Rennie, "The Publication of Sponsored Symposiums in Medical Journals," *New England Journal of Medicine* 327 (1992): 1135–40.

45. Eric G. Campbell, Karen Seashore Louis, and David Blumenthal, "Looking a Gift Horse in the Mouth: Corporate Gifts Supporting Life-Sciences Research," *Journal of the American Medical Association* 279 (1998): 995–99.

46. Haldor Stefansson, "Through the Looking Glass of Image-Advertising in Science" (manuscript, European Molecular Biology Laboratory, 2001).

47. Richard Smith, "Hype from Journalists and Scientists," *British Medical Journal* 304 (1992): 730.

48. Vikki Entwistle, "Reporting Research in Medical Journals and Newspapers," *British Medical Journal* 310 (1995): 920–23; Ian J. Deavy, Martha C. Whiteman, and F. G. R. Fowkes, "Medical Research and the Popular Media," *Lancet* 351 (1998): 1726–27.

49. Craig Horowitz, "Winning the Cancer War," *New York*, 7 February 2000, 27.

50. Theodore Dalrymple, "War against Cancer Won't Be Won Soon," *Wall Street Journal*, 12 June 2000, A-30.

51. H. Gilbert Welch, Lisa M. Schwartz, and Steven Woloshin, "Are Increasing 5-Year Survival Rates Evidence of Success against Cancer?" *Journal of the American Medical Association* 283 (2000): 2975.

52. Dorothy Nelkin, *Selling Science: How the Press Covers Science and Technology* (New York: W. H. Freeman, 1987); the science writer Nicholas Wade is a good example of this proclivity. His book *Life Script: How the Human Genome Discoveries Will Transform Medicine and Enhance Your Health* (New York: Simon and Schuster, 2001) is overrun with enthusiasm, capturing its spirit almost perfectly with the title of his concluding chapter, "Brave New World" (67); see also Miriam Shucham and Michael S. Wilkes, "Medical Scientists and Health News Reporting," *Annals of Internal Medicine* 126 (1997): 976–81, which focuses on five major failings: sensationalism, conflicts of interest, bias, lack of follow-up, and choice of stories not covered.

53. Gina Kolata, "A Thick Line between Theory and Therapy," *New York Times*, 18 December 2001, F-3; see also Trudy Lieberman, "Covering Medical Technologies: The Seven Deadly Sins," *Columbia Journalism Review* (September–October 2001): 24–28; see also Usher Fleming, "In Search of Genohype: A Content Analysis of Biotechnology Company Documents," *New Genetics and Society* 20, no. 30 (2001): 239–53.

54. Elizabeth Pennisi, "Finally, the Book of Life and Instructions for Navigating It," *Science* 288 (2000): 2304.

55. Gail Collins, "Public Interests, a Shot in the Dark," *New York Times*, 29 June 2000, A-25.

56. Steve Jones, *Genetics in Medicine: Real Promises, Unreal Expectations: One Scientist's Advice to Policymakers in the United Kingdom and the United States* (New York: Milbank Memorial Fund, 2000).

57. Quoted in John R. G. Turner, "What's the Forecast?" *New York Times*, 16 April 2000, 7–24.

58. Willard Gaylin, "We Have the Awful Knowledge to Make Exact Copies of Human Beings," *New York Times Magazine*, 5 March 1972.

59. Moore, "Organizing Integrity," 1592–1627.

60. Vincent W. Franco, "Ethical Analysis of the Risk-Benefit Issue in Recombinant DNA Research and Technology," *Ethics in Science and Medicine* 7 (1980): 157.

3. IS RESEARCH A MORAL OBLIGATION?

1. Renée C. Fox, "Experiment Perilous: Forty-five Years as a Participant Observer of Patient-Oriented Clinical Research," *Perspectives in Biology and Medicine* 39 (1996): 210.

2. Ian Gallagher and Michael Harlow, "Health Chiefs? Yes to Human Clones," *International Express*, 1–7 August 2000, 10.

3. W. French Anderson, "Uses and Abuses of Human Gene Therapy," *Human Gene Therapy* 3 (1992): 1.

4. Ronald Munson and Lawrence H. Davis, "Germ-Line Gene Therapy and the Medical Imperative," *Kennedy Institute of Ethics Journal* 2 (1992): 137.

5. Letter to the president and members of Congress sent by the American Society for Cell Biology, March 4, 1999.

6. Glenn McGee and Arthur L. Caplan, "The Ethics and Politics of Small Sacrifices in Stem Cell Research," *Kennedy Institute of Ethics Journal* 9 (1999): 152.

7. Human Embryo Research Panel, *Report of the Human Embryo Research Panel* (Bethesda, Md.: NIH, 1994), 44–45.

8. James F. Childress, "Metaphor and Analogy," in *Encyclopedia of Bioethics*, ed. Warren Thomas Reich, rev. ed. (New York: Simon and Schuster, 1995), 1765–73.

9. George J. Annas, "Questing for Grails: Duplicity, Betrayal and Self-Deception in Postmodern Medical Research," *Journal of Contemporary Health Law Policy* 12 (1996): 297–324.

10. George J. Annas, "Reforming the Debate on Health Care: Reform by Replacing Our Metaphors," *New England Journal of Medicine* 332 (1995): 744–47.

11. Susan Sontag, *AIDS and Its Metaphors* (New York: Farrar, Straus, and Giroux, 1989), 95.

12. Gilbert Meilaender, "The Point of a Ban: Or, How to Think about Stem Cell Research," *Hastings Center Report* 31, no. 1 (2001): 9–16.

13. Onora O'Neill, "Duty and Obligation," in *Encyclopedia of Ethics*, ed. Lawrence J. Becker and Charlotte B. Becker (New York: Garland Publishing, 1992); Richard B. Brandt in *Encyclopedia of Ethics*, 278; and Richard B. Brandt, "The Concepts of Obligation and Duty," *Mind* 73 (1964): 374–93.

14. Hans Jonas, "Philosophical Reflections on Experimenting with Human Subjects" (1969), in *Philosophical Essays: From Ancient Creed to Technological Man*, ed. Hans Jonas (Englewood Cliffs, N.J.: Prentice-Hall, 1974), 129.

15. Ibid., 117.

16. See also Meilaender, "The Point of a Ban."

17. President's Commission for the Study of Ethical Problems in Medicine and Biomedical and Behavioral Research, *Securing Access to Health Care* (Washington, D.C.: Government Printing Office, 1983), 1:22–23.

18. Norman Daniels, "Justice, Health, and Healthcare," *American Journal of Bioethics* 1 (2001): 3.

19. Ibid. See also Ronald Bayer, Arthur L. Caplan, and Norman Daniels, eds., *In Search of Equity* (New York: Plenum Press, 1983); and "European Issue: Solidarity in Health Care," *Journal of Medicine and Philosophy* 17 (1992): 367–477.

20. Ronald Puccetti, "The Conquest of Death," *Monist* 59 (1976): 249–63.

21. Annette T. Carron, Joanne Lynn, and Patrick Keaney, "End-of-Life Care in Medical Textbooks," *Annals of Internal Medicine* 130 (1999): 82–86.

22. Susan Sontag, *Illness as Metaphor* (New York: Farrar, Straus, and Giroux, 1977), 8.

23. Lewis Thomas, *The Lives of a Cell: Notes of a Biology Watcher* (New York: Penguin Books, 1978), 115.

24. Bernard Williams, *Problems of the Self* (Cambridge, Mass.: Harvard University Press, 1976), 94–95; and Eugene Fontinell, *Self, God, and Immortality: A Jamesian Investigation* (New York: Fordham University Press, 2000), chs. 7–8.

25. Hans Jonas, "The Burden and Blessing of Mortality," *Hastings Center Report* 22, no. 1 (1992): 37.

26. Daniel Callahan, *The Troubled Dream of Life: In Search of a Peaceful Death* (New York: Simon and Schuster, 1993), 63.

27. Darrel W. Amundsen, "The Physician's Obligation to Prolong Life: A Medical Duty without Classical Roots," *Hastings Center Report* 8, no. 4 (1978): 23–30.

28. Philippe Ariès, *The Hour of Our Death*, trans. Helen Weaver (New York: Knopf, 1981).

29. Quoted in Lawrence M. Fisher, "The Race to Cash in on the Genetic Code," *New York Times*, 29 August 1999, C-1.

30. William B. Schwartz, *Life without Disease: The Pursuit of Medical Utopia* (Berkeley: University of California Press, 1998).

31. Gilbert Meilaender, personal communication, 2002.

32. E. J. Larson and T. A. Eaton, "The Limits of Advanced Directives: A History and Reassessment of the Patient Self-Determination Act," *Wake Forest Law Review* 32 (1997): 349–93.

33. Carron et al., "End-of-Life Care."

34. L. Scheiderman and N. Jecker, *Wrong Medicine: Doctors, Patients, and Futile Treatment* (Baltimore: Johns Hopkins University Press, 1995).

35. Callahan, *Troubled Dream of Life*.

36. Anthony J. Vita et al., "Aging, Health Risk, and Cumulative Disability," *New England Journal of Medicine* 338 (1998): 1035–41.

37. Gerald J. Gruman, "Cultural Origins of Present-Day 'Ageism': The Modernization of the Life Cycle," in *Aging and the Elderly: Humanistic Perspectives in Gerontology*, ed. Stuart F. Spicker et al. (Atlantic Highlands, N.J.: Humanities Press, 1978), 359–87.

38. Robert Prehoda, *Extended Youth: The Promise of Gerentology* (New York: G. P. Putnam, 1968), 254.

39. Arthur L. Caplan, "The Unnaturalness of Aging—A Sickness unto Death?" in *Concepts in Health and Disease*, ed. Arthur L. Caplan, H. Tristram Engelhardt Jr., and James McCarthey (Reading, Mass.: Addison-Wesley, 1981), 725–37; and Daniel Callahan, "Aging and the Ends of Medicine," in *Biomedical Ethics: An Anglo-American Dialogue*, ed. Daniel Callahan and G. R. Dunstan (New York: New York Academy of Sciences, 1988), 125–32.

40. Timothy F. Murphy, "A Cure for Aging?" *Journal of Medicine and Philosophy* 11 (1986): 237–55.

41. T. B. L. Kirkwood, "Is There a Limit to the Human Life Span?" in *Longevity: To the Limit and Beyond*, ed. Jean-Marine Robine, James W. Vaupel, and Michael Bernard Jeune (Berlin: Springer, 1997), 69–76; and Ali Ahmed and Trygve Tollefshol, "Telomeres and Telomerase: Basic Science Implications for Aging," *Journal of the American Geriatric Society* 49 (2000): 1105–9; and Jim Oeppen and James W. Vaupel, "Broken Limits to Life Expectancy," *Science* 296 (2002): 1029–31.

42. Shiro Horiuchi, "Greater Lifetime Expectations," *Nature* 405 (2000): 744–45.

43. S. J. Olshansky, "Practical Limits to Life Expectancy in France," in *Longevity: To the Limit and Beyond*, 1–10.

44. Ibid.

45. James W. Vaupel, "The Average French Baby May Live 99 or 100 Years," in *Longevity: To the Limit and Beyond*, 11–27.

46. Kirkwood, "Is There a Limit?" 75.

47. Michael R. Rose, "Aging as a Target for Genetic Engineering," in *Engineering the Human Germline*, ed. Gregory Stock and John Campbell (New York: Oxford University Press, 2000), 54.

48. James W. Vaupel et al., "Biodemographic Trajectories of Longevity," *Science* 280 (1998): 855–60; and James R. Carey and Debra S. Judge, "Life Span Extension in Humans Is Self-Reinforcing: A General Theory of Longevity," *Population and Development Review* 27 (2001): 411–36.

49. E. Timmer et al., *Variability of the Duration of Life of Living Creatures* (Amsterdam: IOS Press, 2000), 161–91.

50. Daniel Perry, "The Rise of the Gero-Techs," *Genetic Engineering News* 20 (2000): 57–58.

51. See Callahan, "Aging and the Ends of Medicine," 125–32; Victor R. Fuchs, "Medicare Reform: The Larger Picture," *Journal of Economic Perspectives* 14 (2000): 57–70; David M. Cutler, "Walking the Tightrope on Medicare Reform," *Journal of Economic Perspectives* 14 (2000): 45–56; and Mark McClellan, "Medicare Reform: Fundamental Problems, Incremental Steps," *Journal of Economic Perspectives* 14 (2000): 21–44.

52. John Harris, "Intimations of Mortality," *Science* 288 (2000): 59.

4. CURING, HELPING, ENHANCING

1. Diego Garcia, "What Kind of Values? A Historical Perspective on the Ends of Medicine," in *The Goals of Medicine: The Forgotten Issue in Health Care Reform*, ed. Mark J. Hanson and Daniel Callahan (Washington, D.C.: Georgetown University Press, 1999), 88–100.

2. Christopher Boorse, "On the Distinction between Disease and Illness," *Philosophy and Public Affairs* 5, 1 (1975): 49–68; Christopher Boorse, "Health as a Theoretical Concept," *Philosophy of Science* 44 (1977): 542–73; Robert Wachbroit, "Health and Disease, Concepts of," in *Encyclopedia of Applied Ethics*, ed. Ruth Chadwick (San Diego: Academic Press, 1998), 533–38; Arthur L. Caplan, "The Concepts of Health, Illness, and Disease," in *Medical Ethics*, ed. Robert M. Veatch (Sudbury, Mass.: Jones and Bartlett, 1997), 57–74; H. Tristram Engelhardt Jr., "The Disease of Masturbation: Values and the Concept of Disease," in *Contemporary Issues in Bioethics*, ed. Tom L. Beauchamp and LeRoy Walters (Belmont, Calif.: Wadsworth, 1989), 85–89; and George Khushf, "Expanding the Horizon of Reflection on Health and Disease," *Journal of Medicine and Philosophy* 20 (1995): 461–73.

3. Robert M. Sade, "A Theory of Health and Disease: The Objectivist-Subjectivist Dichotomy," *Journal of Medicine and Philosophy* 20 (1995): 513–25.

4. Boorse, "On the Distinction between Disease and Illness"; Boorse, "Health as a Theoretical Concept"; James G. Lennox, "Health as an Objective Value," *Journal of Medicine and Philosophy* 20 (1995): 499–511; and Tom L. Beauchamp, "Concepts of Health and Disease," in *Contemporary Issues in Bioethics*, 73–79.

5. World Health Organization, "A Definition of Health," in *Contemporary Issues in Bioethics*, 79; and Daniel Callahan, "The WHO Definition of Health," *Hastings Center Studies* 1, no. 3 (1973): 77–88.

6. John Knowles, "Introduction," *Daedalus* 106 (1997): 1–7; and Arthur Barsky, *Worried Sick: Our Troubled Quest for Wellness* (Boston: Little, Brown, 1998).

7. Robert G. Evans, Morris L. Bauer, and Theodore R. Marmor, eds., *Why*

Are Some People Healthy and Others Not: The Determinants of Health in Populations (New York: Aldine de Gruyter, 1994).

8. I drew up the goals for a project, published as "The Goals of Medicine: Setting New Priorities," *Hastings Center Report* 26, s.s. (1996); Mark J. Hanson, "The Idea of Progress and the Goals of Medicine," in *The Goals of Medicine: The Forgotten Issue in Health Care Reform,* ed. Mark J. Hanson and Daniel Callahan (Washington, D.C.: Georgetown University Press, 1999), 137–51; Edmund D. Pellegrino, "The Goals and Ends of Medicine: How Are They to Be Defined?" in *Goals of Medicine,* 55–68; Lennart Nordenfeldt, "On Medicine and Other Means of Health Enhancement: Towards a Conceptual Framework," in *Goals of Medicine,* 69–87; and Fernando Lolas, "On the Goals of Medicine: Reflections and Distinctions," in *Goals of Medicine,* 216–20.

9. Eric Cassell, personal communication, 2000.

10. Daniel Callahan, *False Hopes: Why America's Quest for Perfect Health Is a Recipe for Failure* (New York: Simon and Schuster, 1998); and Daniel Callahan, *What Kind of Life: The Limits of Medical Progress* (Washington, D.C.: Georgetown University Press, 1990).

11. Hippocrates, *The Art* (Cambridge, Mass.: Harvard University Press, Loeb Classical Library, 1923), 193.

12. J. M. McGinnis and W. H. Foege, "Actual Causes of Death in the United States," *Journal of the American Medical Association* 270 (1993): 2207–12.

13. Eric J. Cassell, "Pain, Suffering, and the Goals of Medicine," in *Goals of Medicine,* 101–17.

14. René Descartes, "Discourse on the Method of Rightly Conducting the Reason and Seeking for the Truth in the Sciences," in *The Philosophical Works of Descartes* (Cambridge: Cambridge University Press, 1981), 120.

15. Erik Parens, "Is Better Always Good? The Enhancement Project," *Hastings Center Report* 28, no. 1 (1998): S1–17.

16. Norman Daniels, "Normal Functioning and the Treatment-Enhancement Distinction," *Cambridge Quarterly of Healthcare Ethics* 9 (2000): 309–22.

17. Anita Silvers, "A Fatal Attraction to Normalizing," in *Enhancing Human Traits: Ethical and Social Implications,* ed. Erik Parens (Washington, D.C.: Georgetown University Press, 1998); and Susan Bordo, "Braveheart, Babe, and the Contemporary Body," in *Enhancing Human Traits,* 189–221.

18. Dan W. Brock, "Enhancements of Human Function: Some Distinctions for Policy Makers," in *Enhancing Human Traits,* 48–69.

19. See Allen Buchanan et al., eds., *From Chance to Choice: Genetics and Justice* (New York: Cambridge University Press, 2001).

20. Parens, "Is Better Always Good?"

21. John Harris, *Wonderwoman and Superman: The Ethics of Biotechnology* (Oxford: Oxford University Press, 1992), ch. 7.

22. Michael H. Shapiro, "The Technology of Perfection: Performance Enhancement and the Control of Attributes," *Southern California Law Review* 65 (1991): 11–14; and Nick A. Ghaphrey, "Performance-Enhancing Drugs," *Orthopedic Clinics of North America* 26 (1995): 433–42.

23. Parens, "Is Better Always Good?"

24. Robert Plomin, John C. DeFries, Gerald E. McClearn, and Peter Guffin, *Behavioral Genetics*, 43d ed. (New York: Worth Publishers, 2001), esp. chs. 5 and 6, 156–203; Robert Plomin and Gerald E. McLearn, eds., *Nature, Nurture, and Psychology* (Washington, D.C.: American Psychological Association, 1993).

25. Daniel Goleman, *Emotional Intelligence: Why It Can Matter More Than IQ* (New York: Bantam Books, 1995); Howard Gardner, *Frames of Mind: The Theory of Multiple Intelligences* (New York: Basic Books, 1983); and Richard Roberts, Gerald Matthews, and Moshe Zeidner, "Does Emotional Intelligence Meet Traditional Standards for Intelligence? Some New Data and Conclusions," *Emotion* 1 (2001): 196–231.

26. Gardner, *Frames of Mind*, ix, xi.

27. Goleman, *Emotional Intelligence*.

28. Robert Plomin, "Genetics and General Cognitive Ability," *Nature* 402 (1999): c 27.

29. Jonathan Beckwith, "Simplicity and Complexity: Is IQ Ready for Genetics?" *Current Psychology of Cognition* 18 (1999): 161–69.

30. Daniels, "Normal Functioning and Treatment-Enhancement"; and Ainsley Newson and Robert Williamson, "Should We Undertake Genetic Research on Intelligence?" *Bioethics* 13 (1999): 327–42.

31. Newson and Williamson, "Should We Undertake Genetic Research?" 327.

32. Gerald L. Klerman, "Psychotropic Hedonism vs. Pharmacological Calvinism," *Hastings Center Report* 2, no. 4 (1972): 1–3.

33. See Jacquelyn Slomka, "Playing with Propranolol," *Hastings Center Report* 22, no. 4 (1992): 13–17.

34. Lawrence H. Diller, "The Run on Ritalin: Attention Deficit Disorder and Stimulant Treatment in the 1990s," *Hastings Center Report* 26, no. 4 (1996): 12–18; and Peter D. Kramer, *Listening to Prozac* (New York: Viking, 1993).

35. John A. Robertson, *Children of Choice: Freedom and the New Reproductive Technologies* (Princeton: Princeton University Press, 1994).

36. Glenn McGee, *The Perfect Baby: A Pragmatic Approach to Genetics* (Lanham, Md.: Rowman and Littlefield, 1997); Glenn McGee, "Parenting in an Era of Genetics," *Hastings Center Report* 27, no. 2 (1997): 16–22; and Glenn McGee, "Ethical Issues in Enhancement: An Introduction," *Cambridge Quarterly of Healthcare Ethics* 9 (2000): 299–303.

37. Thomas Murray, *The Worth of a Child* (Berkeley: University of California Press, 1996).

38. See Marcel Verweij and Frank Kortmann, "Moral Assessment of Growth Hormone Therapy for Children with Idiopathic Short Stature," *Journal of Medical Ethics* 23 (1997): 305–9; Leona Cuttler et al., "Short Stature and Growth Hormone Therapy: A National Study of Physician Recommendation Patterns," *Journal of the American Medical Association* 276 (1996): 531–37; Sharon E. Oberfield, "Growth Hormone Use in Normal Short Children—a Plea for Reason," *New England Journal of Medicine* 340 (1999): 557–59; and Otto

Westphal, "Is Short Stature a Psychosocial Handicap?" *Acta Paediatrica Scandinavica* 362, s. (1989): 24–26.

39. Joel Feinberg, "The Child's Right to an Open Future," in *Whose Child? Children's Rights, Parental Authority, and State Power,* ed. William Aiken and Hugh LaFollete (Totowa, N.J.: Rowman and Littlefield, 1980), 124–53.

40. Theresa Marteau, Susan Michie, Harriet Drake, and Martin Bobrow, "Public Attitudes towards the Selection of Desirable Characteristics in Children," *Journal of Medical Genetics* 32 (1995): 796–98.

41. Michel Houellebecq, *The Elementary Particles,* trans. Frank Wynne (New York: Knopf, 2000).

42. Lee M. Silver, "Can You Make My Kid Smarter?" *Time,* 8 November 1999, 68–69.

43. Troy Duster, *Back Door to Eugenics* (New York: Routledge, 1990).

44. Garland E. Allen, "Is a New Eugenics Afoot?" *Science* 294 (2001): 59–61.

5. ASSESSING RISKS AND BENEFITS

1. James D. Watson, "All for the Good," *Time,* 11 January 1999, 91; Watson is by no means representative of most scientists, and many will cringe at his reasoning here. But it is not a trivial matter when he is given a full page in *Time* magazine to express his views.

2. Ibid.

3. Ibid.

4. "Mapping Ourselves," *Wall Street Journal,* 27 June 2000, A-30.

5. Council on Competitiveness (Washington, D.C., 1998), 48.

6. Kirkpatrick Sale,"Ban Cloning? Not a Chance," *New York Times,* 7 March 1997, op ed.

7. Laurence H. Tribe, "Second Thoughts on Cloning," *New York Times,* 5 December 1997, A-31.

8. Richard C. Lewontin, "The Confusion over Cloning," *New York Review of Books,* 23 October 1997.

9. Gregory E. Pence, *Who's Afraid of Human Cloning?* (Lanham, Md.: Rowman and Littlefield, 1998), 172 and 64.

10. Daniel J. Kevles, "Study Cloning, Don't Ban It," *New York Times,* 26 February 1997, A-23.

11. Daniel Callahan, *What Kind of Life? The Limits of Medical Progress* (Washington, D.C.: Georgetown University Press, 1990).

12. Leon R. Kass, "The Wisdom of Repugnance: Why We Should Ban the Cloning of Humans," *New Republic,* 2 June 1997, 17–26; and Sidney Callahan, *In Good Conscience: Reason and Emotion in Moral Decision Making* (San Francisco: San Francisco Harper, 1991).

13. Richard Rhodes, *The Making of the Atomic Bomb* (New York: Simon and Schuster, 1986), 784.

14. Nicholas Rescher, *Risk: A Philosophical Introduction to the Theory of Risk Evaluation and Management* (Lanham, Md.: University Press of America,

1983); National Research Council, *Risk Assessment in the Federal Government: Managing the Process* (Washington, D.C.: National Academy Press, 1983); National Research Council, *Understanding Risk: Informing Decisions in a Democratic Society* (Washington, D.C.: National Academy Press, 1996); Kristin S. Shrader-Frechette, *Risk and Rationality: Philosophical Foundations for Populist Reforms* (Berkeley: University of California Press, 1991); and Larry Gostin, "Public Health Regulation: A Systemic Evaluation," *Journal of the American Medical Association* 283 (2000): 3118–22.

15. D. Ian Hopper, "U.S. Sets Funding Rules on Embryo Cell Research," *Chicago Sun Times*, 23 August 2000, A-10–11.

16. Rhodes, *Making of the Atomic Bomb*, 92–93.

17. Kenneth R. Foster, Paolo Vecchia, and Michael H. Repacholi, "Science and the Precautionary Principle," *Science* 288 (2000): 979.

18. Carl F. Cranor, "Asymmetric Information, the Precautionary Principle, and Burdens of Proof," in *Protecting Public Health and the Environment: Implementing the Precautionary Principle*, ed. Carolyn Raffensperger and Joel A. Tickner (Washington, D.C.: Island Press, 1999), 83–84.

19. Foster et al., "Science and the Precautionary Principle."

20. John Harris and Soren Holm, "Extending Human Lifespan and the Precautionary Paradox," *Journal of Medicine and Philosophy* 27, no. 3 (2002): 355–68.

21. Andrew Jordan and Timothy O'Riordan, "The Precautionary Principle in Contemporary Environmental Policy and Politics," in *Protecting Public Health and the Environment: Implementing the Precautionary Principle*, ed. Carolyn Raffensperger and Joel A. Tickner (Washington, D.C.: Island Press, 1999), 15–35.

22. William J. Broad, "U.S. Tightening Rules on Keeping Scientific Secrets," *New York Times*, 17 February 2002, A-1; and Judith Miller, *Germs: Biological Weapons and America's Secret War* (New York: Simon and Schuster, 2001).

23. Matthew Meselson, "Bioterror: What Can Be Done?" *New York Review of Books*, 20 December 2000, 41.

6. USING HUMANS FOR RESEARCH

1. Susan Lederer, *Subjected to Science: Human Experimentation in America before the Second World War* (Baltimore: Johns Hopkins University Press, 1995), xiv.

2. Matthew Miller, "Phase I Cancer Trials: A Collusion of Misunderstanding," *Hastings Center Report* 30, no. 4 (2000): 34.

3. Lederer, *Subjected to Science*, 1.

4. Ibid., 7.

5. Ibid., 138.

6. Robert J. Levine, *Ethics and Regulation of Clinical Research* (Baltimore: Urban and Schwarzenberg, 1981).

7. George J. Annas and Michael A. Grodin, "Historical Origins of the Nuremberg Code," in *The Nazi Doctors and the Nuremberg Code: Human*

Rights in Human Experimentation, ed. George J. Annas and Michael A. Grodin (New York: Oxford University Press, 1992), 67.

8. Ibid., 84–85.

9. Robert Proctor, "Nazi Doctors, German Medicine, and Human Experimentation," in *Nazi Doctors and the Nuremberg Code,* 28–29.

10. John Miller Turpin Finney, *A Surgeon's Life* (New York: G. P. Putman Sons, 1940), 127.

11. Michael A. Grodin, "Historical Origins of the Nuremberg Code," in *Nazi Doctors and the Nuremberg Code,* 128, 129, 131.

12. Ibid., 133.

13. David J. Rothman, *Strangers at the Bedside: A History of How Law and Bioethics Transformed Medical Decision Making* (New York: Basic Books, 1991), 31.

14. Jonathan Moreno, *Undue Risk: Secret State Experiments on Humans* (New York: W. H. Freeman, 1999), 140–41.

15. Advisory Committee on Human Radiation Experiments, *Final Report of the Advisory Committee on Human Radiation Experiments* (New York: Oxford University Press, 1996), 512–40, 543, 545.

16. Moreno, *Undue Risk;* and Sharon Perley et al., "The Nuremberg Code: An International Overview," in *Nazi Doctors and the Nuremberg Code,* 149–73.

17. Baruch Brody, *Ethics of Biomedical Research: An International Perspective* (New York: Oxford University Press, 1998), 157.

18. World Medical Association, "The Declaration of Helsinki," *Journal of the American Medical Association* 277 (1997): 925–26.

19. Perley, "Nuremberg Code," 160.

20. Brody, *Ethics of Biomedical Research,* 36–37.

21. Henry K. Beecher, "Ethics and Clinical Research," *New England Journal of Medicine* 274 (1966): 1354–60.

22. M. H. Pappworth, *Human Guinea Pigs: Experimentation with Man* (Boston: Beacon Press, 1967).

23. Jay Katz, " 'Ethics and Clinical Research' Revisited: A Tribute to Henry K. Beecher," *Hastings Center Report* 23, no. 5 (1993): 31–39.

24. Moreno, *Undue Risk;* Beecher, "Ethics and Clinical Research"; and Henry K. Beecher, "Some Guiding Principles for Clinical Investigation," *Journal of the American Medical Association* 195 (1966): 1135–36.

25. Jay Katz, *Experimentation with Human Beings* (New York: Russell Sage Foundation, 1972), 84, 37.

26. James Jones, *Bad Blood* (New York: Free Press, 1981); and Allan Brandt, "Racism and Research," *Hastings Center Report* 8, no. 6 (1978): 20–29.

27. David J. Rothman, "Were Tuskegee & Willowbrook 'Studies in Nature'?" *Hastings Center Report* 12, no. 2 (1982): 5.

28. William J. Curran, "Governmental Regulation of the Use of Human Subjects in Medical Research: The Approach of Two Federal Agencies," in *Experimenting with Human Subjects,* ed. Paul A. Freund (New York: George Braziller, 1969).

29. Ibid., 409–30.

30. Ibid., 437.

31. National Commission for the Protection of Human Subjects of Biomedical and Behavioral Research, "The Belmont Report: Ethical Principles and Guidelines for the Protection of Human Subjects of Research" (Washington, D.C.: Government Printing Office, 1978).

32. "United States Regulatory Requirements for Research Involving Human Subjects," *Journal of Biolaw &Business* 1 (1998): 39–44.

33. John H. Evans, "A Sociological Account of the Growth of Principlism," *Hastings Center Report* 30, no. 5 (2000): 31–38.

34. Trudo Lemmens and Alison Thompson, "Noninstitutional Commercial Review Boards in North America," *IRB Ethics and Human Research* 23, no. 2 (2001): 1–12.

35. Francis D. Moore, "Therapeutic Innovation: Ethical Boundaries in the Initial Clinical Trials of New Drugs and Surgical Procedures," in *Experimenting with Human Subjects*, ed. Paul A. Freund (New York: George Braziller, 1969), 365.

36. World Medical Association, "Declaration of Helsinki," *British Medical Journal* 313, no. 7070 (1996): 1448–49.

37. Annas and Grodin, "Historical Origins of the Nuremberg Code," 278.

38. Beverly Woodward, "Challenges to Human Subject Protections in US Medical Research," *Journal of the American Medical Association* 282 (1999): 1947–52.

39. Office of Inspector General, *Institutional Review Boards: A Time for Reform* (Washington, D.C.: Department of Health and Human Services, 1998), 1.

40. Remarks of Jane Henny, commissioner, U.S. Food and Drug Administration, made at a meeting of the Association of American Medical Colleges, Council of Teaching Hospitals, Washington, D.C., 11 May 2000.

41. Donna Shalala, "Protecting Research Subjects—What Must Be Done," *New England Journal of Medicine* 343 (2000): 808–10.

42. Charles Marwick, "New Head of Federal Office Clear on Protecting Human Research Participants," *Journal of the American Medical Association* 284 (2000): 1501. Dr. Koski resigned from that position in fall 2002.

43. Jonathan Moreno, "Goodbye to All That: The End of Moderate Protectionism in Human Subjects Research," *Hastings Center Report* 31, no.3 (2001): 9–17.

44. Woodward, "Challenges to Human Subject Protections," 1947–52.

45. Code of Federal Regulations, "Protection of Human Subjects," Title 45, ch. A, subch. A, part 46.

46. Albert R. Jonsen, "The Weight and Weighing of Ethical Principles," in *The Ethics of Research Involving Human Subjects: Facing the 21st Century*, ed. Harold Y. Vanderpool (Frederick, Md.: University Publishing Group, 1996), 59–82.

47. Brody, *Ethics of Biomedical Research*, 45–48; and 45 CFR 46.

48. Katz, *Experimentation with Human Beings*.

49. Stanley Milgram, "Some Conditions of Obedience and Disobedience to Authority," *International Journal of Psychiatry* 6 (1968): 259–76.

50. David Wendler, "Deception in Medical and Behavioral Research: Is It Ever Acceptable?" *Milbank Quarterly* 74 (1996): 87–114; Mathilda B. Canter et al., *Ethics for Psychologists: A Commentary on the APA Ethics Code* (Washington, D.C.: American Psychological Association, 1994); Allan J. Kimmel, *Ethical Issues in Behavioral Research: A Survey* (Cambridge, Mass.: Blackwell Publishers, 1996); and Patricia Keith-Spiegel and Gerald P. Koocher, *Ethics in Psychology: Professional Standards and Cases* (New York: Random House, 1985).

51. 45 CFR 46, subpart A, §46.111; and Brody, *Ethics of Biomedical Research*, 48–49.

52. Woodward, "Challenges to Human Subject Protections."

53. Gina Kolata, "Ban on Medical Experiments without Consent Is Relaxed," *New York Times*, 5 November 1996, A-1.

54. Loretta M. Kopelman, "Children as Research Subjects: A Dilemma," *Journal of Medicine and Philosophy* 25 (2000): 745–64.

55. Rebecca Dresser, "Mentally Disabled Research Subjects," *Journal of the American Medical Association* 276 (1996): 67–72; William J. Carpenter, Nina R. Schooler, and John M. Kane, "The Rationale and Ethics of Medication-Free Research in Schizophrenia," *Archives of General Psychiatry* 54 (1997): 401–7; and Richard J. Bonnie, "Research with Cognitively Impaired Subjects: Unfinished Business in the Regulation of Human Research," *Archives of General Psychiatry* 54 (1997): 105–23.

56. Alexander Capron, "Ethical and Human-Rights Issues in Research on Mental Disorders That May Affect Decision Making Capacity," *New England Journal of Medicine* 340 (1999): 1433.

57. Advisory Committee, *Final Report on Human Radiation Experiments*, 405.

58. Brody, *Ethics of Biomedical Research*, 37–38.

59. Levine, *Ethics and Regulation of Clinical Research*.

60. Franklin G. Miller, Donald L. Rosenstein, and Evan G. DeRenzo, "Professional Integrity in Clinical Research," *Journal of the American Medical Association* 280 (1998): 1454; Miller, "Phase I Cancer Trials"; and Robert P. Kelch, "Maintaining the Trust in Clinical Research," *New England Journal of Medicine* 346 (2002): 285–87.

61. George J. Annas, "Questing for Grails: Duplicity, Betrayal and Self-Deception in Postmodern Medical Research," *Journal of Contemporary Health Law Policy* 12 (1996): 300, 314.

62. Robert M. Veatch, " 'Experimental' Pregnancy," *Hastings Center Report* 1, no. 1 (1971): 2–3.

63. Peter Lurie and Sidney M. Wolfe, "Unethical Trials of Interventions to Reduce Perinatal Transmission of the Human Immunodeficiency Virus in Developing Countries," *New England Journal of Medicine* 337 (1997): 853–56.

64. Marcia Angell, "The Ethics of Clinical Research in the Third World," *New England Journal of Medicine* 337 (1997): 847.

65. Harold Varmus and David Satcher, "Ethical Complexities of Conducting Research in Developing Countries," *New England Journal of Medicine* 337 (1997): 1003–5.

66. Barry R. Bloom, "The Highest Attainable Standard: Ethical Issues in AIDS Vaccines," *Science* 279 (1998): 187–88.

67. David J. Rothman, "The Shame of Medical Research," *New York Review of Books*, 30 November 2000, 64.

68. National Bioethics Advisory Commission, *Ethical and Policy Issues in International Research—Draft Report* (Bethesda, 2000).

69. Bloom, "Highest Attainable Standard"; and Rothman, "Shame of Medical Research."

70. George J Annas and Michael A. Grodin, "Human Rights and Maternal-Fetal HIV Transmission Prevention Trials in Africa," *Amercan Journal of Public Health* 88 (1998): 560–62.

71. Solomon R. Benatar and Peter A. Singer, "A New Look at International Research," *British Medical Journal* 321 (2000): 824.

72. Ibid., 825.

73. Leonard H. Glantz et al., "Research in Developing Countries: Taking 'Benefit' Seriously," *Hastings Center Report* 28, no. 6 (1998): 38–42.

74. Robert M. Veatch, "From Nuremberg through the 1990s: The Priority of Autonomy," in *The Ethics of Research Involving Human Subjects: Facing the 21st Century*, ed. Harold Y. Vanderpool (Frederick, Md.: University Publishing Group, 1996).

7. PLURALISM, BALANCE, CONTROVERSY

1. Marcia Barinaga, "Asilomar Revisited: Lessons for Today?" *Science* 287 (2000): 1584–85.

2. "Genetics: Conference Sets Strict Controls to Replace Moratorium," *Science* 187 (1975): 931–34.

3. R. J. Jackson et al., "Expression of Mouse Interleukin-4 by a Recombinant Ectromelia Virus Suppresses Cytolytic Lymphocyte Responses and Overcomes Genetic Resistance to Mousepox," *Journal of Virology* 75 (2001): 1205–10.

4. James D. Watson, "Let Us Stop Regulating DNA Research," *Nature* 278 (1979): 113.

5. Charles Weiner, "Is Self Regulation Enough Today? Evaluating the Recombinant DNA Controversy," *Health Matrix: Journal of Law-Medicine* 9 (1999): 289–302; Raymond A. Zilinskas and Burke K. Zimmerman, *The Gene-Splicing Wars: Reflections on the Recombinant DNA Controversy* (New York: Macmillan, 1986); Sheldon Krimsky, *Genetic Alchemy: The Social History of the Recombinant DNA Controversy* (Cambridge, Mass.: MIT Press, 1982); Barinaga, "Asilomar Revisited"; and "SCLR—Asilomar," *Southern California Law Review* 51 (1978).

6. "Researching Violence: Science, Politics, & Public Controversy," *Hastings Center Report* 9, no. 2 (1979): S6.

7. Patricia Jacobs, "Aggressive Behavior, Mental Sub-Normality, and the XYY Male," *Nature* 208 (1965): 1351.

8. Willard Gaylin, Ruth Macklin, and Tabitha M. Powledge, *Violence and the Politics of Research* (New York: Plenum Press, 1981), 100.

9. Barbara J. Culliton, "XYY: Harvard Researcher under Fire Stops Newborn Screening," *Science* 188 (1975): 1284–85.

10. Bernard Davis, "XYY: The Dangers of Regulating Research by Adverse Publicity," *Harvard Magazine*, 1976, 26–30; and Loretta M. Kopelman, "Ethical Controversies in Medical Research: The Case of XYY Screening," *Perspectives in Biology and Medicine* 21 (1978): 196–204.

11. "The XXY Controversy: Researching Violence and Genetics," *Hastings Center Report* 10, no. 4 (1980): S1–31.

12. Ibid.; and Gaylin et al., *Violence and the Politics of Research.*

13. Dr. Farris Tuma, quoted in Eileen O'Connor, "Caution Urged for Brain Research on Violence," *CNN.com Health*, 28 July 2000.

14. Stephanie L. Sherman et al., "Behavioral Genetics '97: ASGH Statement—Recent Developments in Human Behavioral Genetics: Past Accomplishments and Future Directions," *American Journal of Human Genetics* 60 (1997): 1265–75; and Erik Parens, "Taking Behavioral Genetics Seriously," *Hastings Center Report* 26, no. 4 (1996): 13–18.

15. Ruth Hubbard and Elijah Wald, *Exploding the Gene Myth* (Boston: Beacon Press, 1993).

16. E. O. Wilson, "The Attempt to Suppress Human Behavioral Genetics," *Journal of General Education* 29 (1978): 277–87.

17. Ibid., 279.

18. Parens, "Taking Behavioral Genetics Seriously."

19. Albert R. Jonsen, *The Birth of Bioethics* (New York: Oxford University Press, 1998), ch. 4.

20. *Report of the Human Fetal Tissue Transplantation Research Panel* (Bethesda: NIH, 1988), 4.

21. Arthur L. Caplan, "The Short, Exceedingly Strange Debate over Fetal Tissue Transplant Research," *American Journal of Ethics & Medicine* (1994): 24.

22. Curt R. Freed et al., "Transplantation of Embryonic Dopamine Neurons for Severe Parkinson's Disease," *New England Journal of Medicine* 344 (2001): 710–19; and Gerald D. Fischbach and Guy M. McKhann, "Cell Therapy for Parkinson's Disease," *New England Journal of Medicine* 344 (2001): 763–65.

23. Mary Warnock, *Report of the Committee of Inquiry into Human Fertilisation and Embryology* (London: HMSO, 1984).

24. Ethics Advisory Board of the U.S. Department of Health Education and Welfare, *Embryo Research* (Bethesda, 1979), 4.

25. National Bioethics Advisory Commission, *Cloning Human Beings*, vol. 1, *Report and Recommendations of the National Bioethics Advisory Commission* (Rockville, Md., 1997).

26. Committee on Science, Engineering, and Public Policy, *Scientific and Medical Aspects of Human Reproductive Cloning* (Washington, D.C.: National Academy Press, 2002).

27. Gretchen Vogel, "Cloning Bills Proliferate in U.S. Congress," *Science* 292 (2001): 1037.

28. Patient's Coalition for Urgent Research (CURe), *Patient's CURe Overview* (Washington, D.C.: CURe, 2000).

29. Caplan, "Short, Exceedingly Strange Debate"; and Ronald M. Green, "Stopping Embryo Research," *Health Matrix: Journal of Law-Medicine* 9 (1999): 235–52.

30. Gregory Stock and John Campbell, eds., *Engineering the Human Germline* (New York: Oxford University Press, 2000).

31. President's Commission for the Study of Ethical Problems in Medicine and Biomedical and Behavioral Research, *Splicing Life: A Report on the Social and Ethical Issues of Genetic Engineering with Human Beings* (Washington, D.C., 1982), 48.

32. Robert Cook-Deegan, "Germ-Line Gene Therapy: Keep the Window Open a Crack," *Politics and Life Sciences* 13 (1994): 217–48.

33. Joseph Fletcher, "Germ-Line Gene Therapy: The Costs of Premature Ultimates," *Politics and Life Sciences* 13 (1994): 225–27; and Stock and Campbell, *Engineering the Human Germline*. This would seem an instance of the "gambler's principle" at work.

34. Paul Billings et al., "Human Germline Gene Modification: A Dissent," *Lancet* 353 (1999): 1873–75; and this is an instance of a "precautionary principle" at work.

35. Parens, "Taking Behavioral Genetics Seriously."

36. Ibid.; and Robert Pollack, *The Missing Moment: How the Unconscious Shapes Modern Science* (Boston: Houghton Mifflin, 1999).

37. Robert P. Lanza et al., "The Ethical Validity of Using Nuclear Transfer in Human Transplantation," *Journal of the American Medical Association* 284 (2000): 3175.

38. National Bioethics Advisory Commission, *Cloning Human Beings*, 52.

39. Richard H. Nicholson, "The Greatest Happiness," *Hastings Center Report* 31, no. 1 (2001): 8.

40. Leon R. Kass and Daniel Callahan, "Band Stand: Cloning's Big Test," *New Republic*, 6 August 2001, 10–11; Daniel Callahan, "The Ethics of Cloning," testimony given to the Subcommittee on Crime, Committee of the Judiciary, U.S. House of Representatives, June 7, 2001 (Washington, D.C.: Government Printing Office, 2001).

41. Daniel Callahan, *Abortion: Law, Choice, and Morality* (London: Macmillan, 1970).

42. George J. Annas, Arthur L. Caplan, and Sherman Elias, "The Politics of Human Embryo Research—Avoiding Ethical Gridlock," *New England Journal of Medicine* 334 (1996): 1329–32.

43. Zogby International, "Views on Medical Advances, Genetic Testing, Cloning, Nanotechnology," July 6, 2001.

44. National Bioethics Advisory Commission, *Ethical Issues in Human Stem Cell Research*, vol. 1, *Report and Recommendations of the National Bioethics Advisory Commission* (Rockville, Md., 1999), 50.

45. Human Embryo Research Panel, *Report of the Human Embryo Research Panel—Final Draft* (Bethesda: NIH, 1994), 3; and Ethics Advisory Board, *Embryo Research*, 101.

46. Michael J. Meyer and Lawrence J. Nelson, "Respecting What We Destroy: Reflections of Human Embryo Research," *Hastings Center Report* 31, no. 1 (2001): 16–23.

47. Ibid., 19; and "Human Embryo Research," exchange of letters, *Hastings Center Report* 31, no. 4 (2001): 4–5.

48. National Bioethics Advisory Commission, *Human Stem Cell Research*, 51.

49. Eric Juengst and Michael Fossell, "The Ethics of Embryonic Stem Cells—Now and Forever, Cells without End," *Journal of the American Medical Association* 284 (2000): 3181.

50. National Bioethics Advisory Commission, *Human Stem Cell Research*, ii.

51. Francis Fukuyama, "How to Regulate Science," *Public Interest* 146 (2002): 20.

52. Gallup Poll, 30 April–2 May 2000, available at www.gallup.com. "With respect to the abortion issue, would you consider yourself to be pro-choice or pro-life?" 42 percent responded that they considered themselves to be pro-life (48 percent were pro-choice).

53. John H. Evans, *Playing God: Human Genetic Engineering and the Rationalization of Public Bioethical Debate* (Chicago: University of Chicago Press, 2002).

54. Richard Horton, "How Sick Is Modern Medicine?" *New York Review of Books*, 12 November 2000, 50.

55. Weiner, "Is Self Regulation Enough?" 297.

56. Ibid., 300–301.

57. Patients' Coalition for Urgent Research (CURe), "Patients' CURe Overview" (Washington, D.C., 2000).

58. A 26 March 2001 letter to Tommy Thompson, secretary of health and human services, from Stanley O. Ikenberry, president, American Council on Education et al.

59. National Research Council and Institute of Medicine, *Stem Cell Research and the Future of Regenerative Medicine* (Washington, D.C.: National Academy Press, 2001).

60. Lori B. Andrews, *The Clone Age* (New York: Henry Holt, 1999), 206.

61. Robert L. Sinsheimer, "The Presumptions of Science," *Daedalus* 107 (1978): 23–36.

62. Green, "Stopping Embryo Research"; Shannon H. Smith, "Ignorance Is

Not Bliss: Why a Ban on Human Cloning Is Unacceptable," *Health Matrix: Journal of Law-Medicine* 9 (1999): 311–34; Nikki Melina Constantine Bell, "Regulating Transfer and Use of Fetal Tissue in Transplantation Procedures: The Ethical Dimensions," *American Journal of Law & Medicine* 20 (1994): 277–94; David B. Resnik, "Privatized Biomedical Research, Public Fears, and the Hazards of Government Regulation: Lessons from Stem Cell Research," *Health Care Analysis* 7 (1999): 273–87.

63. Thomas I. Emerson, "The Constitution and Regulation of Research," in *Regulation of Scientific Inquiry, Societal Concerns with Research,* ed. Keith M. Wulff (Boulder, Colo.: Westview Press, 1979), 129; and John A. Robertson, "The Scientists' Right to Research: A Constitutional Analysis," *Southern California Law Review* 51 (1978): 1203.

64. David Baltimore, "Limiting Science: A Biologist's Perspective," *Daedalus* 107 (1978): 37–46.

65. Sinsheimer, "Presumptions of Science."

66. Pollack, *Missing Moment,* 177.

67. Hakan Widner, "The Case for Neural Tissue Transplantation as a Treatment for Parkinson's Disease," in *Parkinson's Disease: Advances in Neurology,* ed. Gerald M. Stern (Philadelphia: Lippincott Williams and Wilkins, 1999), 641–49; and Kenneth A. Follett, "The Surgical Treatment of Parkinson's Disease," in *Annual Review of Medicine,* ed. Cecil H. Coggins (Palo Alto, Calif.: Annual Reviews, 2000), 135–46.

68. "News," *Science* 287 (2000): 1672.

69. Green, "Stopping Embryo Research."

70. Elizabeth Heitman, "Infertility as a Public Health Problem: Why Assisted Reproductive Technologies Are Not the Answer," *Stanford Law and Policy Review* 6 (1995): 89–102.

71. National Bioethics Advisory Commission, *Human Stem Cell Research,* ii, 53, 58.

72. David A. Prentice, "No Fountain of Youth," *Regeneration* 6 (2000): 16.

73. "Study: Fat May Be Stem Cells Source," *New York Times,* 10 April 2001, A-15.

74. Sylvia Pagan Westohal, "Beating the Ban: Will Embryonic Stem Cells Made without Embryos Keep Politicians Happy?" *New Scientist* 172 (2001): 5–6.

75. Audrey R. Chapman, Mark S. Frankel, and Michele S. Garfinkle, *Stem Cell Research and Applications: Monitoring the Frontiers of Biomedical Research* (Washington, D.C.: American Association for the Advancement of Science, 1999), x.

76. Glenn McGee and Arthur L. Caplan, "What's in the Dish?" *Hastings Center Report* 29, no. 2 (1999): 36–38.

77. Green, "Stopping Embryo Research," 252; and Ronald M. Green, *The Human Embryo Research Debates* (New York: Oxford University Press, 2001), 165–75.

78. Martha Nussbaum, *Women and Human Development: The Capabilities Approach* (New York: Cambridge University Press, 2000), 179–80.

79. John Rawls, *The Law of Peoples* (Cambridge, Mass.: Harvard University Press, 1999), 131, 133.

80. Amy Gutmann and Dennis Thompson, *Democracy and Disagreement* (Cambridge, Mass: Belknap Press of Harvard University, 1996), 55–63.

81. Louis Menand, "Civil Actions: *Brown v. Board of Education* and the Limits of the Law," *New Yorker*, 12 February 2001, 96.

82. Robert Audi and Nicolas Wolterstorff, *Religion in the Public Square* (Lanham, Md.: Rowman and Littlefield, 1997).

83. Jonathan Moreno, *Deciding Together: Bioethics and the Moral Consensus* (New York: Oxford University Press, 1995), 85.

8. DOING GOOD AND DOING WELL

1. "Pfizer—Life Is Our Life's Work," *International Herald Tribune*, 8 December 2000, 6.

2. William Rothstein, "Pharmaceuticals and Public Policy in America: A History," in *Readings in American Health Care*, ed. William Rothstein (Madison: University of Wisconsin Press, 1995).

3. Jorgen Drews, "Drug Discovery: A Historical Perspective," *Science* 287 (2000): 1960–64.

4. Louis Glambos and Jeffrey L. Sturchio, "The Pharmaceutical Industry in the Twentieth Century: A Reappraisal of the Sources of Innovation," *History and Technology* 13 (1996): 83–100.

5. Ibid., 92.

6. Marcia Angell, "The Pharmaceutical Industry—to Whom Is It Accountable?" *New England Journal of Medicine* 342 (2000): 1902–4.

7. Pharmaceutical Research and Manufacturers of America, *PhRMA Annual Report 2000–2001* (Washington, D.C., 2000), 1.

8. IMS Health, "IMS Health Reports 10 Percent Growth in 2000 Audited Global Total Pharmaceutical Sales to $317.2 Billion" (www.imshealth.com: IMS Health, 2001).

9. Ernst and Young, *The Economic Contributions of the Biotechnology Industry to the U.S. Economy* (Washington, D.C.: Biotechnology Industry Organization, 2000).

10. Bruce Agnew, "When PhRMA Merges, R & D Is the Dowry," *Science* 287 (2000): 1953.

11. "Horn of Plenty," *The Economist*, 21 February 1998, S-5.

12. Pharmaceutical Research and Manufacturers of America, *Pharmaceutical Industry Profile* (Washington, D.C., 2000).

13. Ann-Marie MacIntyre, *Key Issues in the Pharmaceutical Industry* (New York: John Wiley and Sons, 1999), 92 ff.

14. Ian Cockburn and Rebecca Henderson, "Public-Private Interaction in Pharmaceutical Research," *Proceedings of the National Academy of Sciences* 93 (1996): 12726.

15. Jeff Gerth and Sheryl Gay Stolberg, "Drug Makers Reap Profits on Tax-

Backed Research," *New York Times*, 23 April 2000, A-1; and Jeff Gerth and Sheryl Gay Stolberg, "How Companies Stall Generics and Keep Themselves Healthy," *New York Times*, 23 July 2000, A-1.

16. "Changing Marketplace 2000" (2000).

17. Shailagh Murray, "Drug Companies Are Spending Record Amounts on Lobbying and Campaign Contributions" *Wall Street Journal*, 7 July 2000, A-14.

18. Fred Charatan, "Drug Companies Help Pay for Bush Inauguration," *British Medical Journal* 322 (2001): 192.

19. Ernst R. Berndt, "The U.S. Pharmaceutical Industry: Why Major Growth in Times of Cost Containment?" *Health Affairs* 20, no. 2 (2001): 100–114.

20. Pharmaceutical Research, *Pharmaceutical Industry Profile*, 75.

21. Office of Technology Assessment, U.S. Congress, *Pharmaceutical R&D: Costs, Risks and Rewards*, OTA-H-522 (Washington, D.C.: Government Printing Office, 1993), 54–67.

22. Ann-Marie MacIntyre, *Key Issues in the Pharmaceutical Industry* (New York: John Wiley and Sons, 1999), 83.

23. Stephen Hall, "Prescription for Profit," *New York Times Magazine*, 11 March 2001, 59.

24. Gerth and Stolberg, "How Companies Stall Generics."

25. Pharmaceutical Research and Manufacturers of America, *1998 Industry Profile* (Washington, D.C., 1999), 17.

26. Patricia Van Arnum, "Active Pharmaceutical Ingredients: The Opportunities in the Branded Prescription Market," *Chemical Market Reporter* 258 (2000): 14.

27. Rachel Zimmerman, "Drug Spending Soared 17.4% during 1999," *Wall Street Journal*, 27 June 2000, A-3.

28. Sheryl Gay Stolberg, "No Simple Answer to Rising Costs of Drugs for the Elderly," *New York Times*, 3 September 2000, A-26.

29. Henry J. Kaiser Family Foundation, "Understanding the Effects of Direct-to-Consumer Prescription Drug Advertising" (Menlo Park, Calif., 2001).

30. Adam Smith, *The Wealth of Nations* (Buffalo, N.Y.: Prometheus Books, 1991), 118; citing the public's view of apothecaries, Smith also defends their profit, and it is worth quoting him more fully: "Apothecaries' profit is a bye-word, denoting something uncommonly extravagant. This great apparent profit, however, is frequently no more than the reasonable wages of labour. The skill of an apothecary is a much nicer and more delicate matter than that of any artificer whatever; and the trust which is reposed in him is of much greater importance." In those days of course there was no pharmaceutical industry, and the apothecary put together his own drugs from raw material—hence, any onus of high prices fell on him.

31. Baruch Brody, *Ethical Issues in Drug Testing, Approval, and Pricing* (New York: Oxford University Press, 1995), 229.

32. Robert Goldburg, "Bountiful Bogeyman: The Drug Companies—So

Easy to Defend," *National Review*, 25 September 2000; and James Surowiecki, "Big Pharma's Drug Problem," *New Yorker*, 16 October 2000, 98.

33. MacIntyre, *Key Issues in the Pharmaceutical Industry*, 129–32.

34. Ibid., 61–62.

35. Hall, "Prescription for Profit," 100.

36. Angell, "Pharmaceutical Industry—to Whom Is It Accountable?" 1902.

37. Pharmaceutical Research, *Pharmaceutical Industry Profile*, 2000; Dan Baker, "The Real Drug Crisis," *In These Times*, 25 July 1999; Michael A. Heller and Rebecca S. Eisenberg, "Can Patents Deter Innovation? The Anticommons in Biomedical Research," *Science* 280 (1998): 698–701; and Laurie McGinley, "Patent Laws Are Questioned in Drug Study," *Wall Street Journal*, 24 July 2000, A-3.

38. John E. Calfee, *Prices, Markets, and the Pharmaceutical Revolution* (Washington, D.C.: AEI Press, 2000), 33.

39. Patricia Danzon, "Making Sense of Drug Prices," *Regulation* 23 (2000): 61.

40. Geeta Anand, "Immunex Races to Meet Demand for Biotech Drug," *Wall Street Journal*, 20 February 2001, B-1.

41. Congressional Budget Office, *How Increased Competition from Generic Drugs Has Affected Prices and Returns in the Pharmaceutical Industry* (Washington, D.C.: Government Printing Office, 1998).

42. MacIntyre, *Key Issues in the Pharmaceutical Industry*, 129–34.

43. Uwe E. Reinhardt, "Perspectives on the Pharmaceutical Industry," *Health Affairs* 20, no. 5 (2001): 136–49.

44. MacIntyre, *Key Issues in the Pharmaceutical Industry*, 138.

45. Richard G. Frank, "Prescription Drug Prices: Why Do Some Pay More Than Others Do?" *Health Affairs* 20, no. 2 (2001): 115–28.

46. Lynn Etheredge, "Purchasing Medicare Prescription Drug Benefits: A New Proposal," *Health Affairs* 18 (1999): 7–19.

47. John A. Poisal and Lauren Murray, "Growing Differences between Medicare Beneficiaries with and without Drug Coverage," *Health Affairs* 20, no. 2 (2001): 74–85; Shailagh Murray and Lucette Lagnado, "Drug Companies Face Assault on Prices," *Wall Street Journal*, 11 May 2000, B-1; and Bruce Stuart, Dennis Shea, and Becky Briesacher, "Dynamics in Drug Coverage of Medicare Beneficiaries: Finders, Losers, Switchers," *Health Affairs* 20 (2001): 86–99.

48. John K. Iglehart, "Medicare and Prescription Drugs," *New England Journal of Medicine* 344 (2001): 1010–15.

49. Sheryl Gay Stolberg, "Africa's AIDS War," *New York Times*, 10 March 2001, A-1.

50. European Federation of Pharmaceutical Industries and Associations (Efpia), "Non Exhaustive List of Initiatives Carried Out by the Pharmaceutical Industry to Combat Health Problems in the Developing World" (http://www.efpia.org/: Efpia, 2000).

51. Daniel Pearl, "Behind Cipla's Offer of Cheap AIDS Drugs: Potent Mix of Motives," *Wall Street Journal*, 12 March 2001, A-1.

52. Helen Cooper, Rachel Zimmerman, and Laura McGinley, "Patent Pending: AIDS Epidemic Traps Drug Firms in a Vise: Treatments vs. Profits," *Wall Street Journal,* 2 March 2001, A-1.

53. MacIntyre, *Key Issues in the Pharmaceutical Industry,* 177, 179.

54. David B. Resnik, "Developing Drugs for the Developing World: An Economic, Legal, Moral and Political Dilemma," *Developing World Bioethics* 1 (2001): 13–22.

55. MacIntyre, *Key Issues in the Pharmaceutical Industry,* 183.

56. Donald G. McNeil Jr., "Drug Makers and Third World: Study in Neglect," *New York Times,* 21 May 2000, A-1; Meredith Turshen, "Reprivatizing Pharmaceutical Supplies in Africa," *Journal of Public Health Policy* 22 (2001): 198–224.

57. David Noble, *America by Design: Science, Technology, and the Rise of Corporate Capitalism* (New York: Knopf, 1977), 130–31.

58. Ezekiel J. Emanuel and Daniel Steiner, "Institutional Conflict of Interest," *New England Journal of Medicine* 32 (1995): 262–67.

59. David Blumenthal and E. G. Campbell, "Academic Industry Relationships in Biotechnology: A Primer on Policy and Practice," *Cloning* 2 (2000): 129–36.

60. Eyal Press and Jennifer Washburn, "The Kept University," *Atlantic Monthly,* 1 March 2000, 39–40.

61. Ibid., 46.

62. Blumenthal and Campbell, "Academic Industry Relationships."

63. Ibid., 135.

64. "Zero Tolerance Financial Interest Policies Urged by Former NEJM Editor," *Blue Sheet,* 23 August 2000, 5.

65. Hamilton Moses III and Joseph B. Martin, "Academic Relationships with Industry," *Journal of the American Medical Association* 285 (2001): 933–35.

66. National Institutes of Health, *NIH Data Book* (Bethesda, Md., 1990); see also Peter J. Neuman and Eileen A. Sandberg, "Trends in Health Care R&D and Technology Innovation," *Health Affairs* 17, no. 6 (1998): 111–19.

67. Pharmaceutical Research, *Pharmaceutical Industry Profile,* 2000.

68. C. Daniel Mullins, Francis Palumbo, and Bruce Stuart, "The Impact of Pipeline Drugs on Pharmaceutical Spending" (presented at a joint BlueCross BlueShield/Health Insurance Association of America Symposium, 13–14 April 2001, University of Maryland School of Pharmacy [available at www.hiaa.org]).

69. Health Insurance Association of America, *The Impact of Medical Technology on Future Health Care Costs* (Bethesda, 2001); and Health Insurance Association of America, "Press Release: Technology May Account for a Third of Projected Health Spending Increases" (2001; both are available at www.hiaa.org).

70. David M. Cutler, *Technology, Health Costs, and the NIH* (Cambridge, Mass.: Harvard University Press, 1995).

71. Hall, "Prescription for Profit," 45.

72. National Institutes of Health, *A Periodic Evaluation of the Cost-Benefits of Biomedical Research* (Bethesda, 1992).

73. Pharmaceutical Research, *PhRMA Annual Report 2000–2001* and *Pharmaceutical Industry Profile*, ch. 4.

74. Battelle's Medical Technology Assessment and Policy Research Center, *The Value of Pharmaceuticals: An Assessment of Future Costs for Selected Conditions* (Washington, D.C., 1990).

75. Funding First: Mary Woodard Lasker Charitable Trust, *Exceptional Returns: The Economic Value of America's Investment in Medical Research* (New York: Lasker Foundation, 2000).

76. Herbert Pardes et al., "Effects of Medical Research on Health Care and the Economy," *Science* 283 (1999): 36.

77. Ibid., 37.

78. Kenneth G. Manton, Larry S. Corder, and Eric Stallard, "Monitoring Changes in the Health of the U.S. Elderly Population: Correlates with Biomedical Research and Clinical Innovation," *FASEB Journal* 11 (1997): 923–24.

79. Funding First, *Exceptional Returns*.

80. David M Cutler, Mark B. McClellan, and Joseph P. Newhouse, "The Costs and Benefits of Intensive Treatment for Cardiovascular Disease," in *Measuring the Prices of Medical Treatments*, ed. Jack E. Triplett (Washington, D.C.: Brookings Institution Press, 1999), 34–71.

81. Frank R. Lichtenberg, "Do (More and Better) Drugs Keep People Out of Hospitals?" *American Economic Review* 86 (1996): 387.

82. Albert A. Okunade and Vasudera N. R. Murthy, "Technology as a 'Major Driver' of Health Care Costs: A Cointegration Analysis of the Newhouse Conjecture," *Journal of Health Economics* 2 (2002): 147–59.

83. Manton et al., "Monitoring Changes in the Health," 928.

84. Funding First, *Exceptional Returns*, 7; see also Frank R. Lichtenberg, "The Allocation of Publicly Funded Biomedical Research," in *Medical Care Output and Productivity*, ed. David M. Cutler and Ernst R. Bendt (Chicago: University of Chicago Press, 2001).

85. Selma J. Mushkin, *Biomedical Research: Costs and Benefits* (Cambridge, Mass.: Ballinger Publishing, 1979), 9.

86. Cutler et al., "Costs and Benefits of Intensive Treatment," 69.

87. Funding First, *Exceptional Returns*, 1.

88. Kevin M. Murphy and Robert Topel, "The Economic Value of Medical Research" (manuscript, 1999).

89. J. D. Kleinke, while conceding that many better medicines can and do increase costs, argues that the increases are not as important as they are made out to be, and that there are possible reforms that could reduce them ("The Price of Progress: Prescription Drugs in the Health Care Market," *Health Affairs* 20, no. 5 [2001]: 47–59); and Frank R. Lichtenberg, "Are the Benefits of Newer Drugs Worth Their Cost? Evidence from the 1996 MEPS," *Health Affairs* 20, no. 5 (2001): 241–51.

90. David M. Cutler and Mark McClellan, "Is Technological Change in Medicine Worth It?" *Health Affairs* 20 (2001): 11–29.

91. Catherine Hoffman, Dorothy Rice, and Hai-Yen Sung, "Persons with Chronic Conditions: Their Prevalence and Costs," *Journal of the American Medical Association* 276 (1996): 1473–79.

92. American Heart Association, *2001 Heart and Stroke Statistical Update* (Dallas, 2000), 1; idem, *1998 Heart and Stroke Statistical Update* (Dallas, 1997), 10.

93. Murphy and Topel, "The Economic Value of Medical Research."

94. I am indebted to Stuart O. Schweitzer for pointing this out to me; see also Jean Martin, "Research in Biomedicine: Is Anyone Representing/ Advocating the Public Interest?" *European Journal of Public Health* 11 (2000): 459; and "Health Economics and Improved Utilisation of Drugs," *IHE Information* (Sweden) (April 2001): 1–30.

9. ADVOCACY AND PRIORITIES FOR RESEARCH

1. Robert J. Blendon et al., "Americans' Health Priorities: Curing Cancer and Controlling Costs," *Health Affairs* 20, no. 6 (November–December 2001): 222–32.

2. Ibid., 229.

3. Richard H. Shryock, *American Medical Research Past and Present* (New York: Commonwealth Fund, 1947), 44.

4. Stephen P. Strickland, *Politics, Science, and Dread Disease* (Cambridge, Mass.: Harvard University Press, 1972), 35.

5. Elizabeth Brenner Drew, "The Health Syndicate: Washington's Noble Conspirators," *Atlantic Monthly*, December 1967, 76.

6. Senator Arlen Specter, 24 March 1998, in remarks before the U.S. Senate Subcommittee on Labor, Health, and Human Services, and Education and Related Agencies, Committee on Appropriations, Washington, D.C.

7. Judith Havemann, "Crusading for Cash: Patient Groups Compete for Bigger Shares of NIH's Research Funding," *Washington Post*, 15 December 1998, sec. Health, Z10.

8. Rebecca Dresser, "Public Advocacy and Allocation of Federal Funds for Biomedical Research," *Milbank Quarterly* 77 (1999): 257–74.

9. Rebecca Dresser, *When Science Offers Salvation: Patient Advocacy and Research Ethics* (New York: Oxford University Press, 2001), 159–65; Dresser, "Public Advocacy and Allocation"; and David B. Resnik, "Setting Biomedical Research Priorities," *Kennedy Institute of Ethics Journal* 11 (2000): 181–204. Resnik usefully notes drawbacks to a greater lay role.

10. Floyd E. Bloom, "Priority Setting: Quixotic or Essential?" *Science* 282 (1998): 1641.

11. Chris Ham and Louise Locock, "International Approaches to Priority Setting in Health Care," *Health Services Management Center*, Handbook Series 25 (Birmingham, England: University of Birmingham, 1998); Chris Ham,

"Priority Setting in Health Care: Learning from International Experience," *Health Policy* 42 (1997): 49.

12. Paul Belcher and Elias Mossialos, "Health Priorities for the European Intergovernmental Conference," *British Medical Journal* 314 (1997): 1637.

13. Commission on Health Service Research for Development, *Health Research: Essential Link to Equity in Development* (New York: Oxford University Press, 1990).

14. Dean T. Jamison et al., *Disease Control Priorities in Developing Countries* (New York: Oxford University Press, 1993).

15. Report of the Ad Hoc Committee on Health Research Relating to Future Intervention Options, *Investing in Health Research and Development* (Geneva: World Health Organization, 1996, Document TDR/Gen/96.1); see also Christopher J. L. Murray, "Rational Approaches to Priority Setting in International Health," *Journal of Tropical Medicine and Hygiene* 93 (1990): 303–11.

16. Roger Jones, Tara Lamont, Andrew Haines, "Setting Priorities for Research and Development in the NHS: A Case Study on the Interface between Primary and Secondary Care," *British Medical Journal* 311 (1995): 1076.

17. Public Statements of the State, *The Difficult Choices of the Health Service: White Paper on Priority-Setting* (Stockholm: Social Department, 1995); and D. F. Norheim, *Priority-Setting in the Health Service* (Oslo: Center for Medisinsk, 1993).

18. Danish Council of Ethics, *Priority Setting in the Health Service* (Copenhagen: Danish Council of Ethics, 1997).

19. Thomas Bodenheimer, "The Oregon Health Plan: Lessons for the Nation," first of two parts, *New England Journal of Medicine* 337 (1997): 651.

20. Ibid.

21. Carey P. Gross, Gerald F. Anderson, and Neil R. Rowe, "The Relation between Funding by the National Institutes of Health and the Burden of Disease," *New England Journal of Medicine* 340 (1999): 1881; Cayn Donaldson and Gavin Mooney, "Needs Assessment, Priority Setting, and Contracts for Health Care: An Economic View," *British Medical Journal* 303 (1991): 1529; Richard H. Morrow and John H. Bryant, "Health Policy Approaches to Measuring and Valuing Human Life: Conceptual and Ethical Issues," *American Journal of Public Health* 85 (1995): 1356; and Selma J. Mushkin and J. Steven Landefeld, *Biomedical Research: Costs and Benefits* (Cambridge, Mass.: Ballinger, 1979).

22. John Harris, "QALYfying the Value of Life," *Journal of Medical Ethics* 13 (1987): 117; and Jeff Richardson and Erik Nord, "The Importance of Perspective in the Measurement of Quality-Adjusted Life Years," *Medical Decision Making* 17 (1997): 33.

23. Christopher J. L. Murray and Arnab K. Achyara, "Understanding DALYs," *Journal of Health Economics* 16 (1997): 703–30.

24. Jennifer Dixon and H. G. Welch, "Priority-Setting: Lessons from Oregon," *Lancet* 337 (1991): 891–94.

25. Eliot Marshall, "Lobbyists Seek to Reslice NIH's Pie," *Science* 276 (1997): 276.

26. NIH Working Group on Priority Setting, "Setting Research Priorities at the National Institutes of Health," no. 97–4265 (Bethesda, 1998).

27. I use the list presented in a study carried out by the Institute of Medicine and discussed below; because the institute developed it from documents and testimony it received, the list is thus more precise than that presented in the white paper.

28. Gross et al., "Relation between Funding," 693–98.

29. Office of the Director, "Disease-specific Estimates of Direct and Indirect Costs of Illness and NIH Support" (Bethesda: NIH, 1997).

30. Committee on the NIH Priority-Setting Process, *Scientific Opportunities and Public Need: Improving Priority Setting and Public Input at the National Institutes of Health* (Washington, D.C.: National Academy Press, 1998); see also Philip Kitcher, *Science, Truth, and Democracy* (New York: Oxford University Press, 2001); a 1990 study by the Institute of Medicine concluded "that the process for setting research priorities and developing a federal health budget is very fragmented and embedded in a wide range of political considerations." While it recommended a "more uniformly accepted priority setting process," it made no specific recommendations (Floyd E. Bloom and Mark A. Randolph, eds. *Funding Health Sciences Research: A Strategy to Restore Balance* [Washington, D.C.: National Academy Press, 1990], 77).

31. Bruce Agnew, "NIH Embraces Citizens, Council to Cool Debate on Priorities," *Science* 282 (1998): 18; and Dresser, "Public Advocacy and Allocation."

32. Tammy O. Tengs, *Planning for Serendipity: A New Strategy to Prosper from Health Research* (Washington, D.C.: Progressive Policy Institute, 1998).

33. C. Mitcham and R. Frodeman, "The Plea for Balance in the Public Funding of Science," *Technology in Society* 24 (2002): 83–92.

34. Remarks of John Porter at White House Office of Science and Technology Policy's 25th anniversary symposium, Massachusetts Institute of Technology, Cambridge, Mass., 1 May 2001.

35. David Malakoff, "War Effort Shapes U.S. Budget, with Some Program Casualties," *Science* 295 (2002): 952–54.

36. Afschin Gandjour, "Is Subjective Well-Being a Useful Parameter for Allocating Resources among Public Interventions?" *Health Care Analysis* 9 (2001): 437–47; and E. Diener et al., "Subjective Well Being: Three Decades of Progress," *Psychological Bulletin* 125 (1999): 276–302.

10. RESEARCH AND THE PUBLIC INTEREST

1. Associated Press, "World Health Organization Report: U.S. Spends Most on Health; France No. 1 in Treatment," *CNN.com* (20 June 2000).

2. Gerard F. Anderson and Peter Sotir Hussey, "Comparing Health System Performance in OECD Countries," *Health Affairs* 20, no. 3 (2001): 219–32.

3. National Center for Health Statistics, "10 Leading Causes of Death by Age Group—1998" (Bethesda, 2000).

4. Alastair J. S. Wood, "When Increased Therapeutic Benefit Comes at Increased Cost," *New England Journal of Medicine* 346 (2 June 2002): 1819–21.

5. Katharine Levit et al., "Inflation Spurs Health Spending in 2000," *Health Affairs* 21 (January–February 2002): 172–81.

6. Harold Varmus, *NIH Record* 52, no. 2, 25 January 2000.

7. C. Christensen, R. Bohmer, and J. Kenagy, "Will Disruptive Innovations Cure Health Care?" *Harvard Business Review* (2000): 103.

8. Dinah Kim, Robert J. Blendon, and John M. Benson, "How Interested Are Americans in New Medical Technologies? A Multicountry Comparison," *Health Affairs* 20, no. 3 (2001): 194–201.

9. J. D. Kleinke, *Oxymorons: The Myth of a U.S. Health Care System* (San Francisco: Jossey-Bass, 2001), 90.

10. David Leonhardt, "Health Care as Main Engine: Is That So Bad?" *New York Times*, 11 November 2001, C-1, 12.

11. Siddharta Mukherjee, "Fighting Chance: The Case for Funding Curiosity," *New Republic*, 21 January 2002, 16–19.

12. A. L. Cochrane, *Effectiveness and Efficiency* (Abingdon, England: Nuffield Provincial Hospitals Trust, 1972), 86.

13. J. Michael McGinnis, Pamela William-Russo, and James R. Knickman, "The Case for More Active Attention to Health Promotion," *Health Affairs* 21, no. 2 (2002).

Index

abortion: coerced, 95; fetal tissue research and, 170–71; of genetically defective children, 108, 112–13; issues of use of medical knowledge and, 94; as moral decision, 181; moral status of embryo and, 180–87; stem cell research and, 174
absolutizing disease, 61–62
academic researchers. *See* universities and colleges
access to care, as ideal, 5–6
Adams Act (1906), 14
adulthood, needs assessment and, 265–66, 268
adult stem cells, 196–97
Advanced Cell Technology, 175
advance directives, 70
advertising: bonds with researchers targeted by, 49; journals as dependent on, 47–48; by pharmaceutical industry, 201–2, 202, 204, 206, 207, 208, 209; protest advertisements, 193; stock exchange rules for, 260
Advisory Committee on Human Radiation Experiments, 140, 141, 155–56
advocacy groups: celebrity advocates, 189, 240, 274; disease-oriented advocacy, 237, 239–40, 273–74; ethical guidelines for, 240; general types and functions of, 238–40; Laskerism and, 236–38, 239; priority-setting

criticized by, 245; public's support of, 32; stem cell research and, 189. *See also* lobbying
Africa: AIDS as debilitating to societies of, 262; drug trials and availability in, 157–58, 161–62, 215–16, 217
African Americans: fear of medical research among, 136; health improvement of, generally, 262; Tuskegee syphilis study and, 145, 158
Agency for Health Care and Research, 44
aggregate accounting, 229, 230
aging: advocacy groups for, 239; amelioration of, possibilities for, 76–80; biological function of, 75; budgetary focus on, 237; as disease, 74–75; memory enhancement and, 104, 112; pharmaceutical access and, 208, 214–15; research priorities for, 266–67, 268
aging of population: chronic disease and, 225; disability prevalence rate among, 226; health costs and, 225–26; priorities for health care and, 242; social consequences of, 81–82
agricultural research, 14, 27
AIDS/HIV: access to drug trials and, 157; advocacy for, 239; budgets for research, 245; developing countries as debilitated by, 262; drug trials and availability in developing coun-

Compositor:	Binghamton Valley Composition, LLC
Text and display:	Aldus
Printer and binder:	Maple-Vail Manufacturing Group